Inside Fibromyalgia

With

Mark J. Pellegrino, M.D.

INSIDE FIBROMYALGIA
With Mark J. Pellegrino, M.D.
Anadem Publishing, Inc.
Columbus, Ohio 43214
614 • 262•2539
1•800•633•0055
World Wide Web: www.anadem.com

The material in *Inside Fibromyalgia* is presented for informational purposes only. It is not meant to be a substitute for proper medical care by your doctor. You need to consult with your doctor for diagnosis and treatment.

PRINTED IN THE UNITED STATES OF AMERICA

ISBN 1-890018-36-8

Dedication: This book is dedicated to my mom and dad. Thank you for all you do. I love you very much.

Acknowledgments: A special thanks to a wonderful person, Ann Evans, who is a valued friend and reviewer and whose suggestions are most appreciated and helpful.

A special thanks also to an inspirational friend, Chris Marschinke, whose tireless efforts at helping fibromyalgia patients have enriched many lives, including mine.

TABLE OF CONTENTS

INTRODUCTION

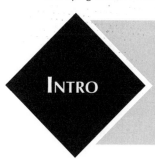

INTRODUCTION

I have fibromyalgia. I'm also a fibromyalgia survivor. When I was 28 years old (a couple of years ago!), I was officially diagnosed with this disorder. I was in the midst of my Physical Medicine and Rehabilitation residency program when I started having persistent and severe pain in my neck and shoulders. One of my residency instructors examined me and discovered my painful tender points, hence my "official" diagnosis.

Since my diagnosis, I have striven to learn as much as I could about fibromyalgia by researching, reading, attending conferences, treating patients, and ultimately, by personal experiences. I've been able to look back and realize that I had various symptoms as a child that probably meant I was at risk for getting fibromyalgia someday. As a patient and a physician, I have come to appreciate how complex this condition really is, and that every individual is affected differently. Some people with fibromyalgia syndrome are hardly bothered by this condition, whereas others are incapacitated because of the pain.

As a medical doctor specializing in Physical Medicine and Rehabilitation, I have treated numerous patients over the years. In my practice, I saw many patients with functional problems that interfered with their ability to complete everyday tasks. These patients required a treatment approach that maximized their abilities so that they could experience a better quality of life.

As my personal and professional interest in fibromyalgia grew, I began to refine my treatment approach and sub-specialize in helping patients with fibromyalgia reach their goals. Over the past twelve years, I have diagnosed and treated over 10,000 people with this disorder. My approach has been to help patients deal with their symptoms, first, by helping them understand fibromyalgia, and second, by encouraging them to use the tools they have learned to ultimately become a fibromyalgia survivor. I have learned to become a fibromyalgia survivor, not from reading medical journals or attending symposiums, but through experiences with the patients that I have come to know and treat over the years. I consider them my colleagues! Today I continue an active clinical practice and am working together WITH fibromyalgia patients to solve OUR problems.

As part of my therapy, I enjoy writing. It helps me accomplish one of my goals: educating people about fibromyalgia. I have published numerous books on fibromyalgia, including *The Fibromyalgia Survivor*. This book, published in 1995, contained detailed strategies for coping successfully with this painful disorder, while maintaining a positive outlook.

Inside Fibromyalgia is an expanded, updated version that combines my philosophy, personal and professional experiences, and hopefully some helpful strategies in understanding and managing fibromyalgia. I have tried to incorporate the most updated research information. I have divided the book into various sections for easy reference. Each section begins with a preview of what each section contains and each chapter ends with a summary of survival strategies. There are various diagrams to help you understand and "digest" the information easier.

There is more than one way to successfully treat pain. Those with fibromyalgia require individual treatment strategies because there is no single universal recipe. My simple philosophy in treating fibromyalgia is to find whatever works. This includes a responsible, successful home program and a good mental outlook. This book will show some ideas and strategies that have worked for me and my patients. I hope you too can become a fibromyalgia survivor!

Mark J. Pellegrino, M.D.& F.M.S. (Fibromyalgia Survivor)

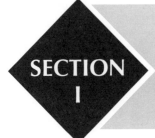

SECTION I

DIAGNOSING FIBROMYALGIA

This section reviews the basics of fibromyalgia, from what it is to how it is diagnosed. The first step in becoming a fibromyalgia survivor is ... having fibromyalgia! This section is a review for the "experienced" person who was diagnosed long ago. For the newly diagnosed person, I think this section will help to provide you with a summary of how you got to your diagnosis and to set a basic framework for where to go from here.

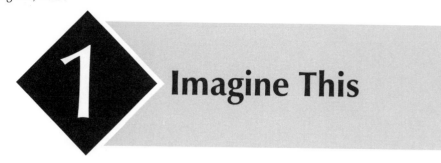

Imagine This

You've been healthy all of your life. Sure, you've had some aches and pains from time to time just like everyone else. If you overexert yourself from playing a game of volleyball, you notice your legs will hurt. If you carry a heavy bag of salt into the basement, you might hurt your back a little. Or you may have had a lot of stress followed by a headache, or did too much on the job and ached. This never stopped you, though. You just took some aspirin, maybe rubbed some muscle creams on the sore areas, or rested a little bit, and you felt better.

One day, you woke up and noticed severe pain in your neck and shoulders. At first you thought, "I must have slept the wrong way." Or maybe you did something the night before that caused some pain. But when you tried your usual remedies such as taking a few aspirin and resting, the pain didn't go away. In fact, the pain got worse and moved around. It spread until you hurt all over.

You saw a doctor and he found nothing wrong. He ran a bunch of tests and they all came back normal. Medicines don't help. Nothing helps the pain. And it's getting worse.

You don't understand it. "How can this be happening to me?" you wonder. "What is wrong with me?" It is like your whole body is on fire. Your nerves seem to be amplifying every pain signal a hundredfold, and you can't ignore the pain. It prevents you from doing simple things that you used to take for granted, things like reaching up, bending over, sleeping, or concentrating. You are having great difficulty doing anything. You can no longer get through your day without pain, you can't work without pain, you can't even function without pain, and no one seems to understand your pain because you look okay. Your life is spinning out of control. It feels like there is no end in sight for your pain.

That's what fibromyalgia does.

Chances are if you are reading this, you aren't imagining this at all; fibromyalgia is a reality for you, and you are not alone...

...and there is hope.

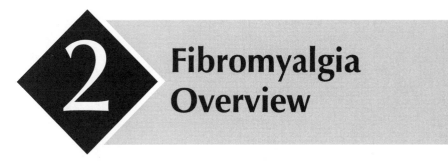

Fibromyalgia Overview

What It Is

Fibromyalgia is a common painful condition of soft tissues, mainly muscles, that causes widespread pain, fatigue, poor sleep, stiffness, as well as other symptoms. It is a chronic condition recognized as a distinct medical entity with characteristic findings. The name fibromyalgia comes from the Latin words "fibro," meaning fibrous tissue such as tendons, ligaments, and bursa; "my," meaning muscle; and "algia," meaning pain. Fibromyalgia used to go by other names including fibrositis, rheumatism, tension myalgia, and myofibrositis. In the past, some physicians used the term "psychogenic rheumatism" to describe what they thought were patients' symptoms that were "all in the head."

Fibromyalgia is very much a "real disease" and not any imagined disorder. The term "fibromyalgia," or "fibromyalgia syndrome," is the medically correct name for this condition, although sometimes the other names are still used. Regardless of the name, we are talking about the same condition.

The pain of fibromyalgia usually consists of generalized aching, a sense of "I hurt all over." Certain parts of the body are particularly painful, and the pain may move around and be accompanied by severe muscle spasms. The muscle pain can fluctuate from day to day and often flares up. It can be aggravated by various physical, environmental, and emotional factors, and the pain can become so intense that it interferes with one's ability to perform daily activities or work. Some people

Fatigue is a major problem that can fluctuate in severity and cause functional limitations, just like the pain. Stiffness, numbness, headaches, poor sleep, chest pain, irritable bowel syndrome, and temporomandibular joint (TMJ) dysfunction are other symptoms and conditions commonly present with fibromyalgia.

with fibromyalgia may have only mild discomfort, and others may be completely disabled by it. Some seem to be like pain magnets and attract all sorts of pain!

In addition to pain, fibromyalgia also causes numerous other symptoms and associated conditions. Fatigue is a major problem that can fluctuate in severity and cause functional limitations, just like the pain. Stiffness, numbness, headaches, poor sleep, chest pain, irritable bowel syndrome, and temporomandibular joint (TMJ) dysfunction are other symptoms and conditions commonly present with fibromyalgia, and each can cause separate problems and limitations as part of the overall fibromyalgia.

What It Is Not

Fibromyalgia can cause symptoms that resemble arthritis or neurological disorders, but it is different from these disorders.

- Unlike arthritis, fibromyalgia does not cause joint swelling or deformities, even though it may cause pain in the tissues or a feeling of swelling around the joint.

- Fibromyalgia does not cause paralysis or progressive neurological problems like Multiple Sclerosis or Lou Gehrig's disease.

- It is not a ruptured disc or a pinched nerve, even though your symptoms may resemble those caused by a pinched nerve.

- It is not a tumor.

It does not turn into one of these conditions, although people with fibromyalgia can certainly get other conditions over time that are unrelated to fibromyalgia. Even though fibromyalgia is not life threatening or crippling, it is very much a painful condition that can cause severe problems. We may look okay on the outside, but we are definitely hurting on the inside.

Who Gets It?

We don't know the exact prevalence of fibromyalgia in the general population, but we do know this: anyone can get it. Millions and millions of people have it worldwide, with about 5% of the overall population estimated to have fibromyalgia. Women are diagnosed more frequently than men, about seven to ten times more. Symptoms usually appear between the ages of 25 and 45. I see a lot of men with this disorder in my practice, although I certainly see many

Fibromyalgia is not a "new" disease or some recent "medical fad."

Fibromyalgia has been around for a long time, even though we have only recently begun to better understand and diagnose this condition.

more women. Children can also have fibromyalgia.

Symptoms may be present for years, even though the diagnosis may not be made until past age 50. Once you are officially diagnosed with the disorder, you continue to have it as you get older; thus the prevalence of fibromyalgia increases in the population as the age increases. According to Dr. Robert Bennett, a fibromyalgia researcher, about 3½ percent of 20-year olds will meet the American College of Rheumatology (ACR) definition of fibromyalgia. Among 70-year olds 12 percent have fibromyalgia. Because fibromyalgia has hereditary components, I frequently see children of a parent who has been diagnosed with fibromyalgia.

Fibromyalgia is not a "new" disease or some recent "medical fad." In reviewing medical literature, it is obvious that fibromyalgia has been around for a long time, even though we have only recently begun to better understand and diagnose this condition. Nearly 100 years ago, Sir William Gower first described the condition of "fibrositis" as a cause of low back pain. At first, it was felt that the pain was caused by fibrous tissue inflammation (hence the term fibrositis). Before we learned that the pain is not caused by an inflammation, a lot of controversy and questions arose regarding the medical legitimacy of fibrositis. Controversies continue to the present day, but those who understand and treat fibromyalgia will agree that it is a legitimate medical condition with unique characteristics requiring individualized treatments.

I don't expect that the controversies surrounding fibromyalgia will disappear as long as there are people who don't understand or believe in fibromyalgia. Not only does it exist, it is a chronic and permanent condition for which there is no cure at this time. A lot can be done for this condition, however, and the challenge is not only to fully understand fibromyalgia, but to minimize its effect on the individual and the community until a cure is found.

Chapter 2 — Survival Strategies

1) Learn what fibromyalgia is. Learn what it isn't.

2) Recognize associated conditions and how they relate to your fibromyalgia experience.

3) Reassure yourself that fibromyalgia does not kill, cripple, or become life-threatening — despite what the pain in your body is telling you.

4) Understand it is clinically and scientifically possible to look good on the outside but be hurting on the inside.

5) Due to hereditary components of this disorder, be attentive to children and other family members and urge them to get treatment early.

6) Try to accept that FMS is a chronic, permanent condition for which there is no cure at this time.

7) Maintain hope that new research is moving in many positive directions.

8) Don't wait for a cure; get treatment for your fibromyalgia now.

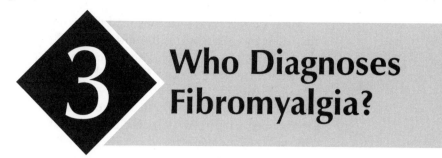

3 Who Diagnoses Fibromyalgia?

Official Diagnosis

Fibromyalgia is an "official" diagnosis which must be made by a doctor. Examples of qualified doctors include M.D.'s (Medical Doctors), D.O.'s (Osteopathic Doctors), D.C.'s (Chiropractors), or N.D.'s (Naturopathic Doctors). According to the Medical/ Legal Guidelines of the Medical Practice Acts, only qualified or licensed doctors can render a medical diagnosis.

Certain medical specialists, particularly rheumatologists and physiatrists (a specialist in Physical Medicine and Rehabilitation), have particular expertise in diagnosing and treating musculoskeletal problems such as fibromyalgia due to their education, training, and experience. A rheumatologist is a specialist in rheumatic conditions, which include a variety of disorders (such as arthritis, lupus, and gout) characterized by inflammation, degeneration, or derangement of connective tissue structures in the body, especially joints, muscles, bursa, tendons, and fibrous tissues. A physiatrist (pronounced fiz-e-AH-trist) is a specialist who deals with the diagnosis, treatment, and prevention of conditions causing pain, weakness, and functional impairment like injuries, stroke, and paraplegia. Both of these specialty programs require additional years of residency training, usually four years, after medical school is completed.

Much of today's research and literature refers to a rheumatologist as the main specialist treating fibromyalgia. I certainly recognize and appreciate the work the rheumatologists have done on fibromyalgia over the years, but as a physiatrist myself, I will be naturally biased and say that my field is uniquely trained and suited in the diagnosis and treatment of fibromyalgia (see Chapter 11).

One does not have to be a specialist in Rheumatology or Physical Medicine and Rehabilitation to diagnose and treat fibromyalgia. There are many knowledgeable physicians who are interested in working with fibromyalgia patients. In fact, I work with many primary care physicians, (i.e., family practitioners and internists) who may have diagnosed fibromyalgia themselves or suspect it and have referred patients to me for further evaluation and recommendations. I think it is important for every patient to have a primary care doctor who is willing to work with her or him in treating this condition.

I also see many patients who refer themselves to me. They may have read about symptoms of fibromyalgia and feel it fits them, and want confirmation or additional evaluation by a specialist. It is not surprising for patients to tell me on their first visit that they were talking to a sister, an aunt, a bank teller, a hairdresser, or a coworker's nephew's fiancée who said they sound like they have fibromyalgia and should get checked out!

Many people have said they read my handout or book or something on fibromyalgia, and it was like reading about their life. They are convinced that they have fibromyalgia even before their evaluation because they read about it and it fit them, and they are usually right. I consider the "read-and-fit" test to be a diagnostic test!

There are many non-physician medical professionals who are knowledgeable and experienced in fibromyalgia, including physical therapists, massotherapists, and nutritionists. Many patients who have been diagnosed with fibromyalgia were first directed to their physician by one of these medical professionals who suspected fibromyalgia. A person "enters the books" when he or she goes to a doctor and receives the official diagnosis of fibromyalgia.

You need an "official" diagnosis, as your pain could be caused by a number of conditions other than fibromyalgia. Diagnosing yourself isn't wise; make sure you see a qualified doctor. Your doctor can determine what tests may be needed to rule out other conditions. I've seen many people who thought they had fibromyalgia but turned out to have something else. You can't pick up a pamphlet and make an official diagnosis on yourself.

Undiagnosed Fibromyalgia

Many people have fibromyalgia but have not been diagnosed yet. It is like the proverbial saying, "if a tree falls in a forest and no one is around to hear it, does it make a sound?" In fibromyalgia talk, it is saying "if someone has symptoms of fibromyalgia and tender points, but no doctor has actually examined the person and made the diagnosis, does this person have fibromyalgia?"

> You need an "official" diagnosis, as your pain could be caused by a number of conditions other than fibromyalgia. Diagnosing yourself isn't wise; make sure you see a qualified doctor.
>
> I've seen many people who thought they had fibromyalgia but turned out to have something else.

The answer is yes. That person has undiagnosed fibromyalgia (this sounds like an oxymoron). Doctors wait for people to come to us with symptoms before making a diagnosis. That is the nature of our work. It would be pretty silly if we went door-to-door asking people if they had any medical problems that they would like treated today. Only the people who seek out medical attention for their symptoms can be diagnosed with fibromyalgia.

However, if we go out into the community, for example, when we perform research projects or studies, we will find fibromyalgia in the community in people who have never gone to the doctor. Or we may find people who have been diagnosed with another problem, but they really have fibromyalgia. Fibromyalgia is probably more like an iceberg, with the tip representing the ones who go to doctors for diagnosis and treatment.

Finding a Doctor

How does one find a doctor who understands fibromyalgia and is willing to treat it? Your doctor should be understanding, knowledgeable, and willing to learn. He or she should be eager to work with you and be open-minded, and also be willing to work with other medical professionals.

Patients have told me how they go about finding these doctors.

1) **Trial and error.** Unfortunately, many patients have had to see a number of doctors before finding one who would work with them. This effort is certainly time consuming, costly, and inefficient, but those who have gone this route are certainly wiser in the end, even if they still hurt!

2) **Word of mouth.** If a friend or family member can put in a good word, your odds of finding a good doctor increase.

3) **References.** Various physician reference agencies are available in your community either through medical organizations or state and local medical societies. These organizations would have names of specialists in Rheumatology or Physical Medicine and Rehabilitation.

4) **Fibromyalgia newsletters and databases on the Internet** have the names of physicians who are interested in treating fibromyalgia, and have been "verified" by patients who have seen these doctors. This technique is a more formalized "word-of-mouth" approach.

5) **Self-research.** Call and ask doctors if they see patients with fibromyalgia, if they are comfortable with treating patients with fibromyalgia, if they accept patients with fibromyalgia and prescribe treatments. You will not likely talk to the doctor himself or herself for this phone interview, but the staff should be very knowledgeable and helpful in getting answers to your questions.

6) **Referral from your primary care doctor.** Perhaps the ideal situation is to have your primary care doctor, whom you trust, make a referral to someone who knows and understands fibromyalgia. If your primary care doctor is agreeable, he/she would appreciate the additional input. This technique ensures that your primary care doctor will continue to be an informed team player in your attempts to optimize fibromyalgia treatments. Sometimes traveling longer distances may be necessary to see a specialist, and it may not be practical for you to follow-up with a specialist on a frequent basis due to the long distance. Following up with your primary care doctor who works closely with your specialist would be an ideal and practical situation.

7) **Networking with other patients.** You can meet them at a local support group, a lecture, a course on fibromyalgia, a health food store, and just about anywhere else! People who have fibromyalgia are everywhere and they love to talk.

Not Everybody Diagnoses Fibromyalgia

There are many doctors including rheumatologists and physiatrists who want nothing to do with fibromyalgia. Working with chronic pain patients can be demanding and challenging. Some physicians do not feel comfortable or talented in this area. Their strengths may lie in treating acute problems or in research. It is better that they recognize that aspect of their personality and let it be known they choose not to see these patients.

But, for whatever reason, some physicians choose to go beyond that. Instead of quietly refusing to see patients with fibromyalgia, they feel it necessary to voice negative opinions regarding fibromyalgia. Examples of these opinions/statements follow....

1) Fibromyalgia simply does not exist.

2) Fibromyalgia is a wastebasket diagnosis used when you don't know what else is wrong.

3) Fibromyalgia is basically a name for depressed ladies with pain.

4) Fibromyalgia is overblown and out of control.

Remember, these statements are made by physicians who have no experience in treating fibromyalgia (because they won't see anybody with it!). Yet they choose to make statements about fibromyalgia under the guise of medical credibility! However, everyone has a right to his or her opinion. We should remember that these people are medical professionals and could consider offering one of the following responses to their opinions. Pick one (or more).

Many doctors want nothing to do with fibromyalgia.

Some physicians do not feel comfortable or talented in this area. Their strengths may lie in treating acute problems or in research. It is better that they recognize that aspect of their personality and let it be known they choose not to see these patients.

1) I'm sorry, I CAN'T HEAR YOU.

2) I'm ignoring you.

3) Are you talking to me? Are you talking to ME?

4) Hey, your shoelaces are untied.

Ultimately, the doctors who are willing to work with you to treat your fibromyalgia have at least one thing in common: they respect your condition, and they respect you. By getting a proper diagnosis of a legitimate condition from a trained physician, you are being validated, and you are being treated with respect.

Chapter 3 — Survival Strategies

1) Learn which types of doctors are the most qualified to diagnose FMS.

2) Work with doctors who have the ability to give you the best care.

3) Network with other FM patients in support groups to find the most "fibro-friendly" health care providers in your area.

4) Become confident that you have an accurate diagnosis of FMS by a qualified physician. This will relieve anxiety when you experience increased pain.

5) Identify your body's pain signals and act on them early, before pain gets out of control.

6) Interview physicians until you find someone that is: knowledgeable, understanding, willing to learn, works well with others, and is compassionate.

7) Expect some doctors to be skeptical of your condition. Choose not to be upset with the doctor. If you can educate him/her then do so. If not, just move on! Your time and energy are too valuable to spend on "nonbelievers."

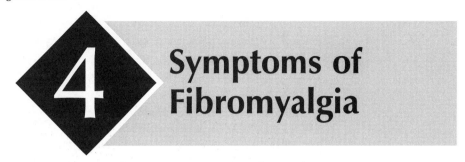

4 Symptoms of Fibromyalgia

Pain

The main complaint with fibromyalgia is pain. Several key phrases describe severe pain: "I hurt all over," "My pain moves around," and "I feel like I've been run over by a Mack truck." Whenever I hear these phrases, I think of fibromyalgia.

The pain may be described as a constant ache, nag, or throbbing. The muscles are not the only painful areas. Other soft tissues, such as ligaments, tendons, and bursa can be painful. Typical pain locations include the head and neck, shoulders (especially between the shoulder blades), low back and hip muscles. Certain areas may cause sharp, stabbing pains. Patients can point to exact areas and note they are very painful to touch.

The pain may appear to wander to different sites; the low back may be sore today, and tomorrow, the neck hurts. These wandering symptoms may lead you to think you are going crazy! I was convinced that there could be no possible physical condition that would cause pain to wander, and therefore I must be imagining things. Once I learned that fibromyalgia can indeed cause wandering pains, I knew I was not as crazy as I thought.

About half of the time, patients report a gradual progression of pain. The pain begins in one location such as the shoulder, but over time other areas become affected until pain is no longer localized but rather generalized throughout the body. Sometimes the onset is so gradual that patients can't even remember the beginning of their pain. Other times, the pain begins after a specific trauma and patients can recall the exact moment when they first had pain. Over half of the patients attribute their symptoms to some type of trauma or severe stress.

Usually a person describes multiple "types" of pain when fibromyalgia is present. Generalized "ache all over" type pain may be accompanied by severe stabbing pains in certain regions, and other areas may have burning or radiating pains. There is usually chronic pain, but often flare-ups occur and certain areas or the whole body become severely painful. Invariably, the pain interferes with everyday activities including work, hobbies, and recreation. Interpersonal relationship problems occur frequently. Almost everyone with fibromyalgia reports disruption of their functional abilities because of pain.

Chest Pain

Chest pain can be of particular concern because patients fear that this may represent heart disease. Usually there is no problem with the heart. Rather, the pain comes from muscles in the chest wall and rib areas, that is, the pectorals and intercostal muscles. The ligaments and tendons around the chest area (sternum or breast plate) can become painful. This is called costochondritis and it can mimic heart pain. Large-busted women and women who have fibrocystic breast disease (painful cysts in the breasts) often have more chest pain with their fibromyalgia. Fear and anxiety triggered by chest pain can make the pain worse.

When I first started seeing people with fibromyalgia, I noticed many had atypical chest pain as their "first" symptom. They may have had a heart work-up at first, which was negative. Ultimately they received a diagnosis of fibromyalgia with associated musculoskeletal chest pain. I published these results in 1989 and have since come to appreciate how common chest pain is in fibromyalgia, whether it is the initial symptom or develops after the fibromyalgia has already been diagnosed.

If you have unexplained chest pain, always get it checked out. If it's found to be related to your fibromyalgia, you can relax a little knowing it's not a heart problem, and focus on managing the fibro-related pain.

Mitral Valve Prolapse

Mitral valve prolapse (MVP), present in fibromyalgia can contribute to chest wall pain. MVP is a condition when one of the heart valves, the mitral valve, bulges excessively during the heartbeat. It can be diagnosed by listening with a stethoscope for a characteristic click-murmur. The diagnosis is confirmed with a sound wave test call an echocardiogram. Although it sounds scary, most doctors feel that MVP is usually a benign condition.

I conducted a study at the Ohio State University which showed that the majority of people with fibromyalgia also had MVP. The mitral valve is mostly connective tissue, not a muscle. This study supports the belief that fibromyalgia involves tissues other than muscles.

Chest pain can be of particular concern because patients fear that this may represent heart disease. Usually there is no problem with the heart. Rather, the pain comes from muscles in the chest wall and rib areas, that is, the pectorals and intercostal muscles.

MVP usually does not cause problems in fibromyalgia patients, but sometimes it can be more severe and cause cardiac problems that require specific medications. Antibiotics may be prescribed before certain surgeries or procedures such as dental work. Atypical chest pain and shortness of breath can occur. Chest pain in fibromyalgia is usually benign, but people with fibromyalgia can have other problems, too, including heart problems. Remember, if you experience new chest pain, consult a physician at once.

Modulating Factors

Certain factors modulate fibromyalgia pain, either worsening or improving it. Physical activities can cause flare-ups in the pain. Performing strenuous activities such as moving furniture or gardening can increase pain even after you've stopped the activity. Too much activity is an obvious cause of increased pain, but too little activity can be just as bad.

I learned first-hand how decreased activities could worsen my fibromyalgia. During my residency, I became involved in so many projects that I was unable to continue my exercise program on a regular basis. Gradually, I noticed increased pain in my low back. My back seemed to go into spasms very easily, even with minimal activity such as bending over to pick-up a tissue. I realized that my body had come to expect a certain physical activity level, and by not keeping up with my program, I became more vulnerable to flare-ups. Once I resumed my regular exercise program, my symptoms improved within a short period of time, and I felt more "stable" in my back. I learned not to neglect my exercises, because I (and my back) would pay the price.

Certain positions that require sustained isometric muscle contractions, such as holding our arms out in front of us for a long time, are not tolerated well by people with fibromyalgia. Our muscles do not like sustained contractions, and they tell us by saying "OUCH!" People who have jobs that require reaching (typing, assembly line work, or driving are examples) will often have increased pain especially in the neck, shoulders, and back.

Weather changes affect our symptoms. Cold, damp weather, and cold drafts or air conditioning drafts are major enemies for us. Likewise, cold water will cause muscle pain to flare-up, and we don't do well in pools where the water temperature is below 90° F.

We tend to do better in warm, dry weather and climates. Many of my patients try to escape to Arizona for "therapeutic" vacations. (I live in Northeast Ohio, which seems like one of the worst places in the world for fibromyalgia!) Hot, humid weather can aggravate the pain whereas hot, dry weather is preferred.

Emotional stress certainly plays a role in fibromyalgia flare-ups. Stress is part of life, but during times of increased stress, we usually experience increased fibromyalgia pain. Most people will experience more pain when they have a flu virus, and sometimes even after getting a flu vaccine. A lot of women notice a flare-up of their symptoms before their period starts and increased premenstrual syndrome (PMS) symptoms. Likewise, the pain symptoms can increase during early menopause.

Sometimes there is no obvious reason why pain flares up. This is common in fibromyalgia, and it can be very frustrating because you may be doing all of the "right" things. Chapter 35 addresses flare-ups and how to handle them.

Fatigue

Next to pain, fatigue is the major complaint in people with fibromyalgia. Fatigue is actually a combination of physical and mental factors. Fibromyalgia muscles already have low energy stores and tire easily. Any activity, whether usual or "out of the ordinary," can cause fatigue. Going shopping at the mall, playing a game of basketball, and walking up several flights of steps are activities that can cause sudden increased fatigue in the muscles.

A steel worker described his leg fatigue at the end of the work day as turning him into a Slow-Mo camera. He felt like his legs were working in super slow-motion with each move requiring detailed concentration.

Fatigue can be unpredictable and strike the muscles suddenly. Another one of my patients described her fatigue as a feeling of driving along and idling at a stop-light when suddenly the car runs out of gas and stalls (she is not an auto mechanic by the way)!

Extreme fatigue has a mental component as well as a physical one. Neurasthenia is a medical term that describes the extreme lack of energy and feeling of mental exhaustion. This mental fatigue makes it hard to concentrate or focus on a task. We feel like we are in a fog.

Concentration and Memory Problems (Fibro-fog)

Fibromyalgia can cause considerable difficulties with our thinking, and this can vary from day to day. These difficulties include forgetfulness, absentmindedness, confusion, short-term memory difficulties, extreme mental fatigue, and something else...but I can't remember what. We refer to these symptoms as "fibro-fog."

We are the people who have to stop and think about which side is right and which side is left. We also are the worst group of people to ever ask for directions, especially since we get lost all of the time!

Many people are extremely concerned that this indicates a deterioration of their brain function or dementia, but that is not the case. We demonstrate normal learning and memory although we process information more slowly because of our fibromyalgia. Part of our fibro-fog problem is that a brain cannot process much information when it is continuously bombarded by pain signals. Monitoring the pain demands so much of our brain's attention that very little attention "space" is available to help us process and retain "routine" information.

> Fibromyalgia can cause forgetfulness, absent-mindedness, confusion, short-term memory difficulties, extreme mental fatigue. We refer to these symptoms as "fibro-fog."
>
> Many people are extremely concerned that this indicates a deterioration of their brain function or dementia, but that is not the case.

Our fibro-fog is one of our most frustrating problems. We can read the same thing over and over and still not understand a word we read. We can see a close relative and suddenly forget her name. We drive past freeway entrances and exits and constantly discover new routes home — inadvertently! Countless times I cannot remember a specific word or person's name, or anything else important! I'm frequently absent of mind (NO, that's not a typo!). On the other hand, fibro-fog is something you can have the most fun with, if you really try. What else can be more exciting than trying to find your misplaced car keys when they're right in your pocket, or wondering how the cereal got in the refrigerator and the milk in the cupboard.

Poor Sleep

Poor sleep is a hallmark in most patients with fibromyalgia. Patients report that the quality of their sleep is poor, and when they awake in the morning they do not feel well rested (non-restorative sleep). You may not have trouble falling asleep, but often your sleep is characterized by frequent awakening especially in the early morning hours, and lack of a deep, sound sleep. Dr. Moldofsky performed studies which demonstrated disruptions of the deep sleep stage in many with fibromyalgia.

I do not have difficulty falling asleep but I usually wake up around 4:00 a.m. I feel ready to conquer the world at that time, but I realize that it is too darn early to get up. So I lay there in bed. Every fifteen minutes I find myself glancing at the clock and never falling back into a deep sleep. When it is finally time to get up, I feel completely exhausted and must use every self-motivation technique as well as great effort to drag myself out of bed.

> Poor sleep is a hallmark with fibromyalgia. Patients report that the quality of their sleep is poor, and when they awake in the morning they do not feel well rested (non-restorative sleep).
>
> Our batteries are not getting recharged adequately during the night.

Many people have trouble falling asleep and wake often. Others suffer from a condition called sleep apnea characterized by irregular breathing and periods of breathing cessation (apnea) during sleep. Whatever the cause(s), a lack of deep sleep certainly contributes to fatigue during the day. Our batteries are not getting recharged adequately during the night.

Stiffness

Stiffness and joint pain are usually present in fibromyalgia. These symptoms are mostly related to pain at the muscle and tendon insertions into the joint area, and not actual joint pathology or inflammation. Morning stiffness is a common complaint, so not only are we sleeping poorly, but when we wake up in the morning we are so stiff that we can hardly move. This stiffness can also occur after prolonged periods of sitting or standing in one position. Usually once we get up and start moving around, we tend to loosen up.

Headaches

We get a lot of tension, migraine, and combined headaches with fibromyalgia. Tension headaches are also called muscle contraction headaches, and they usually begin at the base of the neck and extend upward to the back of the head and frequently into the temples. Many people describe a band-like squeezing headache. Migraine headaches are vascular headaches in which some event triggers the blood vessels to constrict and then dilate. This causes a severe headache that may be located inside the head or behind the eyes and may be accompanied by nausea, vomiting, eye pain, and facial numbness.

Many people with fibromyalgia have headaches with both tension and migraine features. They describe daily tension headache with aching pain, and then on a fairly regular basis, perhaps once a week or twice a month, a severe migraine headache occurs. Various factors can trigger a migraine headache including certain foods, exposure to certain odors, stresses, weather changes, and menstrual cycles.

Frequent severe headaches are particularly tough for patients. Head pain is much more disruptive than pain in other locations, so it will interfere more with work abilities, daily activities, and attempts to interact with others.

Temporomandibular Joint (TMJ) Dysfunction

Over a third of patients with fibromyalgia have pain in the jaw and temple areas related to TMJ dysfunction. TMJ dysfunction can cause a variety of symptoms such as headaches, ringing in the ears, face numbness, and dizziness. Other jaw and "face" symptoms frequently reported include facial twitching, flushing, and a fullness or swelling sensation.

Swallowing Difficulties

Swallowing may be difficult at times, as if a tight band is constricting our throats. This may trouble us if we are having a hard time swallowing a piece of food. These symptoms may fluctuate and seem to worsen if we are more tense and nervous. We have a lot of muscles in the throat for fibromyalgia to bother.

Throat pain and fullness may occur. Many feel hoarse or have problems vocalizing. Still others have a condition called esophageal reflux where acid and stomach contents can "backflow" up to the throat and cause irritation and pain. All these problems are seen more often in people with fibromyalgia.

Neurologic Symptoms

Various neurologic symptoms are present in fibromyalgia. These include numbness or tingling especially in the arms and legs and particularly in the hands or feet. These symptoms can mimic a pinched nerve or carpal tunnel syndrome. Other sensory symptoms include feelings of burning, itching and swelling. Finger swelling is common and rings may become tight on the finger. Any abnormal sensation is known as a paresthesia.

Weakness is a common complaint as well. This weakness is not due to neurologic damage from a pinched nerve, for example, but rather a weakness related to muscle pain and fatigue and overall loss of strength and stamina. If muscles hurt, they prevent us from using them properly, hence we feel weak.

People complain of sensitivity to temperatures and often get hot flashes and cold hands and feet. Some people even develop a condition known as Raynaud's phenomenon, which is characterized by intermittent attacks of red, white or blue discoloration of the fingers or toes. Cold temperatures or stress usually brings on these neurovascular changes.

Other neurologic symptoms include dizziness, light-headedness, and vertigo or spinning sensation. We may have balance problems or lack of coordination. We have to be careful that we don't get up too fast because we are more prone to a drop in blood pressure known as neurally-mediated hypotension. This can cause us to get light-headed and feel like we are going to faint. Fainting is definitely not recommended for those who have fibromyalgia!

Frequently, patients complain of mainly right-sided (or left-sided) pain. If the person is right handed, usually the right side will hurt more, but that's not always the case. Sometimes the non-dominant side will be more painful. The one-sided involvement may be related to neurologic mechanisms which cause one side of the brain to be more sensitive to pain.

Visual Symptoms

Certainly we do not expect our eyes to be spared with fibromyalgia, do we? Up to a third of those with this condition have dry eyes, which may make it impossible to wear contacts. We notice that our eyes are particularly sensitive to smoke or that environments with very dry air cause vision difficulty.

> Up to a third have dry eyes. We notice that our eyes are particularly sensitive to smoke or that environments with very dry air cause vision difficulty.
>
> Eye muscles can get painful or go into spasms with fibromyalgia, so we have difficulty with moving our eyes, focusing, reading and tracking.

Eye muscles can get painful or go into spasms with fibromyalgia, so we have difficulty with moving our eyes, focusing, reading and tracking. Eye muscle spasms combined with dry eyes can cause eye pain and headaches. Many patients have to change their glasses prescriptions frequently because of fibromyalgia-related vision fluctuations. Fibromyalgia does not cause retinal detachments or glaucoma.

A particular visual difficulty experience is what I call "visual overload." This occurs when we try to process a lot of visual information at once. It becomes confusing and overwhelming to us. A common example of this occurs when you are reading a paragraph in a book, and you have read the paragraph three times and still have no clue what you just read. It's like Fibro-fog in the eyes, a combination of cognitive and visual problems.

I have these particular visual difficulties in stores. For example, if I need to find a can of olives and I try to scan all of the colorful cans stacked on a shelf about ten feet high and the length of a football field, I become dizzy and overwhelmed with this visual overload. I am unable to focus and scan and try to spot that can of olives. So, instead of my eyes giving me organized information like "cans of green beans, cans of corn, cans of carrots, cans of olives," they give me jumbled bits of information like this: "bright-yellow label, cans of corn, don't they come in frozen boxes, too?, little girl smiling, green and orange design on a can, that one isn't centered, what's behind this box?, don't forget you have to get ice-cream, too, my back is getting sore, did I know that guy? WHAT AM I LOOKING FOR AGAIN?"

Leg Pains

Many people develop leg pains and cramps, especially in the calves, or an intense feeling of restlessness in the legs. This sensation occurs particularly when you lay down at night and is often not relieved until you move the leg or literally get up and walk around. This is called restless leg syndrome. Nocturnal myoclonus is another leg problem that consists of involuntary jerking of the legs during sleep. The nighttime leg symptoms are usually worse if you have been more active and on your feet during the day.

These conditions are felt to be related to a neurologic mechanism where there is difficulty "turning off the switch" when you are trying to relax. Your throbbing leg pains are blocked out during the day by all the other sensory bombardments (from the eyes, ears, muscles, etc.). At night, all these other sensory inputs disappear as we lay down, turn off lights, and tune out noise. The leg pains and other sensations are no longer blocked out — and we feel them.

Allergies

Many patients with fibromyalgia have allergies or sensitivities. These may be due to environmental substances such as dust or pollen, or they may be medications or foods. We are hypersensitive to odors, noises, weather changes, bright lights, various chemicals, food additives, and more. We get a lot of nasal congestion, sinus headaches, nausea, itching, and rashes. We probably have a dysfunctional allergy and immune system responsible for these problems.

I am particularly sensitive to smells. Cigarette smoke, perfumes and colognes, and incense will often make me nauseated and cause my eyes to water. Particular enemies are the plug-in scents and those most annoying perfume and cologne inserts in magazines.

Irritable Bowel Syndrome or Spastic Colon

About half of the patients describe frequent bouts of constipation and/or diarrhea accompanied by abdominal pain, bloating and upset stomach. Irritable bowel syndrome may have been a problem in the past, or it may be an ongoing problem as part of the overall fibromyalgia. Many patients with severe gastrointestinal symptoms require specific medicines and treatments "separate" from the fibromyalgia treatments.

Irritable Bladder

The sister of irritable bowel syndrome causes symptoms of a bladder infection with frequent painful urination, but a urine test does not reveal any evidence of infection. Some people have been found to have benign microscopic blood in the urine. Severe bladder problems may require a urologic evaluation.

Pelvic Pain

Both sexes may report pelvic pain, but it is more common in women. The low back, sacroiliac, and pelvic muscles may be particularly painful. Women may develop endometriosis (painful uterine tissue growing in various locations of the pelvic cavity) or vulvodynia (painful, itching vulva and vaginal region). Irritable bowel syndrome can refer pain to the pelvic area.

Depression

Depression is commonly seen in conditions that cause chronic pain such as fibromyalgia. Up to half of patients become clinically depressed over the course of their fibromyalgia. Symptoms of low self-esteem, frequent crying spells, feeling of helplessness, and a bleak outlook are common. Some people have been diagnosed with depression before they were diagnosed with fibromyalgia.

Anxiety Disorder and Panic Attacks

Many people experience episodes of extreme anxiety and near panic. They may feel their heart racing, their chest tightening and find it difficult to get their breath. There may be a feeling of impending doom. We appear to be extremely sensitive to adrenaline, the main hormone that causes anxiety and panic attacks.

We frequently have "silent" anxiety attacks. I say silent because to the outside world nothing is apparent. When we first encounter a stressful situation, we look calm, cool and collected. But on the inside we feel like a runaway train is rushing through our blood vessels.

Fibromyalgia Personality

I think people with fibromyalgia have a certain type of personality. People with fibromyalgia tend to be compulsive, highly organized, perfectionists, time-oriented, and anxious. We like to do things ourselves because we know it will get done exactly the way we want. We cannot trust others to "get the job done right," so we end up doing almost everything ourselves. It really bothers us when others do not respect the details and time as we do.

Because we are so compulsive, we are not satisfied with just getting a job done; we want it to be the best job ever done. Consequently, no matter what we do, whether at work or home, we are always putting pressure on ourselves to do the best that we can. Even if we would change our job to testing recliner chairs, we would still be stressed out because we would want to be the best recliner chair testers ever!

This long chapter has pointed out various symptoms and associated conditions seen with fibromyalgia. Believe it or not, there are still more symptoms and associated conditions. I've only mentioned the most common ones. I didn't describe all possible symptoms because I wanted to have room in this book to write about other things!

Chapter 4 — Survival Strategies

1) Learn which symptoms are associated with fibromyalgia.

2) Monitor those symptoms and decide if you need help from a doctor.

3) Reduce anxiety about your pain and condition through self- education.

4) Review these symptoms with your doctor.

5) Compile a symptom log to track causes of your pain.

6) If you have unexplained chest pain, check it out.

7) Work towards a stable baseline by identifying and controlling modulating factors.

8) Recognize the role that emotional stress and mental fatigue have on your pain level. Eliminate as many stresses as possible.

9) Accept fibro-fog as a chance for comedic relief instead of creating an environment of frustration.

10) Become less compulsive, less organized, less of a perfectionist, less time-oriented, and less anxious.

11) Relax!

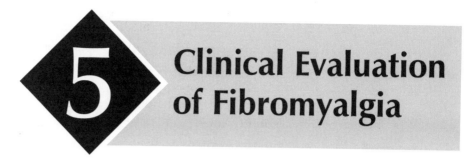

5 Clinical Evaluation of Fibromyalgia

The medical evaluation of the fibromyalgia patient includes a history and a physical exam. The medical history is an account of events in a patient's life that have relevance to the particular problem that brings the patient to see the doctor. It is a discussion between you and the doctor about why you are seeing the doctor. Your chief complaint when you see the doctor is usually PAIN! Lots of it!!

The medical history is not simply an unprompted narrative by the patient. If given the chance, many people with fibromyalgia could talk for hours about what's wrong with them! Rather, the medical history is more of a specialized form of information-gathering. Knowing which questions to ask is one of the most important tools in making the diagnosis of fibromyalgia. For this reason, your physician should be properly trained to work with fibromyalgia patients. As I ask questions, I record and evaluate the symptoms, but this is not the only data I need. The patients' feedback about their condition is also critical to this fact-finding mission. Think of your medical history as your "fibromyalgia resume." Its purpose is to highlight the most relevant facts, background information, and symptoms in the same way a resume does for a job interview.

There are consistent features in the medical history of someone with fibromyalgia. When I take the history of a patient who is complaining of pain, I note key features. Below are types of questions that I might ask and typical answers given by people with fibromyalgia.

1) Where is the pain?

Typical answers: "I hurt all over." "I ache all over, but I have severe headaches and neck pain." "My back hurts me especially, but so do my head, shoulders, arms, hips, legs, hands, and feet."

Most people with fibromyalgia will complain of generalized pain but may have regions that are relatively more painful. People can literally hurt everywhere on their body.

2) When did the pain start?

Typical answers: "I've had pain since I was young, I remember having growing pains as a kid." "Years ago my back started to hurt, but then it seemed to spread to other areas over time." "It started after I got mono in college." "It began in 1985 when I had a lot of stressful things happen to me." "My pains began at 1:48 p.m. on April 15, 1993 when I was sitting at a red light and was rear-ended by another car."

Sometimes the pain onset is so gradual that patients cannot remember the beginning of the pain. Other times, the pain began after a trauma and the exact moment is remembered.

3) What caused your pain?

Typical answers: "A motor vehicle accident." "A work injury." "A stressful event." "I don't know, nothing that I can relate to."

Over half of patients attribute their symptoms to trauma or severe stress. The rest cannot identify any specific cause.

4) What aggravates your pain?

Typical answers: "Any weather change, especially cold, damp weather." "Air-conditioning drafts will aggravate my pain." "If I bend or lift or overdo any activity." "Stress."

5) What helps your pain?

Typical answers: "Heat feels good." "If I lay down and rest this usually helps." "I get my husband (or wife) to massage my muscles." "If I move around and try to stay active."

Modulation factors were described in the last chapter. Helpful clues are obtained when people describe what makes the pain worse or better.

6) Describe the pain.

Typical answers: "I feel like I've been run over by a Mack truck." "It is a dull ache but often there are sharp pains." "It is a constant pain that radiates up and down my arms and legs."

Usually a person describes multiple "types" of pain when fibromyalgia is present.

7) How has the pain interfered with your life?

Typical answers: "I can barely work, and when I get home I am so exhausted I can hardly do anything." "I used to exercise three days a week, and now it is too painful to try to move." "My husband (wife) complains that I never want to do anything with him anymore."

Nearly everyone with fibromyalgia will report some disruption of their abilities due to pain (activities of daily living, work, hobbies, recreational activities, interpersonal relationships).

Sometimes the pain onset is so gradual that patients cannot remember the beginning of the pain. Other times, the pain began after a trauma and the exact moment is remembered.

8) What has been done for this pain?

Typical answers: "I've tried everything, and nothing seems to work." "I've seen my family doctor and he has prescribed medicines." "I've tried to do stretches and take walks."

Various treatments including medicines and therapies usually have been tried before I first see a patient. Many patients may have found a fairly successful home program, but their fibromyalgia still flares up from time to time.

9) Do you have symptoms other than pain?

Typical answers: "Yes doctor, in fact I wrote things down so I wouldn't forget them. Where is my list? Here it is. I have fatigue, difficulty sleeping, irritable bowel syndrome, depression, anxiety, headaches, TMJ problems..."

Many associated symptoms and conditions associated with fibromyalgia contribute to the patient's pain or may interfere with the treatment and recovery. These associated conditions may require separate treatment approaches altogether in addition to the overall fibromyalgia treatments.

When giving their histories, patients may say one thing but they really mean something else. Sometimes I have to read deeper into what people are telling me. Let me share some examples of what you may say, and what you really mean!

What You Say . . .	What You Mean . . .
It's a terrible toothache.	My teeth are the only part of me that doesn't hurt.
I used to walk 3 miles a day.	It hurts me to drive for 3 miles.
I used to have a photographic memory.	Doctor, my brain is out of film.
I used to go on vacations.	The only things that travel now are my pains.
Do you see many people with fibromyalgia?	I sure hope I don't know more about this condition than you do!

Patients may minimize their pain in a doctor's office. They may be embarrassed to admit it, or worry that the doctor may think it isn't real. Your pain is REAL, so tell us about it.

A detailed history of the pain and other symptoms of fibromyalgia enables the doctor to think about fibromyalgia as a possible diagnosis. The history is only part of the clinical exam, however, and not sufficient alone to diagnose fibromyalgia. The physical exam must be done and must be consistent with fibromyalgia.

Physical Exam

The purpose of the physical examination is to detect any abnormalities or patterns of abnormal changes that help the physician determine the diagnosis. An abnormality detected by a physician during the physical exam is called an objective finding. It is one that is verifiable and reproducible by the examining physician. It would also be found by another knowledgeable physician who examines the same patient.

Many patients will complain that previous doctors have examined them and found nothing wrong. They may have been told that their exam was normal, and this causes confusion and frustration because the patients are hurting, but the doctor is telling them that they are normal. The physical examination in the fibromyalgia patient is NOT normal. Fibromyalgia patients have characteristic abnormalities, particularly tender points.

Tender Points

The main findings on physical examination are the tender points. Tender points are areas in the soft tissue (the muscles, tendons, and/or ligaments) that are very sensitive and painful when pressed. These tender points are found in distinct loca-

These signature areas include:

1) The occiput. This is in back of the head where the suboccipital muscles connect to the skull.

2) Low cervical muscle. This is along the neck muscle in front of the fifth, sixth, and seventh cervical vertebrae.

3) Trapezius muscle. This broad muscle extends from the neck to the shoulder. The tender point is in the mid point of the upper part of the muscle.

4) Supraspinatus muscle. This muscle is located at the top of the shoulder blade and the tender point is located near the spine.

5) The second rib. This costochondral area is right below the collarbone.

6) Lateral epicondyle. This is located at the top of the forearm and is also called the "tennis elbow" area.

7) Outer gluteus maximus. This is the buttock muscle and should be painful in the upper outer portion.

8) Greater trochanter. This is part of the femur or thigh bone which has a knobby protrusion right below the hip joint, covered by a bursa (fluid-filled sac).

9) Medial knee. This painful area is right above the inside of the knee.

tions of the body. They do not move around and can be found in multiple locations of the body.

The presence of tender points is the main criterion used to identify fibromyalgia. According to a landmark study by the American College of Rheumatology published in 1990 (Frederic Wolfe, *et al*), fibromyalgia is diagnosed when an individual has a history of widespread pain present for at least three months, and at least 11 of 18 positive tender points in characteristic locations (*see figure*). The pain is considered widespread when all of the following are present: Pain is in both sides of the body, pain is above and below the waist, and pain is along the spine.

These are "signature" areas that distinguish individuals with fibromyalgia from those with chronic muscle pain from other causes. The 18 tender points are located in nine areas of the body, both sides, in pairs.

These signature areas include: 1) The occiput. This is in back of the head where the suboccipital muscles connect to the skull. 2) Low cervical muscle. This is along the neck muscle in front of the fifth, sixth, and seventh cervical vertebrae. 3) Trapezius muscle. This broad muscle extends from the neck to the shoulder. The tender point is in the mid point of the upper part of the muscle. 4) Supraspinatus muscle. This muscle is located at the top of the shoulder blade and the tender point is located near the spine. 5) The second rib. This costochondral area is right below the collarbone. 6) Lateral epicondyle. This is located at the top of the forearm and is also called the "tennis elbow" area. 7) Outer gluteus maximus. This is the buttock muscle and should be painful in the upper outer portion. 8) Greater trochanter. This is part of the femur or thigh bone which has a knobby protrusion right below the hip joint, covered by a bursa (fluid-filled sac). 9) Medial knee. This painful area is right above the inside of the knee.

Positive Tender Point

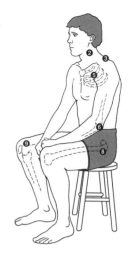

A positive tender point is one that is painful upon palpation with enough pressure to cause my thumbnail to blanch (about 4 kilograms of force). Palpation is the art of using the sense of touch to feel for abnormalities. The tips of the fingers and thumb are the medical examiner's most sensitive "instruments" for examining the soft tissue for the presence of painful tender points. I prefer to use my thumb for palpating. The patient may indicate pain by saying "ouch" or grimacing, or by trying to withdraw and avoid the pressure. The area must hurt or be painful to be positive, it can't just be "tender."

While we are on the subject of tender points, I want to call to attention one of my pet peeves: the name "tender point." By definition, a tender point is positive when it is painful. If it is just tender, it is not a positive tender point. Why don't we call them painful points? I explain to my patients that sometimes things aren't logical! I call these areas painful tender points.

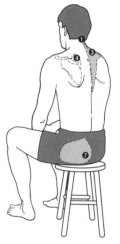

Painful tender points can be found in essentially any muscle, but usually are present in larger muscles such as the neck, shoulder, back and hips. Examining for painful tender points is a process of "mapping out" the soft tissues to determine where the painful areas are, both in the designated signature areas, and in areas that are painful, but not part of the designated eighteen tender points. Mapping helps in the diagnosis of fibromyalgia and helps determine the response to treatments.

Ropey muscles

What exactly do these tender points feel like? Fibromyalgia muscles have a peculiar consistency that feels like ropey bands or nodules. This band-like or ropey consistency is an important abnormal finding in fibromyalgia. Sometimes these taut ropey bands involve a larger area and form a fibromyalgia nodule, a firm lump that can be palpated within the muscle. This tightness, ropiness, or nodular consistency represents localized muscle spasms that can be detected with palpation by an experienced physician. These ropey muscle findings can vary in size depending on how much of the muscle is in a spasm. Usually the painful tender points will have palpable localized spasms.

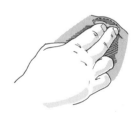

Normal muscle has a texture of firm gelatin. Imagine that you take this firm gelatin and put some grapes and strands of carrots and a couple chunks of pineapple, and when you palpate the gelatin fruit salad, you can imagine the lumpy, bumpy consistency (grapes and chunks) and ropey consistency (carrot strands). This is what the fibromyalgia muscles feel like.

People with fibromyalgia are painful all over with palpation compared to someone without fibromyalgia. Indeed, studies have indicated that people with fibromyalgia are sensitive to painful stimuli throughout the body, not just in the American College of Rheumatology defined locations (Granges and Littlejohn, 1993). The tender points are more painful than "control" areas, or areas expected to be less sensitive or painful. Example of control areas are the inside of the forearms, the front of the legs below the knees, and the back of the hands.

Many patients do not realize they have so much muscle pain until their muscles are palpated on exam. Painful tender points may not be spontaneously painful. "Latent" tender points are common, and they usually aren't so latent immediately after the exam! The spontaneously "active" tender points are what the patients notice and what ultimately brings them to the doctor.

The "11 of 18" criterion has been agreed upon for academic and research purposes to enable a consistent fibromyalgia diagnosis using a "gold standard." In the clinical setting, however, fewer tender points may be present and still indicate fibromyalgia (Wolfe, 1994). Indeed, many patients with fibromyalgia have fewer than 11 painful tender points in characteristic locations, but have other typical symptoms. If I find 10 of 18 painful tender points on someone with a typical history of fibromyalgia, I don't say, "You have nothing wrong with you!" I make the diagnosis of fibromyalgia if it best fits the overall exam.

Tender point counts can differ from exam to exam on the same patient. It would not be unusual for someone to have 14 of 18 positive on the first exam, and on the follow-up exam a month later, 12 of 18 are positive. The pattern and numbers of tender points are important in the diagnosis, but the exact locations and total numbers are less important when following a patient over time. I map out the painful areas and document them. The patients may improve but still have the same number of positive tender points (or even more!). More tender points may have become "latent" with treatment instead of remaining "active," hence the overall improvement despite the same tender point count.

The number of tender points do not correlate with the severity of the overall pain. People with 11 of 18 positive tender points can have worse pain that those who have all 18 points positive.

While we cannot compare tender points among different patients, we can look at the tender points in a given patient and correlate them to the severity of his/her pain. For example, someone whose tender point score decreased from 14 to 11 of eighteen after treatment will usually report less pain overall. Individual tender point scores are more meaningful than scores for the entire population, especially when correlating responses to treatment.

Regional Fibromyalgia

Many people have regional pain and clustering of painful tender points, that is, fewer than 11 of 18 designated ACR tender points. I believe that regional fibromyalgia is part of the fibromyalgia spectrum, and is essentially synonymous with a condition called myofascial pain syndrome. My own view is that the 11 of 18 tender points in the ACR criteria is an excellent diagnostic tool to be used as a guideline for generalized fibromyalgia, but there are many patients (including those with regional fibromyalgia) who have fewer than 11 painful tender points on a given examination date. Chapter 10 will discuss regional fibromyalgia and myofascial pain syndrome in more detail.

Trigger Points

If pressing on a particularly painful tender area causes pain, numbness, or tingling to radiate or spread to another area, this spot is called a trigger point. A trigger point is another typical finding in patients with fibromyalgia and was first described by Dr. Janet Travell. If I were to press on an area in your mid-trapezius muscle and you felt numbness radiating down your entire right arm into the hand, that area in the trapezius muscle would be called a trigger point. It could also be a painful tender point as well.

These trigger points can cause confusion since they may mimic a pinched nerve. Rather, the trigger areas in the muscles are causing radiating symptoms to distant locations. *(see figure below)*

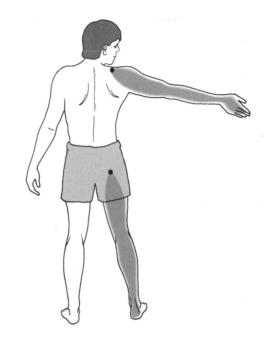

Trigger points arise from shared neurologic links between seemingly unrelated body parts. These seemingly unrelated parts actually shared a common neurologic tissue during the body's early fetal development. After these tissues divided and formed specialized parts, a common sensory neurologic link remained and can "communicate" (refer pain) in certain situations. For example, if a man is having a heart attack, he may experience numbness in the left arm. There is no problem with the left arm, per se. Rather, the heart muscle is being damaged, and because it has sensory connections to the left arm, it sends referred symptoms down the left arm. The injured heart muscle acts as a trigger point in this situation.

The human body has hundreds of potential trigger points. They can develop wherever fibromyalgia pain develops and are very common after trauma to muscles. Trigger points can cause numbness, headaches, dizziness, ringing in the ears, jaw pain, sciatica, and many other symptoms. If trigger points are spontaneously irritated, they may cause constant symptoms. If pressing on these trigger points during the exam causes them to be "activated," the physician may be able to reproduce some of the patient's subjective complaints such as referred pain and numbness. This valuable information can help distinguish between symptoms caused by a trigger point and those caused by a pinched nerve.

Other Exam Findings

Other physical exam abnormalities can be present in fibromyalgia. These include:

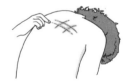

1) **Dermatographism** (Latin for "skin writing"). Scratching with a finger along the skin will cause a red mark or rash to form in patients with dermatographism. This phenomenon is most pronounced in the skin overlying painful muscles. This is thought to be due to dysfunctional autonomic nerves that "overreact" to the pressure and cause a low grade skin irritation.

2) **Decreased skin sensation.** Light touch and pin prick sensations may be decreased in fibromyalgia patients. Affected body parts include hands, feet, arms, legs, and face. Only one side of the body may be affected. Patients still feel these sensations, but they are not "normal." This is felt to be caused by an autonomic nervous system dysfunction.

3) **Goosebumps.** This frequent finding is another result of a dysfunctional autonomic nervous system. These are usually noticed in the legs during the palpation of painful tender points, but can be seen in the arms also. These goose bumps are medically known as piloerections (this has nothing to do with Chapter 31!).

4) **Decreased range of motion**. Still another physical exam abnormality is decreased joint range of motion due to painful, tense muscles. Full joint flexibility depends on the muscles' ability to relax and allow the joint to move.

Tight painful muscles prevent the joints from moving freely through their range.

The physical examination of a person with fibromyalgia should NOT reveal the following abnormalities:

1) "True" weakness (from nerve damage)

2) Loss of reflexes

3) Joint swelling, heat, or inflammation

4) Atrophy or wasting of muscles

5) Abnormal muscle tone

If any of these physical findings are present, a condition in addition to, or other than, fibromyalgia must be present. I've mentioned various physical exam abnormalities in a person with fibromyalgia. The most important and meaningful findings are the painful tender points in characteristic locations. It is this abnormal pattern of painful tender points that enables doctors to objectively identify fibromyalgia.

In case you are wondering, I've found that some tender point locations are more commonly "positive" than others. Based on my experience, I award the top two tender point pairs to the trapezial and cervical areas. The least common two tender point pairs are the medial knee and costochondral areas. Many people achieve a perfect tender point score, 18 of 18 (remember we are perfectionists). I tell people that the tender point test is one test they don't want to ace! But most do, anyway! What is the most common tender point score? I would have to say, 14 of 18, which happens to be my score.

Chapter 5 — Survival Strategies

1) Understand the importance of your medical history and physical exam.

2) Realize the doctor needs a brief version of your history and is looking for specific pieces of information.

3) Review the questions most likely to be asked in the doctor's office.

4) Prepare a list of questions and concerns. Write them down.

5) Realize the clinical findings of tender points are important in confirming this diagnosis.

6) Learn to recognize and identify the 18 characteristic tender points.

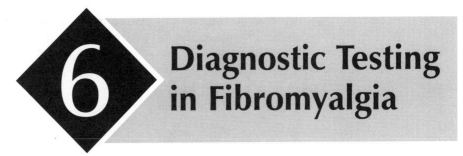

6 Diagnostic Testing in Fibromyalgia

You would expect a condition that is so painful and causes so many symptoms and associated conditions to have numerous abnormal lab tests and X-rays, right? Well, the answer is: not really. We know that a lot of measurable abnormalities are present in fibromyalgia, but no single lab test or X-ray is considered diagnostic. In fact, routine labs and other tests are usually normal. There are specialized tests in which fibromyalgia patients may test positive, but these tests are not considered routine, nor are they positive in all patients with fibromyalgia.

In the last chapter, I described objective tender point abnormalities in a typical pattern that were characteristic findings in fibromyalgia, the 11 of 18 painful tender points. These tender points are found through physical examination, not laboratory tests or X-rays. If characteristic tender points are present on exam in a patient with widespread muscle pain for more than three months duration, fibromyalgia is fairly straightforward. Few conditions cause chronic widespread muscle pain like fibromyalgia. But numerous conditions cause overlapping symptoms and can mimic fibromyalgia. Examples of these conditions include polymyalgia rheumatica, rheumatoid arthritis, lupus, hypothyroidism, myopathy, osteoarthritis, multiple sclerosis, mononucleosis, blood disorders, and more. Other times, fibromyalgia coexists with one of these other conditions, either being "caused" by this other condition or coincidentally present along with this other condition. Many conditions mimicking fibromyalgia can be ruled out by a careful history and physical examination. Certain specialized laboratory and other types of testing may be helpful also.

Although many lab tests are normal in fibromyalgia, this does not mean nothing is wrong. A normal test result simply means the particular test did not detect any abnormality. If an X-ray, a test to look at bones, is normal, it does not mean that fibromyalgia is not present. Rather, it means the X-ray of the bones was normal.

Likewise, an abnormal test does not necessarily mean a particular condition is present. Your doctor has to correlate this test abnormality with your clinical examination. For example, if a magnetic resonance image (MRI) of the brain shows abnormal white spots suggesting Multiple Sclerosis, but the person has a completely normal neurologic examination and no symptoms whatsoever, the doctor would not diagnose Multiple Sclerosis without more evidence.

Any diagnostic test in medicine has its limitations. Each test measures something specific; it may detect something, quantify something, or observe something. Depending on what test is being done and what is being measured, the physician might be able to make certain diagnoses or rule them out. Physicians, however, cannot rule out a diagnosis based on a particular test if the test is not "measuring" that particular diagnosis. In other words, a blood sugar lab test won't show a broken bone.

Another concept to understand with medical testing is that not everyone with a particular disease will test "abnormal" for it, and conversely, some normal people without the disease will test "positive" for it. When an individual has a disease but tests normal, we call this test a false negative, which means it should have tested positive. When a test is positive, but the person really doesn't have the disease that is being tested, we call this test a false positive, which means it should have tested negative.

A common example of a false positive in fibromyalgia is a positive ANA (antinuclear antigen), which is a screen for lupus. Many people with fibromyalgia have a positive or elevated ANA result, yet they do not have the clinical disease of lupus. In these people, the high ANA is a false positive. Most of you will tell me you have had a billion tests done before your diagnosis of fibromyalgia was made. Many times you go to another doctor and proceed to have yet another billion tests done. The results are always the same: normal! You just happen to have fibromyalgia, and various lab studies, electrical studies, X-rays and other radiographic imaging are normal because these tests look for other conditions which you don't have.

Below is a brief review of some common categories of testing that may be done to evaluate the cause of your pain or rule out specific conditions other than fibromyalgia. Some tests are very expensive, others are invasive. In fibromyalgia, various tests can show abnormalities. Certain laboratory studies, specialized radiographic studies, and some electrical studies can be abnormal but are not necessary to diagnose fibromyalgia. These specialized tests are not routinely done for fibromyalgia, because they are more often used in research centers. The following is a summary of some of these tests. You and your doctor need to decide what testing may be needed, if any. Don't assume that any test abnormalities are due to fibromyalgia or some serious problem. Your doctor will guide you through the test results.

Laboratory Tests

In patients with persistent pain, laboratory studies are often done to look for any abnormalities in the body's electrolytes, muscle enzymes, bone enzymes, or other areas that might provide clues to the source of pain. Useful laboratory screening tests include erythrocyte sedimentation rate, serum creatinine kinase, complete blood count, thyroid function tests, and perhaps tests for rheumatoid factor and antinuclear antibody (Goldenberg 1987). If a patient has true muscle inflammation (not from fibromyalgia), the sedimentation rate might be elevated. If the patient has anemia, the hemoglobin and hematocrit on the complete blood count might be low. There are hundreds of lab tests that measure the body's major functions, but your physician will select the ones that will give the most useful information for your particular problem.

Although many lab tests are normal in fibromyalgia, this does not mean nothing is wrong. A normal test result simply means the particular test did not detect any abnormality.

Physicians cannot rule out a diagnosis based on a particular test if the test is not "measuring" that particular diagnosis. In other words, a blood sugar lab test won't show a broken bone.

I usually order screening lab tests in patients who have not had any recent blood work if I suspect fibromyalgia. Remember, some people can also have another condition present that is causing fibromyalgia, and the clinical exam is revealing "only" the fibromyalgia.

Routine screening lab tests that I order include:

1) **Complete blood count with differential and platelets.** This checks for anemia, abnormal white blood counts, or platelet abnormalities that could signal a blood disorder, a bone marrow problem, iron deficiency, and more.

2) **Sedimentation rate.** This is considered a nonspecific marker for inflammation. If it is high, additional testing might be necessary to look for conditions such as rheumatoid arthritis, lupus, or myositis.

3) **Thyroid function studies.** This measures for abnormal thyroid problems, such as hypothyroidism or hyperthyroidism, and can also determine if the person has "relatively" low levels of thyroid although still within the normal range.

4) **Vitamin B_{12} level.** If fatigue, numbness, and tingling are problems, I frequently order this test to make sure it is not low, as Vitamin B_{12} deficiency can cause these symptoms. Many people with fibromyalgia have a "low normal" B_{12} level, that is, it is still within the normal range but at the lower end.

Certain laboratory studies have been found to be abnormal in fibromyalgia. These tests are not considered "routine" labs, but specialized labs. Here is a summary of these labs.

Serotonin. Serotonin is a neurotransmitter and a hormone. It is important in the brain's ability to control pain, maintain an upbeat mood or outlook, be motivated, and concentrate on a task. It has been described as the "brightness switch" of the brain, and a low serotonin level is equivalent to turning down the brightness switch on your brain's TV.

Serotonin is usually low in patients with fibromyalgia. One place that serotonin is stored is in the platelets of the blood, and Dr. I. Jon Russell discovered that serotonin storage in the platelets of fibromyalgia patients is low compared to normal people. Low serotonin is also closely related to clinical depression, so it is not surprising that many people with fibromyalgia will also have clinical depression at some time during the course of their syndrome.

Substance P. This is a small protein neurotransmitter that is found mainly in the spinal column. It has several purposes; one is the transmission of pain signals (think P for pain). Substance P can also help block pain signals. It is not unusual for neurotransmitters (small proteins) to perform different, seemingly opposite functions. One portion of the substance P molecule produces pain while another blocks the pain sensation and controls its severity.

Dr. Russell has also discovered that substance P is significantly high in the spinal cord fluid of patients with fibromyalgia, and because fibromyalgia causes so much pain this likely means that the "bad" function of substance P is overriding the good.

Nerve growth factor (NGF). NGF is another small protein that causes the growth and repair of nerves. Dr. Alice Larson found that NGF in spinal fluid of fibromyalgia patients is significantly elevated compared to normal people. Excesses of NGF are probably contributing to pain, perhaps causing hypersensitization of the nerves.

The regeneration (growth/repair) of nerves is actually a painful process. For example, patients who have had nerve trauma or spinal cord injury will often experience severe burning, tingling type pain that corresponds to the attempted regeneration of the nerves. NGF may be producing this type of pain in people with fibromyalgia, even though there has been no obvious nerve injury.

Neuropeptide Y. This small protein is a breakdown product of the hormone norepinephrine, a primary brain hormone. Dr. Daniel J. Clauw has found levels of neuropeptide Y to be low in patients with fibromyalgia, particularly when a stress, such as the tilt-table test described later in this chapter, is applied to the autonomic nervous system. This finding suggests that the autonomic nervous system is dysfunctional, particularly when it is stressed. Among other things, this dysfunction causes low blood pressure, fast heart rate, and anxiety.

Growth hormone. The "master" hormone in the body is growth hormone, secreted by the pituitary gland. Growth hormone's many functions include buildup of proteins, breakdown of fatty tissues, and enhanced metabolism. In the blood stream, growth hormone breaks down to various particles. One of them is IGF 1 (insulin-like growth factor 1). Dr. Bennett has been researching growth hormone in patients with fibromyalgia and has found that the IGF 1 levels (and hence growth hormone levels) are low in many patients. Low growth hormone may contribute to various fibromyalgia symptoms including fatigue, feeling cold, and lack of motivation.

Thyroid antibodies. Thyroid studies, as previously mentioned, are usually normal in patients with fibromyalgia. A number of people with underactive thyroid or relatively low functioning thyroid may have thyroid labs that are normal (false negative lab results). Looking at the microsomal thyroid antibodies may provide an additional clue as to whether there is a condition known as autoimmune thyroiditis. Dr. Arflott Bruusgaard performed a study that found 16% of people with fibromyalgia have positive thyroid antibodies. Does this mean that these people have a thyroid problem in addition to fibromyalgia? Remember, fibromyalgia has many subsets, and one may cause thyroid problems that need specific treatment.

Cortisol. This hormone is our natural steroid hormone secreted in response to stress. Different researchers have found that the adrenal glands in people with fibromyalgia produce less cortisol than normal. Having fibromyalgia and its associated elevated stress may ultimately wear down our stress response mechanisms to the point where our adrenal glands have a hard time producing enough corti-

Substance P is a small protein neurotransmitter that is found mainly in the spinal column.

Dr. Russell has also discovered that substance P is significantly high in the spinal cord fluid of patients with fibromyalgia.

sol. Too little cortisol means an inability to handle the body's stresses well, causing us to be at risk for infection, fatigue, and anxiety.

Magnesium. Magnesium is a mineral that plays a major role in key body functions. A primary role of magnesium is to help the muscles manufacture energy molecules known as ATP. Dr. Thomas Romano performed a study that found low magnesium levels in the muscles of patients with fibromyalgia. Measurement of the total body magnesium level is usually within the normal range, but selectively deficient in muscles, probably reducing the muscles' energy metabolism abilities and increasing their pain and spasm. When muscles relax, they require energy (ATP). Muscle relaxation is an active, not passive, process. Anything that decreases ATP in the muscles will decrease the muscles' ability to relax, and thus, increase muscle spasms.

Antipolymer Antibody (APA). Antipolymer antibodies are complex proteins that were first discovered in the blood of some women who had silicone breast implants (Dr. Tenenbaum's research). The APA is thought to be a marker for an immunological response and has been found to be high in a subset of patients with fibromyalgia. A recent study by Dr. Russell Wilson, *et al*, found that 61% of people with severe fibromyalgia had positive APA reactivity, and 30% of those with mild fibromyalgia had increased APA. The APA reactivity appears to correlate with severe fibromyalgia and may someday be used as an objective laboratory marker in the diagnosis and assessment of certain types of fibromyalgia. More research is needed, but this test has some exciting potential!

Radiographic Imaging

X-rays. X-rays are pictures that tell us whether the bones have normal density, whether there is a fracture, whether the bones are in proper position, or whether any bony diseases are present. X-rays do not "see" muscles or discs. There may be abnormal positioning of the bones on the X-ray that gives us clues that something has occurred in the soft tissues such as the muscles, ligaments, or discs. An example is a cervical spine X-ray taken shortly after a whiplash injury that shows "straightening." A normal cervical spine has a curvature called a lordosis. If a whiplash has occurred and spasms have resulted, the cervical spine may tighten up. X-rays may show a straightening or a reversal of the normal cervical lordosis.

Often X-rays will show "incidental" abnormalities such as some arthritis changes, disc deterioration, or calcifications. However, X-rays of anyone over the age of 29 will show bony changes from wear and tear, especially in weight bearing bones (spine, knees, and hips). We must not misinterpret these X-ray changes, particularly normal aging changes, as the "cause" of the pain. Normal aging changes are usually not painful.

Sometimes the X-rays reveal conditions such as osteoarthritis, osteoporosis, scoliosis, or calcified tendons, that indicate something else is present in addition to, or instead of, fibromyalgia.

Computerized tomography (CAT scan). A CAT scanner uses thousands of small X-ray beams to take picture "slices" of the part being tested. A computer generates an image that combines all these slices to form a "whole" picture of that body part. This picture can show brain white and gray matter, blood, ruptured discs, fractured bones, and more. A CAT scan can be taken of the head to look for a brain hemorrhage, for example, after a concussion. It can evaluate the spine for any ruptured or herniated disc.

In fibromyalgia, the CAT scan is almost always normal. If it is abnormal, something else is present.

Magnetic resonance imaging (MRI). This specialized imaging is accomplished by placing the patient in a powerful magnetic field, then beaming radio waves into the field, which causes tissue particles to orient themselves in a specific pattern in the magnetic field. The images generated by the MRI machines are remarkably sharp and give detailed pictures of the anatomy of the spine, soft tissues, and organs, depending on what part is being scanned.

This testing is a valuable tool in the diagnosis of tumors, disc herniations, and ligament tears, but in fibromyalgia the routine MRIs are usually completely normal.

Bone scan. This specialized imaging study uses labeled calcium particles injected into the patient's blood stream. These particles are taken up by the bone. If the bone is inflamed in a particular area, more of these particles will accumulate there and show up as a "hot spot." Although we feel like our muscles have a bunch of "hot spots," our bone scans are usually normal.

Myelogram. A myelogram is performed when a dye is injected into the spinal column in the low back. The dye fills up the spinal fluid spaces that surround the spinal cord and nerve roots, and when an X-ray picture is taken, the dye shows up on the film and gives an anatomical view of the spinal cord and nerve roots. Any abnormality within the spaces, particularly a protruding or herniated disc, can be detected. A myelogram can also detect severe narrowing of the spinal column called spinal stenosis.

The myelogram is no fun at all, and in patients with fibromyalgia, it is usually normal. Some fibromyalgia patients have been found to have narrowing of their cervical spinal column, called cervical spinal stenosis.(see later in this chapter)

SPECT Scan. This is a specialized imaging of the brain. SPECT stands for Single Photon Emission Computerized Tomography and examines brain function by measuring brain blood flow. Drs. James Mountz and Laurence Bradley have identified abnormalities in patients with fibromyalgia. Specific parts of the brain that process pain, the thalamus and caudate nucleus, have shown decreased blood flow on the SPECT scan. If these parts of the brain do not function well, the result may be more pain. This research may lead to a better understanding of the brain's role in inhibiting pain.

Positron Emission Tomography (PET). A PET scan can be another sensitive test for pinpointing brain abnormalities by measuring the rate of glucose metabolism. Glucose metabolism correlates with the activity of a cell. Active cells use glucose as food, and active cells are functioning cells.

An injection of a tracer glucose is given to the patient, and after thirty minutes or more, the PET scan is taken to study the glucose metabolism in different regions of the brain. Dr. J.C. Hsieh coordinated a study of PET scanning in patients with fibromyalgia and found increased glucose activity in specific parts of the brain, namely the anterior cingulate cortex.

Cervical CAT Scans, MRI and Myelograms. A subgroup of people with fibromyalgia were found to have a higher incidence of cervical spinal stenosis (narrowing of the cervical spinal canal) and Arnold-Chiari malformation (birth defect where the lower part of the brain protrudes into the cervical spinal canal). Many of these conditions don't cause any noticeable symptoms. This stenosis can cause compression of the cervical spinal cord and perhaps contribute to the neck and shoulder pain of fibromyalgia. Some patients have noted improvement in their fibromyalgia symptoms following surgery to relieve the spinal stenosis. Cervical cord compression in fibromyalgia needs to be studied further.

Electrical Studies

Whereas laboratory studies measure the presence and quantity of a particular unit, and X-rays show the bone anatomy, electrical studies measure the function of certain body organs. Persons with chronic or persistent pain may undergo various electrical studies to look for any measurable functional abnormality.

Electroencephalogram (EEG). In the waking individual with fibromyalgia, who has various electrodes attached to the scalp and hooked to a machine that measures electrical currents and activities of the brain's nerves, this testing will be normal. Even with a severe, splitting headache, the EEG should be normal, since headaches usually do not cause changes in our brainwaves. The EEG can detect seizures or damage to the brain, neither of which is part of fibromyalgia.

Dr. Stuart Donaldson in Canada did a research study looking at EEGs in patients with fibromyalgia after a trauma. He found an increase in the low frequency brain waves (the theta waves) in these patients. This increase in theta activity means the brain is functioning in a "slow" mode and may explain some of our fibro-fog. This testing may help clarify how the pain causes the brain's electrical patterns to change.

Another EEG test, the sleep study, measures brain activity during various sleep cycles. In fibromyalgia, many people will demonstrate a characteristic sleep abnormality where the deep part of sleep, stage IV sleep, is abnormal. Harvey Moldofsky, M.D. has done the important pioneer research studies on these types of abnormalities in fibromyalgia.

Electromyelogram (EMG). This specialized test measures the function of nerves and muscles. Since people with fibromyalgia often have numbness and weakness, this test is commonly performed to look for any nerve irritation. Small electrical shocks resembling static shocks are given to stimulate the nerves and record the function. A needle electrode is inserted into different muscles to measure if they are working properly. Electrodiagnostic testing can help identify certain problems such as a radiculopathy, carpal tunnel syndrome, neuropathy, or myopathy.

Unless a person with fibromyalgia has one of these conditions, the electrodiagnostic testing will be normal. Many people with fibromyalgia can also get carpal tunnel syndrome, which is very common. However, fibromyalgia does NOT cause carpal tunnel syndrome, nor does it cause any typical electrodiagnostic abnormality.

This test may be ordered to be sure there is no nerve damage other than fibromyalgia symptoms.

Electrocardiogram (EKG). This test measures the electrical function of the heart and may be ordered in individuals with chest pain. Chest pain is common in fibromyalgia, but EKGs are usually normal because the chest pain is not due to cardiac muscle or heart involvement. Rather, the chest and rib muscles and the soft tissues around the ribs are the usual source of the pain.

Tilt-table testing. This testing is one way to investigate the autonomic nerve function in people with fibromyalgia. The autonomic nerves control blood pressure and heart rhythm, and Dr. Daniel J. Clauw has performed tilt-table testing which involves monitoring blood pressure, pulse, and the EKG.

An individual having a tilt-table test lies down flat on a table and is monitored. The table is then slowly tilted up and the blood pressure, pulse, and EKG are continuously monitored for any changes. In people with fibromyalgia, about 25% have a significant drop in blood pressure and an increase in pulse rate. These abnormalities are felt to represent dysfunctional sympathetic nervous system activity causing inability to respond to stress. In the case of the tilt-table, the stress is gravity acting upon the body.

Many tests have shown some abnormalities in people with fibromyalgia. I have not mentioned every test. Ongoing studies are showing additional abnormalities and giving us some clues as to the pathology of fibromyalgia. Some additional research is discussed in Section II: Understanding Fibromyalgia. With ongoing research, we may some day see a specific test that is accepted as a good marker for fibromyalgia. Such a test does not exist at this time.

Putting It All Together

As I've emphasized, fibromyalgia is not a diagnosis that is made by performing some specialized test. Nor is it a diagnosis that cannot be made if there is no specialized test to detect it. Diagnostic tests such as laboratory studies, X-rays, or electrical studies are not necessary to make a diagnosis of fibromyalgia. There are various test abnormalities present in fibromyalgia, but there is no single lab test that indicates fibromyalgia 100% of the time. The key diagnostic test remains the physical exam finding of the painful tender points.

Chapter 6 — Survival Strategies

1) You will not die from fibromyalgia — you may just wish you would!

2) Fibromyalgia is not a wastebasket diagnosis. Your condition is real. Your pain is legitimate.

3) Find a trained M.D. who is "fibro-friendly." That can help increase your confidence in the diagnosis. Be clear in your mind that there isn't some hidden condition and you just haven't found the right doctor.

4) Expect X-rays and bone scans to be normal.

5) Consider with your doctor which tests are appropriate, and worth the investment of time, money, and personal energy. Question whether the data is *really* needed.

6) Remember that tests should be done to evaluate the cause of your pain or rule out other conditions, not to confirm something you already know.

SECTION II

UNDERSTANDING FIBROMYALGIA

This section focuses on what I know about fibromyalgia today. First I describe "normal" pain, then move on to abnormal pain. Chronic pain is "abnormal" pain and it includes fibromyalgia. Emotional aspects contribute to all types of pain and I've discussed these aspects well. Confused? I hope it will be more clear when you finish this section. If it is, you've accomplished an important part of being a Fibromyalgia Survivor: you've understood it (or at least some of it)! I know this section is complicated, but hopefully it helps. I'm not trying to stress you out!

Our knowledge of this complicated condition continues to change and evolve as more and more research is done and clinical experience is accumulated. Understanding fibromyalgia is really half the battle...so go forth and win knowledge!

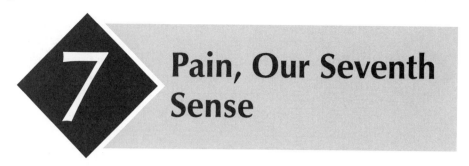

7 Pain, Our Seventh Sense

Pain is a bad word. All we have to do is watch any TV commercial or look in a magazine and we will see multiple advertisements constantly telling us that pain is bad and we need to do something about it. Every year we spend billions of dollars on medicines and devices for our pain. If you factor in medical costs, lost wages, and Workers' Compensation, we are spending probably 100 billion dollars a year in treating pain.

Pain may be a warning that something is wrong, and it may invoke fear that something is terribly wrong with our bodies, such as a heart attack or cancer. But pain is essentially a part of living. In fact, the average person experiences pain every day, and the average American over 45 has at least two painful conditions (Dr. Ernest W. Johnson). I think Dr. Johnson, my mentor at Ohio State University, says it best: "Pain is a part of living. It is an expected and necessary part of our interface with the environment. Pain is a privilege, a reminder of being alive."

This is for "normal" pain, though. Pain in fibromyalgia is different than the everyday aches and pains. As we will learn in the next chapter, it is amplified pain that can't be ignored. It is *not* a privilege! In this chapter, we'll try to understand regular "normal" pain.

I find it fascinating to look back in history and see how pain was viewed. In prehistoric times, pain was believed to be caused by demons entering the body through wounds and swimming around, and the treatment was to open new wounds to allow fluids with the demons to escape. During the Renaissance, the heart was perceived as the pain center. It wasn't until the 1800's that the nervous system was understood to be the cause of the pain. We now know that pain is a complicated process of the nervous system, and in fibromyalgia, pain gets even more complicated.

Seventh Sense

We are all familiar with our usual five senses: sight, smell, taste, touch, and hearing. Likewise, we have attributed ESP (extrasensory perception) as a sixth sense. I affectionately describe pain as our "seventh sense." Pain travels through the same nerves that convey our sense of touch, but we fibromyalgia people know that we can have severe pain without touching anyone or having anybody touch us! So, when we talk about regular pain, I like to think of it as "meet your seventh sense." When we talk about fibromyalgia pain, I think we should say "delete your seventh sense, it's gone awry!"

Normal Pain

Pain is a normal built-in process to give us information about our body and the world it is in. Acute pain warns us that something is wrong and tells us that we had

> The normal transmission of pain begins at pain sensitive cells called nociceptors. Nociceptors are programmed to respond to specific noxious or painful stimulations that could be potentially harmful to the body.

better do something about it — fast. Not feeling pain would be dangerous to our health. We wouldn't be able to tell if we were having a heart attack, a broken bone, appendicitis, or a ruptured brain aneurysm.

The normal transmission of pain begins at specialized nerve endings of skin, muscles, bones, and other tissues. These specialized nerves are pain sensitive cells called nociceptors. Nociceptors are programmed to respond to specific noxious or painful stimulations that could be potentially harmful to the body. When you drop a pan on your foot, you activate the foot nociceptors and initiate a chain reaction.

The nociceptors release chemicals called neurotransmitters, which create tiny electrical currents that travel up the nerves into the spinal cord via a nerve relay system. The neurotransmitters are the chemical messengers. Once the signal reaches the spinal cord, specialized nerve tracts called spinal neurons relay the signals upward to the brain. The spinal neurons are highly specialized and dynamic in their responses. Spinal neurons can respond to nociceptive stimuli and transmit this information upward, but they can also block pain signals, sensitize them, or desensitize them. After the spinal neurons process the signals, it relays them up to the brain.

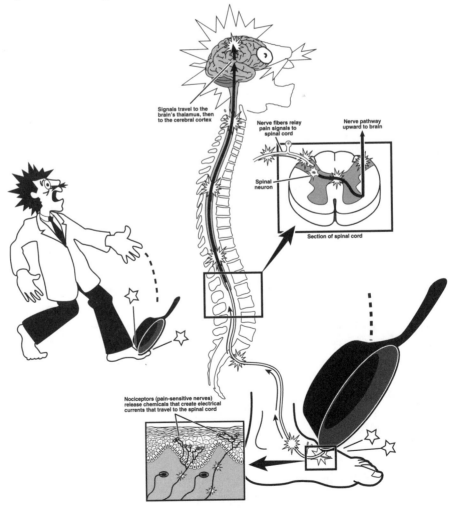

It isn't until the signals reach the brain that a phenomenon called nociperception occurs, which is when the brain detects pain, and therefore, you first perceive the original signal (the pan falling on your foot) to be painful. This whole process happens in milliseconds. Normally, the pain signal travels at a speed of 112 m.p.h., so you will feel pain immediately when you drop a pan on your foot. The pain signals are closely connected to your motor nerves, too, which enables an immediate physical reaction to pain. For example, if you put your hand on a hot stove, you reflexively move your hand off of the stove. If you drop a pan on your foot, the motor neurons reflexively tell your mouth to open and say something like "Darn, I wish I hadn't dropped the pan on my foot."

The brain perceives pain and it interprets the incoming pain signals from the spinal cord centers. Specifically, the information relayed to the brain deals with: What type of pain is it? Pain can be perceived as a burning, numbness, tingling, ache, stabbing, tearing, itching, swelling, crawling or a combination. Where is the pain? How intense is the pain? Is the body still being injured? Why did you drop a pan on your foot? Did you think your foot was a stove?

The process of getting the pain signals from the nociceptors to the brain is fairly constant and universal in all normal humans. That is not to say that the neurologic system is constant, unchanging, and always produces the exact same response in everyone. We know that the nervous system in the spinal cord is dynamic and has a lot of variations from individual to individual. It would be like saying that all humans are equipped with a radio broadcasting system representing the nerve endings and spinal cord. This radio system has multiple channels representing different neurologic pathways to the brain. Whenever signals are broadcast, our brains receive these signals at once, but each of us gets signals through different channels. Our radios are always turned on and we each always have an "open" channel for our pain to be relayed, but we are not all using the same channel at any given time.

Even though the signals get to our brain in a fairly constant way, we aren't saying that all individuals perceive pain the same way. In fact, part of what makes us unique is that we each perceive pain differently, uniquely. Using the radio station analogy, that would mean that we all receive the pain radio signals to our brain fairly equally, but some of us interpret the pain with a more "country" flavor while others give it a more "rock-n-roll" component, and still others interpret their pain to have a more "oldies" feel. I imagine the radio station for fibromyalgia would be something like "no rhythm with the blues."

The unique individual component of pain is interpreted at two centers of the brain known as the limbic system and the cerebral cortex. The limbic

Part of what makes us unique is that we each perceive pain differently, uniquely.

system is a structure that includes the thalamus and hippocampus, amygdala, locus ceruleus, and cingulate gyrus. It is a complex unit that gives an "emotional component" to pain. Fear, anxiety, and depression can modulate one's perception of how bad pain is, and one's pain threshold can be elevated or lowered based on emotional responses generated by the limbic system.

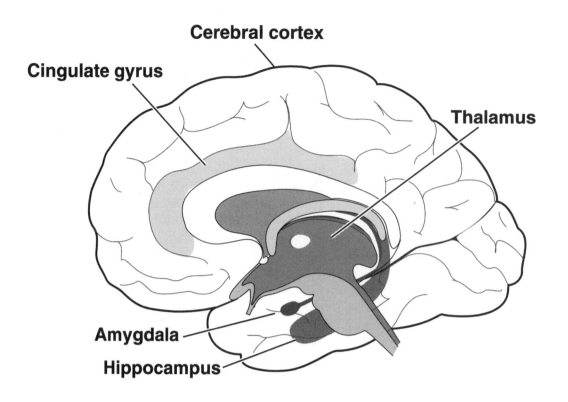

The cerebral cortex is the intelligence center of the brain where pain information is ultimately interpreted, processed, responded to, and stored. It is the most advanced part of our brain that makes us human. The cortex ultimately completes our sensory and motor pain experience with the emotional aspect contributed from the limbic system. In our cortex, we experience, learn, behave, and memorize in unique ways as a result of pain experiences. Individual brain responses to pain are shaped by factors such as genetics, learned responses and previous experiences.

Childhood experiences with pain will influence how pain is perceived later in life. What is the first thing we do when a child cuts his knee? We say, "Oh no, you've got a boo-boo, let me put a Band-Aid on it." And then, every grown-up who sees the Band-Aid says to the child "Oh you poor thing, you've got a boo-boo, let me kiss it. How does it feel?" The child learns at a very young age that pain hurts, but one can be rewarded with attention and other good things! Cultural differences also contribute to a child's pain learning experience. Pain experiences can have both "negative" components (it hurts!) and "positive" ones (get attention, get candy).

It doesn't take long for people to recognize a pattern that if they hurt and look like they hurt, other people will immediately notice the pain. In fact, people can learn that acting like they have pain (pain behaviors) even if no pain is present will still cause other people to react as if pain were present. A person can learn to signal pain behaviors to others to indicate pain. A facial grimace, a groan, or grabbing one's back may be signals to call others' attention to pain. These are examples of pain behaviors that can be learned, and sometimes they are used to avoid undesired chores such as taking out the garbage or visiting in-laws!

Another example of how pain can be perceived and learned differently is the expectation of what happens from the pain. For example, most mothers will tell me that giving birth is the worst pain they have ever experienced, yet many mothers have been pregnant many times. Why is that? Quite simply, despite the severe pain during delivery, the outcome of their pain was good, that is, a new life was born. This is a highly positive reward to experiencing severe pain. On the other hand, an individual with chronic muscle pain with no end in sight may experience the pain as the worst imaginable. Nothing good is expected from this never-ending pain. In our culture we have learned that pain is bad, and we have learned "responses" to pain. The pain isn't less real because of our perceptions and learned responses. As we will see, the pain is physiologically worse in fibromyalgia.

Differences in Pain Between Men and Women

There are sex differences in the perception of pain. According to recent research (Dr. William Isenberg), women are more sensitive to pain than men, but are better able to cope with it, recover more quickly, and are less likely to let pain control their lives. Men tend to cope poorly with pain and suffer in silence. It is probably a macho thing, literally, because Dr. Isenberg's research suggests that the presence of the hormone testosterone (at higher levels in men) increases pain tolerance. Women (with their high estrogen and low testosterone) have a lower pain threshold, but their sensitivity to pain probably increases their awareness of potential health problems and they seek health care sooner than men.

Another factor that may cause sex differences in pain is that women have a bigger corpus callosum. The corpus callosum is the part of the brain that connects the right and left halves of the brain. A bigger corpus callosum means that women connect both sides of the brain better. Thus, the female brain halves can work together simulta-

Individual brain responses to pain are shaped by factors such as genetics, learned responses and previous experiences.

Childhood experiences with pain will influence how pain is perceived later in life.

The child learns at a very young age that pain hurts, but one can be rewarded with attention and other good things!

neously better than those of men, who are suffering with small corpus callosums and use only one side of the brain at a time. These differences allow women to incorporate more information simultaneously when solving a pain problem and use their keener sense of pain as a call to action to overcome pain.

The International Association for the Study of Pain (IASP) defines pain as an unpleasant sensory or emotional experience associated with actual or potential tissue damage (Merskey and Bogduk, 1994). This definition states that pain can be present whether or not there is tissue damage. Pain is always subjective and unpleasant, by definition. Pain is difficult to measure, standardize, or reproduce because its perception is influenced by multiple factors such as personal beliefs, education, culture differences, learned experiences, and genetics. But we know pain exists even if we can't always measure it. In fibromyalgia, our seventh sense has to work overtime!

Chapter 7 — Survival Strategies

1) Understand that your pain is "real" even if it can't always be scientifically measured.

2) Consider how you perceive pain.

3) Identify which factors influence your pain the most. Is it personal beliefs, education, cultural differences, learned experiences, or genetics, or a combination?

4) Change the way you think about pain by working on the areas you have identified.

5) Remember that your pain is different than that of others. The exact same pain response is not produced in each person. We each perceive it differently.

6) Measure your pain against yourself — not other people. Their pain data will not compare to yours.

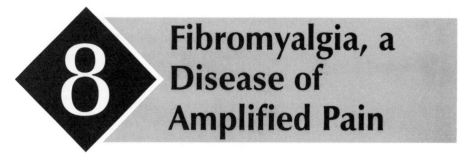

8 Fibromyalgia, a Disease of Amplified Pain

In the last chapter, I described "normal" pain, if there is such a thing. A normally functioning pain pathway will act as our seventh sense to continuously monitor the body and its environment. Different types of pain can be identified, but the two main types are acute and chronic.

Acute pain can be a brief warning signal such as touching a hot stove with no damage done to the tissue. Or there could be tissue damage as occurs with any number of conditions including muscle strains, ligament sprains, bone fracture, ruptured disc, skin burn, or a pinched nerve. In acute pain, healing is the body's expected outcome, and hopefully the pain will be able to go away completely. The healing may take anywhere from a few days for a muscle sprain to many months for a ruptured disc. Where surgery is required, hopefully the problem is corrected, and when healing is complete, the pain is gone.

When persistent, acute pain signals are sent through the normal pain pathways, the body has various adaptive mechanisms designed to tolerate or reduce the pain. Here are some examples.

Reflexes. One way to avoid pain is to perform a variety of complicated and protective reflexes. When you quickly withdraw your hand after touching a hot stove, you are performing an automatic motor reflex in response to the pain. If you move your hand quickly away from a painful source, the tissue damage can be minimized.

Muscle spasms. These often occur around a painful inflamed area. Protective muscle spasms act as a splint to "guard" the painful or unstable area and prevent further damage or movement. For example, someone with a low back disc herniation may develop protective spasms of the back muscles as an involuntary attempt to minimize movement and prevent damage of the inflamed disc area. As we very well know, these muscle spasms themselves are very painful. The body figures if it doesn't want a painful area to move, it will make that area even more painful so one will not even think about moving it!

Accommodation. This mechanism is one in which the body tries to tolerate persistent pain signals. The body releases its own pain medications, endorphins, which are small neurotransmitters that inhibit pain. This desensitization process makes it harder for pain signals to activate the pain pathways to the brain because the body has made it more difficult for these signals to reach the pain threshold. This is the point of no return, when pain signals are "strong" enough to activate the pain pathways. The body has accommodated these pain signals by decreasing their intensity and therefore, decreasing the chance of reaching pain threshold.

An example of accommodation is when you step into a hot tub (or cold pool). At first your skin actually hurts, but then the sensation becomes tolerable even though the water temperature hasn't changed. Another good example occurs when a husband ignores his wife's repeated request to take out the garbage. The words are still coming out of the wife's mouth, but the husband has been able to accommodate the words and not respond to them!

The gate control theory of Melzack and Wall. In 1965, Dr. Melzack and Dr. Wall described the gate control theory of pain. They observed that pain signals traveled in small diameter nerve fibers. Large diameter nerve fibers carry different types of sensory signals (touch and pressure) and can inhibit the signal transmissions of the smaller nerve fibers carrying pain. They proposed a gate mechanism in the spinal cord where the large and small nerve fibers converge. If signals from both the large fibers and small fibers arrive at the gate at the same time, the nerve signals from the large fiber will inhibit the small fibers, thus closing the gate for the small fiber transmission and opening the gate for the large fiber transmission. Only the large fiber signals, touch and pressure, are able to pass through the gate and travel upward to the brain. Small fiber signals, pain, are blocked at the closed gate.

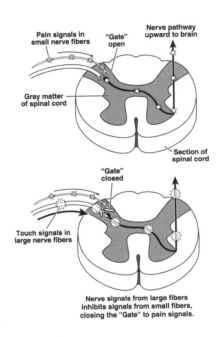

We can take advantage of this gate mechanism to control our persistent, acute pain. If we bruise or burn our hand, we will often blow on it or rub it. This blowing and rubbing sensation travels up the large nerve fibers and blocks out the pain signals traveling up the smaller fibers. If our legs are very painful from an injury, we may walk around to reduce the pain. The pressure and motion signals from walking will travel up the large nerve fibers and block the smaller fiber pain signals.

"Fight or Flight" response. This occurs when the body senses an injury and releases its adrenaline hormones (epinephrine and norepinephrine) to heighten the body's abilities to fight off the threat or take flight to evade it. The body and brain are put in a state of heightened awareness, and pain is lessened. If acute pain signals persist, the body can sustain this response for a while before fatigue sets in.

A good example of this response is the athlete who plays in spite of an injury. The pain from the injury may not be noticed because the athlete is in his "game mode" which is similar to this heightened awareness state. After the game, the painful injury is noticed much more as the adrenaline response wears off. The adrenaline temporarily blocked the acute pain.

Chronic Pain ("Abnormal" Pain)

If there is a progression of tissue damage, or the pain signals persist even though the "acute" injury has subsided, chronic pain may result. Many conditions can give rise to chronic pain, and the key is that permanent changes occur in the pain pathways either from tissue damage or abnormal neurologic changes. The pain pathways become "abnormal," leading to persistent pain. Chronic pain can result at any part of the pain pathway: the nociceptors, neurotransmitters, nerves, spinal cord, or brain:

Nociceptors. Neuropathy, burns, inflammatory conditions (*e.g.*, rheumatoid arthritis) and causal-

Muscle spasms act as a splint to "guard" the painful or unstable area and prevent further damage or movement.

Accommodation. Mechanism in which the body tries to tolerate persistent pain signals. Endorphins are small neurotransmitters that inhibit pain.

gia (burning pain) are examples of conditions that cause damage to the nociceptors and increase pain signal transmission up through the pain pathway.

Neurotransmitters. Various neuromuscular disorders including myasthenia gravis, myotonia, and tetanus can cause chronic pain by interfering with the neurotransmitter mechanism.

Nerves. Carpal tunnel syndrome, radiculopathy (pinched nerve in neck or back), shingles, and thoracic outlet syndrome (pinched nerve in underarm) are some conditions that can cause chronic pain by irritating the nerves.

Spinal cord. Spinal cord injuries and spinal stenosis can cause chronic pain by damaging spinal cord pain pathways. Multiple Sclerosis is an example of a condition that causes demyelination, or loss of the nerve's fatty insulation (myelin) which can lead to chronic pain.

A rare syndrome called congenital insensitivity to pain causes the person to be completely unresponsive to pain. This condition is felt to be related to problems in the spinal cord. Insensitivity to pain is not a good thing. In fact, people with this problem usually die young because of damage and complications to the body when pain was not perceived.

Brain. Brain problems that can cause chronic pain include Multiple Sclerosis, strokes, aneurysms, and brain tumors. These conditions can disrupt brain nerve signals and affect how pain is perceived.

Fibromyalgia Pain

Many conditions can lead to permanent changes in the pain transmission mechanism and result in chronic pain that overwhelms the body's pain defense mechanisms. One such condition is near and dear to all of us, fibromyalgia. Fibromyalgia may not cause destruction along the pain pathways as can other conditions I have mentioned. However, fibromyalgia does cause chronic abnormal changes along all the pathway components and this results in chronic pain via both peripheral (from skin, muscles and nerves) and central (from spinal cord and brain) neurologic mechanisms. The end result of fibromyalgia's abnormal changes appears to be a state of pain amplification that causes severe generalized pain. Fibromyalgia is ultimately a disease of amplified pain.

Dr. Robert Bennett has written and presented excellent information that explains why we hurt with fibromyalgia (*e.g.*, 1999 review article in Mayo Clinical Proceedings). If we trace the pain signals through the various parts of the pain pathway (from the nociceptors to the nerves to the spinal cord to the brain) in people with fibromyalgia, we find various abnormalities along the way. Many studies have shed light on different points along the complete pain pathway. I want to briefly summarize some of these different abnormalities and possible problems encountered by fibromyalgia pain signals on the path to the brain.

Nociceptors. Pain originates from the nociceptors (those specialized pain nerve endings). Trauma is a common trigger of fibromyalgia. Tissue injury, damage to the muscles and soft tissues, activates the nociceptors. Some studies have suggested that microscopic injury occurs in specific parts of the muscles (for those who aren't totally lost by now and want the medical names: muscle spindles, intrafusal fibers, and calcium pumps). Localized tissue injury probably activates arachidonic acid (a biologic protein), which turns into "bad" prostaglandins, which cause inflammation and pain (called Cox-II prostaglandins).

In addition to trauma, autoimmune factors may be another pain nerve activator. Perhaps autoimmune processes create the APA (antipolymer antibody, see Chapter 6) which acts as an irritant and activates the nociceptors chronically to the point where they become "permanently" sensitized and irritated. As a result, biochemical, hormonal, and red blood cell changes occur that interfere with the cells' ability to receive adequate supplies of oxygen, glucose, and other nutrients. Blood flow, energy formation, and the cells' electrical and neurologic harmony are all disrupted. Since the nociceptors remain "faulty," the electrical and neurological balance remains abnormal, and the nociceptors continue to be activated. Pain-producing neurotransmitters are released and accumulate as long as the nociceptors stay activated at the peripheral level (skin and muscles, especially).

The pain signals may be interpreted as an itching, burning, swelling, or tingling at one end of the spectrum, or, at the other end, knife stabbing, burning, or throbbing. One nociceptor can signal different pain signals and sensations depending on its level of irritation – the more irritated it is, the more severe the pain.

These changes can become permanent and cause the nerves to become sensitized to the point where they are easily activated to send pain, even in the absence of any noxious stimulus. In other words, persistent pain signals can *spontaneously* arise from peripheral nerve endings and bombard the rest of the pain pathway. So, instead of waiting for outside stimulation such as trauma, pressure, temperature, or touch to signal the nociceptors, these nociceptors send pain signals on their own, without any outside help. This "spontaneous" pain is what we complain about the most!

Nerves. The nerves, especially the sensory nerves and the autonomic nerves, "wonder what is happening" because they are getting bombarded by all of these signals from the nociceptors. At first, they try to diminish these painful signals by using accommodation and gate mechanisms. However, the signals persist, and they, too, undergo a sensitization process. They become hypersensitized and react with an exaggerated response instead of a normal or diminishing response (accommodation). Now we get even more pain, numbness, swelling, burning, and other sensations. Some of the hypersensitization may be mediated by nerve growth factor, which has been found in higher levels in fibromyalgia. A high nerve growth factor may indicate the nerves are trying to regenerate or repair themselves. But instead of repairing the nerves so they act normal again, the opposite seems to happen. Nerve growth factor is probably enhancing the nerves' abilities to transmit pain to the spinal cord. More pain results, not less.

Spinal cord. At the spinal cord level, the fibromyalgia begins to take control. It is here that additional changes occur to perpetuate the pain and spread it to different levels. Spinal cord nerves are bombarded by continuous stimulation from the peripheral nerves, causing a progressive increase in electrical signals to be sent up to the brain. This phenomenon is called "wind-up," and is the neurologic mechanism for the amplification of pain. Once this wind-up phenomenon occurs, a central sensitization results in which various types of sensory signals, not just pain, will arrive in the spinal cord, become amplified, and be sent to the brain as pain. The spinal cord becomes more sensitized to sending pain, lots of it. Once this happens, the spinal cord is not able to properly sort out and filter various sensory signals.

As a result, different sensory signals such as touch, pressure, temperature, and joint movement all become amplified and sent up the pain pathways, resulting in pain signals instead of the appropriate touch, pressure, temperature, or joint motion signals. Unfortunately for the person with fibromyalgia, the spinal cord is now "wired" to interpret nearly all sensory signals as pain, severe pain! We can still appreciate touch, pressure, temperature, joint movement, and other non-pain signals, but pain contaminates these signals, and we feel the pain.

Another key change at the spinal cord level is an increased formation of Substance P and other neurotransmitters (see Chapter 6). Substance P's primary role at the spinal cord level is to transmit pain signals and to sensitize the spinal cord so it is readily available to transmit pain. When Substance P reaches high concentrations (as it does in fibromyalgia), it can migrate up and down the spinal cord, away from the initial location of the pain signal. As a result, multiple levels of the spinal cord undergo sensitization and send increased pain signals, leading to a "generalization" of the fibromyalgia. This spreading of pain explains how one can develop generalized fibromyalgia from an initial regional area of pain. A common example of this occurs following a motor vehicle accident where a particular body part, such as the neck, was injured. Over time, the pain begins to involve the mid-back, low back, and ultimately the whole body even though these areas were never injured. The Substance P-induced spinal cord changes can explain this migration of pain from the neck to the entire body.

Brain. Our poor brains have no chance, do they? Any pain memory stored in the past will be re-awakened by this process. Fibromyalgia is notorious for causing previously injured areas to hurt more once it develops. This previously injured area may have settled down and become essentially pain-free, but the pain memories remained, although inactive. Thanks to the fibromyalgia pain amplification process, the inactive memories were reactivated. The pain centers of our brain, the limbic system and the cerebral cortex, are continuously fed these amplified signals from the spinal cord. Changes occur: serotonin levels decrease, brain waves change, sleep stages are affected, blood flow and glucose metabolism are affected.

The brain gets overwhelmed with these pain signals and spends a lot of attention and energy monitoring the pain. Fibro-fog occurs. Emotional components are "attached" to pain, including fear, depression, anxiety, anger, hopelessness, and helplessness, which can further amplify the pain.

Brain plasticity is probably occurring. Plasticity is an adaptive capability of the brain that modifies its own neurologic structural organization and functioning. The mechanisms include sprouting (growing of new nerve fibers), unmasking (activating previously "quiet" nerve pathways), and hypersensitization (increasing the responsiveness of the nerves). The brain makes these changes to enhance its ability to perceive pain, brain amplified pain. Alas, we have completed the full circle!

Fibromyalgia Pain Summary

To summarize, fibromyalgia changes our pain pathways. It may start off as a peripheral irritant, but eventually it becomes a self-perpetuating process that affects the entire pathway from the nociceptors to the brain. The main problem, in a nutshell, is amplified pain. What comes in at a signal of a level 1 does not end up in the brain as a signal of a level 1 as it would in people without fibromyalgia. Our pain signal of a level 1 gets amplified and magnified, and by the time it reaches our brain, it is a level 10. Other nonpainful signals get thrown into this pain amplification pathway and arrive at our brain as pain signals. These are not your everyday aches and pains, these are severe pains that cannot be ignored. This severe, chronic pain can completely disrupt one's life. And by the way, while all of this is happening, we continue to look completely normal on the outside.

To use the radio station analogy, we now have a Fibromyalgia (FM) station that plays continuously. This station picks up everything – rock and roll, country, R&B (representing different sensory signals) and plays these different types of music. But pain music is also played and it distorts the other sounds. The volume is stuck on high and you can't turn off the music. The result: an FM station that plays blaring pain music all day, all night, all the time!

Chapter 8 — Survival Strategies

1) Validate that you have a real condition: fibromyalgia causes chronic, amplified pain that is severe and cannot be ignored.

2) Understand that uniquely perceiving pain does not mean the pain is imaginary; the pain pathways become abnormal in fibromyalgia and cause you to perceive more pain.

3) Keep a pain diary of different types of pain you feel, what causes them, and what you do that helps them.

4) Educate those you care about how you can look normal yet hurt so badly. Their pain data will not compare to yours.

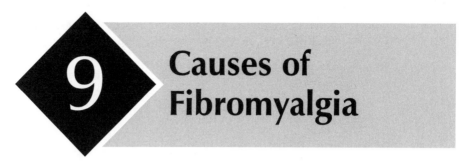

9 Causes of Fibromyalgia

In 1993, I wrote in my first book, *Fibromyalgia: Managing the Pain*, that "the exact cause of fibromyalgia is unknown." At that time, a lot of research had been done that shed light on various contributing factors. Since that time, additional research has uncovered significant clues to what causes fibromyalgia and how fibromyalgia develops. Areas such as genetics, trauma, infectious; and autoimmune, biochemical, and neurologic mechanisms are helping us to refine our knowledge about what causes fibromyalgia. All of us involved with fibromyalgia, either by treating it or having it, have come to appreciate how complicated this condition is. Fibromyalgia has different types and subsets. More than one factor may be involved in causing it. Causes may be recognized, but the exact mechanism of how fibromyalgia develops from this cause is not fully known. Most importantly, there is more than one way to get fibromyalgia; it is an "end point" condition with multiple ways leading to it.

Think of fibromyalgia as a theme park, for example, the Magic Kingdom park in Orlando, Florida. The Magic Kingdom has various sections including Main Street, USA, Adventure Land, Frontier Land, Liberty Square, Fantasy Land, Tomorrow Land, and Mickey's Star Land. Think of these various sections as different subsets of fibromyalgia. However, with fibromyalgia you do not have lots of fun and adventure and meet famous cartoon characters! Now think of the different roads and highways that lead to this theme park. These represent the different ways that one can get to fibromyalgia, there are some direct paths via the main highways, and there are some back routes through smaller roads that represent indirect pathways. There are many direct and indirect ways to get to fibromyalgia, and once you are there, you may end up in a specific subset.

I think we can say a number of causes of fibromyalgia are known at the present time. Yet I continue to read in the scientific literature statements such as "the cause of fibromyalgia is not currently known...," or "future research will hopefully discover the cause of fibromyalgia...." I think one of our inherent problems is that we try to be TOO scientific when we really need to be more practical and logical. We are allowed to use common sense along with our scientific research. A couple of inherent "problems" arise when talking about the cause of any condition, not just fibromyalgia. Let's review these "proof vs. probability" and "cause vs. mechanism" problems.

Proof Versus Probability

Causality is the relationship between a cause and its effect. In medicine, we speak of whether or not something causes a particular medical condition. We can ascribe a degree of causality. That is, at one end of the spectrum, we can say that a cause and effect relationship happens with absolute certainty. At the other extreme, the cause and effect relationship is only a remote possibility. Absolute certainty implies that scientific proof has been established with 100% certainty. However, scientific causality in medicine is rarely established to that degree. As Thomas Edison once said, "We do not know one millionth of one percent about anything."

Much of the time, scientific discovery happens by accident. As an example, the drug minoxidil was "accidentally" discovered to promote hair growth in balding people. The original use of this drug was to treat hypertension. A side effect was noted: hair growth. After further research proved minoxidil causes hair growth, this product became available as a topical solution for treatment of hair loss. Minoxidil is still used in pill form to treat hypertension.

Most of what we treat in medicine does not have causes or treatment effects established with absolute certainty by scientific studies. If we waited for scientific proof to be established for everything we treated, doctors would not be able to treat most of the medical conditions known to us today. We have to recognize and acknowledge that our clinical practices are not based on absolute certainty principles, but rather on probability principles.

Most of what we treat in medicine does not have causes or treatment effects established with absolute certainty by scientific studies. If we waited for scientific proof to be established for everything we treated, doctors would not be able to treat most of the medical conditions known to us today. We have to recognize and acknowledge that our clinical practices are not based on absolute certainty principles, but rather on probability principles.

Probability means that the causality is more likely than not. It does not mean 100% absolute certainty, but 51% or more certain. Our clinical practices are based on principles of reasonable probability within a reasonable degree of medical certainty. We can't wait around for scientific proof to accidentally be discovered; we need to diagnose, treat, and determine causes now.

To use the argument that we do not have scientific proof, and therefore something cannot cause a condition such as fibromyalgia is a ridiculous "defense." It may be difficult to establish scientific proof in medical research, but that does not mean we can't establish probable relationships between cause and effect with well-designed research studies. Dr. Muhammad Yunus, *et al*, reported a number of research techniques that can establish causality within a reasonable degree of medical certainty (Fibromyalgia Consensus Report Additional Comments, 1997). Examples of such research techniques include:

1) **Consistent clinical pattern**. This means that doctors who treat a condition regularly note a relationship between cause and effect.

2) **Case control studies**. These studies measure a response or outcome to a particular stimulus or treatment using a controlled subject population.

3) **Dose response relationships**. These studies measure a relationship between a specific quantity or dose and an outcome or response.

4) **Biologic plausibility**. This technique often relies on research of animals and use of a logical extrapolation to similar biologic human models. This also involves understanding biologic responses that can be measured at the present time, and then logically extrapolating what would happen over time.

There has been a lot of controversy regarding cigarette smoking and lung cancer. Is there a scientific causality? If we look at the different types of researches, it can be concluded that scientific causality has not been established with absolute certainty between cigarette smoking and lung cancer. Yet, there has been a consistent clinical pattern observed: Doctors who treat people with lung cancer note that many of them are heavy cigarette smokers. There are case control studies and dose response relationships that suggest that the more one smokes, the more one is at risk for developing lung cancer. There is also biologic plausibility data that allows us to logically conclude, for example, that if there are over two dozen carcinogens in smoke, and carcinogens can cause cancer, then smoking can cause cancer. Even if it can't be proved that a single one carcinogen causes lung cancer consistently, it is plausible to assume that many carcinogens will do it.

With fibromyalgia, there are no scientific studies that establish causality with absolute certainty. There are many studies and patterns that establish scientific causality to within a reasonable probability. Doctors have to use the best of our clinical experience and research in evaluating and treating conditions. As Dr. Sackett said, "Good doctors use both individual clinical expertise and the best available external evidence, and neither alone is enough."

Cause Versus Mechanism

Another difficulty in determining cause is determining the difference between cause and pathological mechanism. In fibromyalgia, the cause would be WHY fibromyalgia developed. The pathologic mechanism would be HOW fibromyalgia developed. Let me give you a couple of examples to explain.

Someone throws a baseball and it accidentally hits your nose and breaks it (great example, huh?). The cause of your broken nose (the WHY) is the baseball hitting your nose and injuring it. The pathological mechanism of the injury (the HOW) is that high amounts of compressive force impacted the nasal bones, causing them to fracture. A fairly simple example, right?

Here is a more complicated example. You have allergies, and you are exposed to ragweed and develop a lot of congestion and sinus drainage. You then get a sinus infection and require an antibiotic. The pathologic mechanism (HOW) is that the body's allergic system was activated causing increased secretions. The increased secretions trapped more dirt and germs, and eventually a bacteria was able to establish itself in this sinus fluid and cause an infection. What was the cause (WHY)? The main overall cause was the ragweed which lead to the problem to begin with, and the secondary cause was bacteria which directly lead to the sinusitis. That particular sinusitis wouldn't have happened, however, without the ragweed.

Many times, it is difficult to determine if an abnormal research finding is part of the cause or the mechanism of fibromyalgia. Changes occur after fibromyalgia has developed, so an abnormality can be one of the consequences of fibromyalgia. It is like asking what came first, the chicken or the egg? The ongoing research challenge in fibromyalgia is to sort out the information into the proper categories and ultimately try to determine what comes first, and what happens after it develops. I often tell my patients that their fibromyalgia happened because "the sun, the moon, and the stars lined up just right for them!" Now that's pretty scientific, don't you think?

I have compiled a list of probable causes of fibromyalgia. This list is based on my experiences and understanding of the current literature. My opinions on these probable causes may not be shared by everyone. My list of probable causes is as follows:

1) Genetics

2) Trauma

3) Connective tissue disease

4) Infection

5) Catastrophic stress

6) Chemical exposure

Genetics

Physicians who see patients with fibromyalgia can recall a number of patients who are relatives. I have seen numerous family members, mother-daughter, sister-sister, sister-brother, etc. who have the typical symptoms and findings of fibromyalgia. Several members of my family have fibromyalgia, through four generations! I also see numerous patients who tell me they have family members known to have it (their family history is positive for fibromyalgia). Many adult patients state they had pain as a child. These observations support the notion that fibromyalgia can be inherited, or at least the tendency to develop fibromyalgia is inherited.

Several studies on the hereditary aspects of fibromyalgia have been published. Dr. George Waylonis and I published a study in 1989. We studied seventeen families and as many first degree relatives as we could gather up, and concluded that a number of family members had fibromyalgia in a pattern that suggested an autosomal dominant mode of inheritance. This means that if one parent has fibromyalgia, then 50% of the offspring has a chance of getting fibromyalgia, whether they are male or female. There appeared to be a variable latent stage which means that the fibromyalgia could develop at different ages in different offspring. There also appeared to be variable transmission, it could "skip a generation." My study found a high percentage of fibromyalgia in men with a positive family history, nearly equal to the women. This is much different than the people who present to the doctor's office, because more than six times as many women than men will be diagnosed with fibromyalgia. Men DO have fibromyalgia, but they take a different course than women. We have to go out and look for them because they do not tend to come to us to be diagnosed.

Dr. Dan Buskila from Israel performed a study looking at 60 children of 21 mothers with fibromyalgia. He found a number (23%) of the offspring, most of them female, to have fibromyalgia. When he looked at the males with fibromyalgia, he found the ones who were under 18 had fibromyalgia almost as frequently as the women under 18. He concluded that fibromyalgia had a major genetic component that possibly fit the autosomal dominant mode of inheritance, especially among males and females under age 18. Dr. Buskila did another study looking at people with fibromyalgia and many of their relatives, and found that 45% of them reported widespread musculoskeletal pain resembling fibromyalgia.

Other studies have supported an inherited pattern to fibromyalgia. Dr. Muhammad Yunus performed Human Leukocyte Antigen (HLA) studies in fibromyalgia. HLA are genetically determined molecules that are found in virtually all cells. HLA genes can be markers for certain diseases, and the results of Dr. Yunus' HLA study suggests a genetic role in fibromyalgia.

I believe that the current literature, combined with accumulated clinical experience, supports a genetic cause of fibromyalgia. A "common sense" approach would be to recognize that fibromyalgia is so common in the general population of the entire world that there must be some type of common genetic make up that leads to it. Another logical conclusion from all of the available information is that people are genetically predisposed to getting fibromyalgia. I think a number of people are programmed genetically to develop fibromyalgia over time, probably independent of the environment. However, for a number of others, an environmental trigger must occur (*i.e.*, the other causes listed here) for the fibromyalgia to develop.

Who is at risk genetically to develop fibromyalgia? I think the following can be considered at risk.

1) A child with one or both parents with fibromyalgia.

2) A child of one or both parents with a connective tissue disorder such as
   rheumatoid arthritis or lupus.

3) A child with a sibling who has fibromyalgia.

4) A child with a first degree relative who has fibromyalgia.

Just because someone is a risk does <u>not</u> mean he or she will automatically get fibromyalgia. The right "trigger" may never happen. If a child at risk does become symptomatic with fibromyalgia, there's a lot that can be done. Don't assume that someone will get fibromyalgia or that it will be bad if they do.

Genetics play a role in pain sensitivity. Dr. George Uhl found that differences in pain perception were due to variations on the surface of nerve cells, specifically on the molecule called the mu opiate receptor. The mu receptor works by bonding with natural chemicals called peptides that help diminish the sensation of pain.

Individuals who have lots of these receptors have more ability to diminish pain; they have less pain. But those who have reduced mu receptors (too few mu's!) cannot diminish the pain as well, and even small stimuli can cause severe pain. The number of these receptors is controlled by the action of the mu opiate receptor gene.

Those with fibromyalgia, or at risk for it, may be genetically mu deficient. I believe with additional research we will be able to further clarify specific genes causing pain, and develop genetic-specific medicines to control pain.

Trauma

Fibromyalgia caused by trauma is called posttraumatic fibromyalgia. Trauma causes tissue injuries, and not everyone completely recovers from a trauma. In predisposed injuries, a physical trauma can trigger the development of fibromyalgia. Physicians who treat fibromyalgia regularly report that the majority of fibromyalgia patients attribute the onset of fibromyalgia symptoms to a traumatic event. In my own private practice, I reviewed 2,000 fibromyalgia patients seen from 1990 to 1995. Of those, 65% reported the onset of their symptoms after a traumatic event. The most common trauma reported was a motor vehicle accident, and the second most common trauma was a work injury.

The story is always the same. Basically, a person is pain-free, then has a trauma, then develops pain that never disappears. Eventually that person is diagnosed with fibromyalgia. I've seen many people with no previous pain develop fibromyalgia right before my eyes following a trauma, despite my best treatment efforts to heal the trauma. This type of clinical experience screams for a logical conclusion based on common sense: Fibromyalgia must have been caused by the trauma.

The science of fibromyalgia and trauma is evolving. In 1996, a Vancouver fibromyalgia consensus group published a consensus report in the *Journal of Rheumatology*. In this report, the current knowledge of fibromyalgia was reviewed (in 1994), and a statement was made that at the present time, there is no conclusive scientific proof as to whether or not trauma causes fibromyalgia. This statement is truthful, as expected, because scientific proof is rarely established for any condition treated in medicine. However, a lot of good research has been published on trauma and fibromyalgia which I believe shows reasonable probability that trauma is a cause.

The mechanism by which trauma leads to fibromyalgia appears to be peripheral triggers from the trauma that mediate biochemical and neurologic changes, first in the muscle and then in the central nervous system (spinal cord and brain). Once the trauma sets the process in motion, eventually it leads to fully developed fibromyalgia syndrome.

The research that has been done so far uses scientific principles to support clinical probability. Let's review some of these techniques that support the probable relationship between fibromyalgia and trauma.

Consistent clinical pattern. Various researchers of fibromyalgia including Dr. Romano, Dr. Greenfield, Dr. Waylonis, Dr. Modolfsky, Dr. Wolfe, and Dr. Simons have published papers on clinical observations and clinical patterns of patients who developed posttraumatic fibromyalgia or posttraumatic myofascial pain syndrome.

Case control study. Dr. Buskila (*Journal of Rheumatology*, 1997) published case studies on patients who had whiplash injuries to the cervical spine and an injury to the lower extremity and found that fibromyalgia developed thirteen times more in people who had a neck injury. This study showed a relationship between cervical spine injury and the onset of fibromyalgia, as well as showing that a regional injury can evolve into generalized fibromyalgia syndrome.

Biologic plausibility. Dr. Bennett has described how it is biologically plausible for a regional injury to lead to generalized fibromyalgia following a trauma.

Many other studies have been published. I have reviewed a few of them here.

The mechanism by which trauma leads to fibromyalgia appears to be peripheral triggers from the trauma that mediate biochemical and neurologic changes, first in the muscle and then in the central nervous system (spinal cord and brain). Once the trauma sets the process in motion, eventually it leads to fully developed fibromyalgia syndrome. The fibromyalgia may be regional where the injury occurred, or it may spread and become generalized over time and cause pain in areas that were never injured in the first place. There is a lot of controversy regarding trauma and fibromyalgia. To me, the clinical and scientific evidence support trauma as the second most common cause of fibromyalgia.

Rheumatic and Connective Tissue Diseases

Many people get fibromyalgia associated with another disease, particularly rheumatic and connective tissue diseases. After genetics and trauma, I believe this type of disease is the most common cause of fibromyalgia. Conditions in this category that can lead to reactive fibromyalgia include rheumatoid arthritis, lupus, polymyalgia rheumatica, and autoimmune disorders (thyroiditis, Sjogren's syndrome, and systemic reaction to silicone breast implants). The reverse is not true, though. That is, fibromyalgia does not turn into rheumatoid arthritis, lupus or other inflammatory conditions.

The immediate cause of the secondary or reactive fibromyalgia is the primary disease. However, the exact cause of most of these primary diseases is not fully understood. Theories for the cause of various rheumatic and connective tissue diseases include genetic susceptibility, infections, and certain stresses or exposures. The fact that the exact cause for the primary disease might not be known does not prevent one from stating that it is the cause of the secondary fibromyalgia. The cause should be the most immediate and direct one responsible, and in this case, the primary disease.

One could debate the "original" cause just as one could debate the theory of creation of the universe. What happened first? For example, we could say that fibromyalgia was caused by trauma. But what caused the trauma? It was a car that had run a stop sign. But what caused the car to run the stop sign? The driver was not paying attention. But what caused the driver not to pay attention? The driver was using a cell phone. But what caused the driver to use the cell phone? Somebody needed milk. And so on. Do I sound like a 2-year-old?

We can recognize more than one cause of a condition, and some are more direct than others. For the purposes of being very practical and logical, let's just say that the majority of the cause "weight" goes to the event closest to the development of the fibromyalgia. Rheumatic and connective tissue diseases in themselves cause specific symptoms and have specific measurable pathologies. Fibromyalgia, once it develops, becomes a separate entity and will often have a course independent of the original primary disease. For example, people with rheumatoid arthritis who have secondary fibromyalgia, can have the rheumatoid arthritis in remission, but be in a severe fibromyalgia flare-up that is more disabling to them than the rheumatoid arthritis ever was.

All of the rheumatic and connective tissue diseases may actually be variations of autoimmune diseases. Autoimmune diseases can involve any system in the body, but the joints and connective tissue seem more vulnerable. Up to 5% of the adult population has an autoimmune disease, over two-thirds of those are women. Autoimmune disorders occur when the immune system begins to attack the body. Fibromyalgia can develop as a consequence of these primary diseases if the autoimmune/inflammatory mechanism sets the "fibromyalgia cascade."

Many women with silicone breast implants develop symptoms and findings consistent with fibromyalgia. Various reports have been published which describe musculoskeletal manifestations following silicone breast implants (Dr. Cuellar, et al; Dr. Cohen, et al; and Dr. Bridges et al). The APA described in Chapter 6 was initially detected in women who had developed musculoskeletal complaints following silicone breast implants. I have seen a number of women in my practice who got fibromyalgia secondary to the implant. Whether the silicone caused an autoimmune-like condition which subsequently led to fibromyalgia, or whether the fibromyalgia resulted directly from the silicone exposure is not known for certain. Allergic-type reactions can be closely related to autoimmune reactions; either could lead to fibromyalgia.

Infection

Like trauma, infection is one of those causes of fibromyalgia that just screams for common sense. I've seen hundreds and hundreds of people whose basic story goes like this: "I was fine, I got a virus, I developed fatigue and pain, and I've never been the same since." The logical thinking in this scenario is that fibromyalgia was not present before the viral infection. There may have been a hereditary predisposition or a vulnerability, but fibromyalgia was not present. The virus caused the condition to develop and it has been present since the virus and continues to be present. This is a straightforward infectious cause.

The mechanism by which an infection leads to fibromyalgia is probably related to inflammatory or autoimmune changes caused by the infection that starts the "fibromyalgia cascade" permanent changes occurred in the body, and these changes caused fibromyalgia to develop.

Not all infections are as straightforward. Many people who have fibromyalgia get a viral infection and find it worsens the fibromyalgia. People with active viral infections are at risk for additional infections, particularly bacterial infections which can create additional problems. Some people with fibromyalgia are more vulnerable to any type of infection because the fibromyalgia renders them more immunocompromised or more at risk for infection. The physician needs to sort out the various possibilities to determine whether an infection is the cause, a consequence, or an aggravator of the fibromyalgia.

The mechanism by which an infection leads to fibromyalgia is probably related to inflammatory or autoimmune changes caused by the infection that starts the fibromyalgia cascade. The actual clinical infection resolves and is long gone, yet fibromyalgia symptoms continue. Sometimes, the infecting virus or bacteria may hang around and create a persistent low grade infection which activates the autoimmune responses, thereby "triggering" the fibromyalgia. Many times though, the infection has long disappeared, but permanent changes occurred in the body, and these changes caused fibromyalgia to develop.

Various viral infections can cause fibromyalgia. The Epstein-Barr virus which causes infectious mononucleosis is one. Cytomegalovirus causes a syndrome similar to infectious mononucleosis. Different strains of the Influenza virus can also result in fibromyalgia. The Adenoviruses, especially Type II, cause common colds, bronchitis, and various upper respiratory infections, and may lead to fibromyalgia. Reactive fibromyalgia has been described in patients with AIDS and hepatitis. Sometimes viral titers can be directly measured to demonstrate that an acute infection has occurred. This concentration can be correlated with the clinical development of fibromyalgia. Many times, though, the exact offending virus is not known, but we can still categorize the fibromyalgia as one that was caused by an infection, probably a viral infection, if it fits clinically.

Bacterial infections can also cause fibromyalgia. I have seen patients who have developed fibromyalgia after sepsis (blood infection) and salmonella infections, one who, I felt, had gotten it from a Listeria infection. Some research studies found microplasma incognitus and chlamydia pneumonia in patients with fibromyalgia and chronic fatigue syndrome (Dr. Garth Nicholson, and Dr. Darryl See). These infectious organisms may be causing some of the symptoms. Indeed, some of the patients improve with antibiotic therapy. Gulf War Syndrome, in part, may have been related to infections from one of these bacteria. Symptoms of Gulf War Syndrome include fatigue, headaches, depression, joint and muscle pain, sleep disorders, and poor memory (sound familiar?).

Fibromyalgia can be caused by yeast and parasite infections. I have seen some patients who developed it following a severe Candida yeast infection, and others following parasite infections such as Giardia. Most of the time, yeast or parasite infections occur in patients after the fibromyalgia has already developed. These infections may aggravate the preexisting fibromyalgia or cause it to flare up. Fibromyalgia may predispose us to these infections by interfering with our immune function. On the other hand, these infections can sometimes cause the fibromyalgia by "triggering" the fibromyalgia cascade. Many of the symptoms of a chronic Candida yeast infection such as fatigue, irritable bowel syndrome, bloating, allergies, altered immune response, and skin conditions overlap with fibromyalgia symptoms. This can make it difficult to "separate" the two conditions and determine cause and effect relationships.

As I've mentioned, some infections come in, do their damage and disappear. The infectious agent is no longer present in the body and thus can't be detected at a later point in time. Other infectious agents may hang around in the body and establish a chronic infection, one that perhaps can be detected with blood tests. What remains to be seen is whether these chronic infections can be eradicated with antibiotic treatment and, if so, will the fibromyalgia symptoms disappear? Or has the fibromyalgia already established itself as a separate entity which does not disappear with the antibiotic treatment? Hopefully, we will have these answers in the near future.

Catastrophic Stresses

Catastrophic stresses are synonymous with emotional trauma. These are not your everyday stresses, rather, they represent more severe stresses which can cause fibromyalgia. The mechanism is probably very similar to a physical trauma, only instead of a tissue injury, there is a stress injury that may disrupt the hypothalamic-pituitary-adrenal hormone regulation (the stress hormones). Dr. Leslie Crofford has described stress hormone abnormalities after a severe stress. Once fibromyalgia develops following such an emotionally stressful event, it can be exacerbated by additional stress. Catastrophic stresses or emotional traumas can include death of a loved one, serious illness in a loved one, history of abuse, severe illness, and more. A special type of stress that causes fibromyalgia is war. Researchers have evaluated war veterans with rheumatic conditions and have described conditions that appeared identical to fibromyalgia. Posttraumatic stress syndrome was commonly diagnosed in men who had fought in the Vietnam War. It is not surprising to find that many people who have been diagnosed with posttraumatic stress syndrome also meet the criteria for fibromyalgia.

Acute severe stresses can create changes in the hormones, behavior, sleep, and pain responses which ultimately establish a chronic feedback loop that amplifies pain and perpetuates fibromyalgia. The primary cause in this situation is the stress which leads to the fibromyalgia cascade.

Chemical Exposure

I've seen a number of patients who have developed fibromyalgia after chemical exposure. Usually they have inhaled fumes from these offending chemicals which include petroleum oils, paint thinners, cleaning solvents, dyes, or gases/fumes from burning products. Most of the time, these patients are treated at the hospital, but have lingering symptoms and ultimately develop fibromyalgia. The mechanism whereby these chemical exposures cause fibromyalgia appears to be an allergic and/or autoimmune response that escalates and sets off the fibromyalgia cascade.

Acute severe stresses can create changes in the hormones, behavior, sleep, and pain responses which ultimately establish a chronic feedback loop that amplifies pain and perpetuates fibromyalgia. The primary cause in this situation is the stress which leads to the fibromyalgia cascade.

Many people with fibromyalgia are sensitive to chemicals, drugs, and environmental allergens like pollen, dust, and molds. A condition known as chemical sensitivity syndrome occurs when one becomes chronically fatigued and ill from exposures to various substances. An autoimmune mechanism is probably involved. Perhaps this condition is a subset of fibromyalgia. Various researchers have suggested that symptoms of Gulf War Syndrome could have been triggered by various chemical exposures including smoke, fire, diesel fumes, oil, vaccines, and preventive drugs. The body's immune system reacted adversely to these chemicals in many who developed Gulf War Syndrome.

Possible Causes/Probable Mechanisms of Fibromyalgia

This group of conditions may be causes or mechanisms. They probably all have mechanisms in the development of fibromyalgia (the HOW) and particularly subsets of fibromyalgia. In addition, they can be part of the cause of fibromyalgia (the WHY). At this time, I do not think these entities are consistently direct causes, rather they contribute indirectly to fibromyalgia. These entities include:

1) Hormonal disorders

2) Neurologic conditions

3) Cervical spinal stenosis

4) Arthritic conditions such as osteoarthritis, osteoporosis, and scoliosis

Hormonal Disorders

Various neuroendocrine dysfunctions (abnormalities of neurotransmitters and hormones) can cause problems. Concentrations of these substances are either too low or they are present in normal amounts but are not functioning properly. A number of people have low thyroid, low growth hormone, low cortisol, low estrogen as reported by various researchers. Some people do better with thyroid, growth hormone, or cortisol replacement therapy. A subset of women experience aggravation of fibromyalgia symptoms when estrogen levels become relatively low as can occur during certain phases of the menstrual cycle and during menopause. Some of these women improve with estrogen supplementation even if the fibromyalgia does not disappear. Further research will hopefully answer a key question: Are the hormonal disturbances the result of fibromyalgia, or are they the cause of the ongoing problem?

Neurologic Conditions

I see a number of people with multiple sclerosis, diabetic neuropathy, and postpolio syndrome who also meet the criteria for fibromyalgia syndrome. Did the neurologic condition cause the fibromyalgia? Or is the fibromyalgia coincidentally present in addition to the neurologic condition? A possible mechanism (or cause) is a neurologic "trigger" that leads to pain amplification and ultimately, fibromyalgia. In addition, neurologic conditions cause weaknesses, muscle imbalances, and changes in muscle tone that create chronic mechanical stresses on the body tissues. These altered biomechanics, over time, can create a posttraumatic type of fibromyalgia.

Cervical Spinal Stenosis

Fibromyalgia patients may have spinal cord compression from cervical spinal stenosis which causes some of their symptoms. Dr. Michael Rosner has pioneered neurosurgery to relieve or decompress the tight spinal canal patients with fibromyalgia. Dr. Rosner believes that some people have fibromyalgia because they have cervical spinal stenosis, a condition where the base of the skull and the top of the spinal canal are too narrow, causing pressure on the spinal cord. Symptoms of severe cervical spinal stenosis include pain and numbness in the arms, headaches, difficulty concentrating, wobbly gait, and exaggerated reflexes. Dr. Rosner reports a number of patients have improved fibromyalgia symptoms following this surgery.

If surgery corrected all the symptoms, the person may not have had "true" fibromyalgia, rather, the patient had cervical cord compression from stenosis that caused symptoms mimicking fibromyalgia. It's certainly possible for fibromyalgia to coexist with a neck problem. It's also possible that a neck problem such as cervical spinal stenosis can lead to reactive fibromyalgia. We know that neck injuries can lead to fibromyalgia, so it is logical to conclude (biologic plausibility) that problems affecting the cervical spinal cord and nerves in the neck area could possibly cause the condition.

Dr. Thomas Milhorat and associates described an interesting Substance P abnormality in patients with a condition known as syringomyelia (a painful cyst in the spinal cord). They found that Substance P was increased in the spinal cord below the cyst, and decreased at the level of the cyst. This suggests that anything which puts a pressure on the cervical spinal cord can lead to changes in Substance P that increases pain (remember, people with fibromyalgia have high levels of Substance P).

People who have neck injuries and neck arthritis may develop a "traffic jam" that causes more pressure in the cervical spinal cord and interferes with the Substance P distribution and pain control, ultimately causing fibromyalgia symptoms. More research is needed to clarify this.

Rheumatologic Conditions

Everyone gets osteoarthritis (wear and tear of the bones) with age, but not everyone gets fibromyalgia, so I don't think we can say osteoarthritis causes fibromyalgia. However, in people with fibromyalgia, osteoarthritis can cause it to worsen or flare up. Both need to be treated. Osteoporosis (thinning of the bones) can cause bone compression, ligament sprains, muscle strains and sprains, and biomechanical changes that are all likely to aggravate fibromyalgia.

I see fibromyalgia commonly in individuals with scoliosis. The two conditions co-exist, but I believe they are part of a genetic mechanism whereby a person inherits the tendency to have both. The scoliosis creates altered biomechanical stresses on the spine which can be an additional mechanism for developing fibromyalgia. People who have fibromyalgia do not develop scoliosis as part of the fibromyalgia, but people with scoliosis are more at risk for developing fibromyalgia. As our understanding of various causes, mechanisms, and overlapping relationships between these two increase, we may be able to revise my list.

Unknown Causes of Fibromyalgia

One of my pet-peeves is the liberal use of the phrase, "the cause of fibromyalgia is unknown." This implies that we don't know anything about the causes. I have had attorneys suggest to me that if the cause is unknown, then perhaps we are not even sure that fibromyalgia exists. We know many causes, and I've described several in this chapter. We may not know the specific cause for any particular individual, but every single person with fibromyalgia has a cause, whether we know it or not. Just because we may not know the cause doesn't mean fibromyalgia isn't there. Fibromyalgia is a big world with many parts yet to be discovered. What knowledge we have empowers us, but let's not get too comfortable and arrogant about what we know, because we really know very little of the "big picture!"

Chapter 9 — Survival Strategies

1) Remember that medicine and science are not just black and white—there's a lot of gray area.

2) Accept the fact that medicine does not know what causes fibromyalgia. At this time there is no cure.

3) Realize that even if fibromyalgia cannot be cured, a certain level of "healing" or reduction of symptoms can be achieved.

4) Consider that there may be a genetic predisposition to fibromyalgia. If this is true, patients may end up with fibromyalgia some time during their life.

5) Stop wasting time and energy assigning blame (to accidents, people, doctors) and being angry about the event that triggered your fibromyalgia. If you are genetically predisposed to fibromyalgia or had it your entire life—it's possible an event would eventually trigger the cycle.

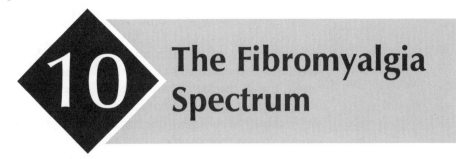

10 The Fibromyalgia Spectrum

As a senior resident at the Ohio State University in 1988, I gave a lecture on fibromyalgia at the Physical Medicine Grand Rounds. One of my lecture slides was entitled "Fibromyalgia, A Spectrum of Conditions?" I discussed how fibromyalgia appears to be a "broader" condition with specific subsets. Fibromyalgia was in that area between normal and disease, the "gray" area. Some of the subsets were closer to normal, involving regional pain only or milder symptoms without numerous associated conditions. Some subsets were closer to abnormal, with some features of connective tissue or rheumatic diseases but were not quite "there." Today I'm convinced fibromyalgia is indeed a "broader" condition with various subsets. I believe this information is helpful in explaining why everyone's symptoms are different even though they all have fibromyalgia. This chapter addresses how the fibromyalgia spectrum is part of the big picture in understanding fibromyalgia.

Fibromyalgia has been viewed as a discrete medical entity, and appropriately so. We have long recognized, however, that many conditions overlap it, and various conditions exist that can lead to secondary fibromyalgia. Dr. Muhammad Yunus has developed the concept of Dysregulation Spectrum Syndrome (DSS) to describe how conditions overlap. Dr. Yunus describes DSS as representing various associated conditions that share similar clinical characteristics and pathologic mechanisms with fibromyalgia. Ten conditions are in the DSS umbrella: fibromyalgia, chronic fatigue syndrome, irritable bowel syndrome, tension headaches, migraine headaches, primary dysmenorrhea, periodic limb movement disorder, restless leg syndrome, temporomandibular pain syndrome, and myofascial pain syndrome. He predicts other entities will be added to this list in the future.

According to Dr. Yunus, conditions in DSS share a number of characteristics:

1) Patients with different conditions sharing similar profiles

2) Common shared symptoms, such as pain, poor sleep, fatigue, and female predominance

3) Hypersensitivity to pain

4) No "diagnostic" pathology that can be measured

5) Shared psychological complaints such as depression and anxiety

6) Shared common genetic factor likely

7) Common neurohormonal dysfunctions

8) Treatments directed at the central nervous system leading to improvement

9) TMJ dysfunction

Dr. Yunus' concept includes fibromyalgia as a member of a bigger DSS family.

I have discussed the fibromyalgia spectrum with my patients to help them understand the various subsets possible. I do not see fibromyalgia as a member of a bigger family, but as the main condition. It is the "founding father" and keeps its name. If fibromyalgia is the founding father, then the various overlapping conditions and subsets become the children. The name, fibromyalgia, remains, but different subsets have unique characteristics, and together, they become the fibromyalgia spectrum.

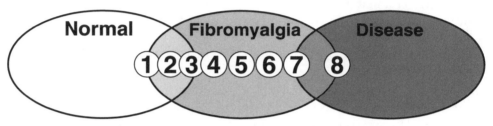

1 **Predisposed state**
2 **Prodromal state**
3 **Undiagnosed fibromyalgia**
4 **Regional fibromyalgia**
5 **Generalized fibromyalgia**
6 **Fibromyalgia with particular associated conditions**
7 **Fibromyalgia with coexisting mild disease**
8 **Secondary fibromyalgia reactive to disease**

The diagram above shows the concept of the fibromyalgia spectrum. The fibromyalgia entity partially overlaps with the normal entity on one side and the disease entity on the other side. Within the fibromyalgia entity are eight subsets. The first subset is in the most "normal" portion of fibromyalgia, and the eighth subset is in the most "diseased" portion of fibromyalgia. Each number represents a distinct subset with distinct characteristics. The eight subsets of the fibromyalgia spectrum are:

1) Predisposed state

2) Prodromal state

3) Undiagnosed fibromyalgia

4) Regional fibromyalgia

5) Generalized fibromyalgia

6) Fibromyalgia with particular associated conditions

7) Fibromyalgia with coexisting mild disease

8) Secondary fibromyalgia reactive to disease

An individual can move up this spectrum — from a lower numbered subset to a higher numbered subset, but once she/he is in a particular subset, they do not return to a lower numbered subset. One can achieve a remission, but stays in that subset. In other words, there is no going back. Let's review the features of each subset.

Subset 1: Predisposed state. The individual is asymptomatic. Clinical fibromyalgia is not present in this state. The individual is at risk for developing fibromyalgia due to hereditary factors, which may include one or both parents with fibromyalgia or a rheumatic/connective tissue disease, or a sibling or first degree relative with fibromyalgia.

Subset 2: Prodromal state. Prodromal means preceding, or the state leading to the condition. Clinical fibromyalgia is still not present. There are no widespread pain or painful tender points. The individual is not asymptomatic, however. Associated conditions common with fibromyalgia may be present in this stage, such as headaches, restless leg syndrome, fatigue, irritable bowel syndrome. Pain may be present at times, but intermittently (not chronic, persistent pains). Even though the individual may have one or more associated problem condition(s), widespread persistent pain is not present, so therefore fibromyalgia is not yet present. Typical fibromyalgia pain must be present before we can diagnose clinical fibromyalgia, no matter how many associated conditions may be present, but those who have numerous associated conditions are at risk.

Subset 3: Undiagnosed fibromyalgia. Chronic pain is now present, either regional or generalized in nature. This is the point of no return. The person has painful tender points which may or may not meet the American College of Rheumatology-defined 11 of 18. The person in this stage usually has milder symptoms and has not yet seen a doctor or been officially diagnosed with fibromyalgia. If this individual were to see a knowledgeable physician, that diagnosis would be made.

Subset 4: Regional fibromyalgia. Individuals in this stage have been diagnosed with fibromyalgia, but not generalized. Chronic pain is limited to one or a few areas such as the upper body or the low back. The symptoms may wax and wane. Usually, this subset is triggered by a trauma. I believe myofascial pain syndrome is part of this regional fibromyalgia, and both terms are essentially synonymous. Myofascial pain syndrome has become familiar through the work of Dr. Janet Travell and Dr. Robert Simons.

Myofascial pain syndrome is defined by painful muscles and the presence of trigger points and taut bands of muscle fibers which are ropey and painful when palpated. An involuntary shortening of the fibrous muscle band can create a local twitch response. Some of those who work with myofascial pain syndrome will argue that it is a separate distinct entity from fibromyalgia. I disagree. The similarities between myofascial pain syndrome and fibromyalgia are far greater than their differences. They both have trigger points, tender points, ropey muscles, sympathetic nerve dysfunction, ATP abnormalities, peripheral and central mechanisms, regional and generalized versions, and associated conditions. Sound familiar? The treatments are essentially the same. As our clinical experience has evolved and our knowledge and research have become more refined, I think it is clear that myofascial pain syndrome is a part of the overall fibromyalgia spectrum.

Individuals with regional fibromyalgia, over time, often develop generalized fibromyalgia. Or they can remain in this stage indefinitely. Identifying the regional stage early and treating it can definitely help to prevent progression.

Subset 5: Generalized fibromyalgia. Individuals in this stage have widespread pain and tender points. They will usually meet the American College of Rheumatology defined 11 of 18 criteria, but as previously explained, one can still have generalized fibromyalgia with fewer tender points. Various associated conditions seen with fibromyalgia can be present—sleep disorder, irritable bowel syndrome, depression, fatigue, and so on, but these associated conditions are not taking a life of their own so to speak, but are part of the whole and managed with the overall fibromyalgia treatment. Regional fibromyalgia can progress to this subset. Various causes of generalized fibromyalgia include genetic factors, trauma, infections, and more, but secondary fibromyalgia from a primary disease is not included in this subset.

Subset 6: Fibromyalgia with particular associated conditions. People in this group have developed associated conditions that are giving them particular problems which appear as "separate" entities requiring separate attention. Some of these particular associated conditions include irritable bowel syndrome, fatigue, tension/migraine headaches, and depression. None of these conditions in themselves have "classic" disease laboratory markers or cause tissue destruction, yet they may require treatments in addition to the overall fibromyalgia treatment. Another associated condition is dysautonomia (dysfunction of the small nerves) which can cause symptoms of hypoglycemia, hypotension, cardiac arrhythmia, irritable bowel syndrome, and vascular headaches.

Myofascial pain syndrome and fibromyalgia both have trigger points, tender points, ropey muscles, sympathetic nerve dysfunction, ATP abnormalities, peripheral and central mechanisms, regional and generalized versions, and associated conditions. The treatments are essentially the same. I think it is clear that myofascial pain syndrome is a part of the overall fibromyalgia spectrum.

Subset 7: Fibromyalgia with coexisting disease. Individuals in this category have a specific disease, and also have fibromyalgia. The disease doesn't necessarily cause fibromyalgia, but it can aggravate it if it's already present. Examples of diseases that can be present and worsen the fibromyalgia symptoms include:

- Hormonal problems (hypothyroidism, low estrogen, low growth hormone, and low cortisol).

- Infectious problems (yeast, parasite or viral infections).

- Low grade rheumatic or connective tissue disease (lupus, autoimmune disorders. Dry eyes syndrome described by Dr. Don Goldenberg may be part of a low grade Sjogren's syndrome).

- Arthritic conditions (cervical spinal stenosis, osteoarthritis, osteoporosis, scoliosis).

- Neurologic conditions (multiple sclerosis, polio sequelae, neuropathy, head injury residuals) For example, people who have both diabetes and fibromyalgia will often have more painful fibromyalgia because the diabetes caused the nerves to be more sensitive. Diabetes is a common cause of neuropathy, or damage to the small nerves, which is painful in itself and even more so with fibromyalgia. One needs to keep the diabetes under good control to help the pain.

- Lung conditions. I see a number of people who have fibromyalgia along with a lung problem such as emphysema, asthma, chronic bronchitis, or heavy tobacco use. Cigarette smoking can increase fibromyalgia pain. The nicotine in the smoke causes constriction of the blood vessels, decreasing blood flow, oxygen, and nutrients to the muscles, thereby increasing pain and spasms. Also, carbon monoxide in smoke enters the bloodstream and binds to the hemoglobin molecules in the blood. This blocks oxygen from binding to the hemoglobin, further decreasing oxygen availability to the muscles (and increasing pain). Stop smoking and your muscles will feel better!

These diseases exist concurrently with fibromyalgia but probably do not cause it. Any of these diseases can progress from a mild to a more severe state, and fibromyalgia worsens as the disease worsens. The physician determines if the disease is coexisting with and aggravating fibromyalgia (subset 7), or if a disease caused the fibromyalgia (subset 8).

Subset 8: Fibromyalgia reactive to disease. Individuals in this category have secondary fibromyalgia. They have a primary disease (*e.g.*, lupus, rheumatoid arthritis) and fibromyalgia developed as a result of this disease. People in this subset probably wouldn't have gotten fibromyalgia if they never had the primary disease. The primary disease requires treatment, and fibromyalgia may improve with this treatment. However, the fibromyalgia often requires its own treatment, and can continue to be a major problem even when the primary disease is treated or in remission.

I find that the fibromyalgia spectrum provides a useful clinical model for me when evaluating and treating my patients. It helps me to "organize" them better! When I diagnose fibromyalgia, I try to be as specific as possible about what the cause is and what subset it fits. This helps me to better explain fibromyalgia to the patients and to individualize their treatment programs. Of course, if I've diagnosed fibromyalgia it would be subset 4 or greater. The patient wouldn't be seeking a medical consultation for subsets 3, 2, or 1. If possible, I note the cause. Each subset can have flare-ups or remissions within it, and I note that as well, if appropriate. Subsets 1, 2, and 3 are useful in appreciating the progression of fibromyalgia through the spectrum, and can be helpful when advising patients and family members who have specific concerns and questions.

Let's review some patient profiles to determine the subset they fit into in the fibromyalgia spectrum.

Patient #1. Mary is a 25-year-old receptionist with severe neck and shoulder pain. She had always been very active with aerobics and bicycling and had never had any pain requiring treatment until after a motor vehicle accident on April 7, 1998, when she was rear-ended and suffered a whiplash injury. The pain never went away, and when I saw her I found numerous painful tender points and trigger points with localized spasms in the neck and shoulder muscles.

Mary has regional fibromyalgia (subset 4). She was most likely predisposed to fibromyalgia and a traumatic event triggered the development of her regional fibromyalgia. She "leaped" from predisposed state (subset 1) to regional fibromyalgia (subset 4).

Patient #2. Martha is a 30-year-old housewife. She was diagnosed with fibromyalgia five years ago, and she was at a stable baseline with her home program of stretches, exercises, and using a hot tub. In the past year, she has been having increasing pain and fatigue and difficulty managing her fibromyalgia. She reports that in the past year she has been getting frequent yeast infections. She is on birth control pills and has had a couple of bladder infections requiring antibiotics in the past year. Her more recent history is otherwise unremarkable.

Martha has fibromyalgia with a coexisting disease, chronic yeast infection (subset 7). Her birth control pills, antibiotic treatment, and perhaps fibromyalgia have contributed to the chronic yeast infection. In turn, the yeast infection has aggravated her fibromyalgia.

Patient #3. Jamie is a 38-year-old school teacher. She has lupus, diagnosed when she was thirteen years old, and has been on various medications since then. She has been in remission for a number of years, but has developed widespread pain. Her sedimentation rate is not elevated to suggest active inflammation. Her clinical exam does not reveal any joint inflammation or active lupus findings, but she does have sixteen of eighteen positive painful tender points.

Jamie has secondary fibromyalgia from a disease (subset 8). In her case, the lupus is in remission, but her fibromyalgia is causing her problems and needs to be treated.

Patient #4. Jamie's 12-year-old son has been complaining of leg pains. The pains occur at nighttime, and Jamie has to rub the legs and use warm compresses. The pediatrician told her his pains were growing pains. Jamie's son gets occasional headaches, and sometimes he feels exhausted. He plays many sports, and if he works out a lot his muscles are very sore for several days. On exam, there are no areas of pain or painful tender points.

Jamie's son is probably in a prodromal state (subset 2). He is at risk because his mother has fibromyalgia and a connective tissue disease, and he has some associated conditions with intermittent pains, but has not developed the persistent widespread pain or painful tender points yet.

Patient #5. Bob is 42 years old and has an awful lot of pain for his age. His pains are more severe than everyday pain, and sometimes he has had to miss work. He is an assembly line worker. He mentions this to his primary care doctor when he is there for his yearly physical. He is examined and found to have twelve of eighteen positive painful tender points.

Bob had undiagnosed fibromyalgia (subset 3) until he became official, "entering the books" with generalized fibromyalgia (subset 5) after he saw his primary care doctor.

Fibromyalgia Spectrum Test

Let's see how well you have been paying attention in the chapter! I'm going to test your knowledge on the fibromyalgia spectrum. Below are three case histories for you to review and then determine which subtype of the fibromyalgia spectrum each case fits. The answers follow.

Case 1: Peggy is 52 years old and works as a secretary. For about ten years, she has been bothered by pains in her neck, shoulders, and upper back. In the past two years the pain has become more widespread. She has difficulty sleeping and has extreme fatigue. She also has irritable bowel syndrome. Recently she switched to a different computer at work and has been typing a lot more than usual. After a couple weeks on this new computer, she noticed pain and numbness in her wrists and hands. This pain awakens her at night and she has to shake her hands to relieve the symptoms.

She has noticed weakness in her hands, particularly when holding her coffee cup or trying to grip a pen. Since she developed these hand symptoms, she is noticing more pain throughout her arms, neck and shoulders.

Assuming this lady has fibromyalgia, what subtype does she have?

Case 2: Patty is a 32-year-old housewife. Eight years ago she was diagnosed with fibromyalgia syndrome and has managed this condition well with a regular program of stretching and exercises. She used to play tennis a lot, but since she developed fibromyalgia, she stopped playing regularly. Even before she was diagnosed with fibromyalgia, she was always prone to getting tendinitis or bursitis in various joints. Recently she accepted an invitation from a few of her friends to join a tennis league. She started playing tennis again once a week and within a few weeks noticed increased pains in her shoulders, forearms, hips, and knees. Her doctor diagnosed her with tendinitis and bursitis.

Based on this information, what subtype of fibromyalgia does Patty have?

Case 3: Tom is 39 years old and started to hurt all over the past several months. He has had various aches and pains in the past, but nothing like this. His wife thinks he is worried about turning 40. Tom thinks something else is going on because he never had this severe muscle pain before. He also has headaches and stomach cramps. He wakes up every night at 4:00 a.m.; he used to sleep through the night. He is also has a harder time concentrating at work where he owns a printing company. He saw his doctor and his exam was normal except for various painful and sore muscles and 9 of 18 positive tender points. Laboratory studies were normal.

What is Tom's diagnosis? If he has fibromyalgia, what subset does he have?

Answers to Test Questions:

Case 1: Subset 7, fibromyalgia with co-existing disease. Peggy has fibromyalgia and carpal tunnel syndrome. When she developed carpal tunnel syndrome, this condition caused her fibromyalgia symptoms to flare up, causing neck, shoulder, and arm pain, as well as unique carpal tunnel symptoms (the hand numbness, pain, and weakness). Peggy's carpal tunnel syndrome was caused by repetitive typing. The carpal tunnel syndrome did not cause the fibromyalgia, nor did the fibromyalgia cause the carpal tunnel syndrome. These two conditions coexist.

Case 2: Subset 6, fibromyalgia with particular associated condition. Patty has fibromyalgia and a long history of tendinitis and bursitis, which are associated conditions in this case. Fibromyalgia can lead to painful tendons and bursas, particularly in the shoulders, forearms, hips, and knees. Usually the tendinitis and bursitis are not "true" inflammations, but they hurt just as bad. When Patty resumed playing tennis, she aggravated this tendinitis and bursitis, the associated conditions of her fibromyalgia.

Case 3: Subset 5, generalized fibromyalgia. This is a trick question! Even though Tom had fewer than eleven of eighteen designated tender points as defined by the American College of Rheumatology, his history and exam are still consistent with generalized fibromyalgia. Remember, one can have fewer than eleven of eighteen tender points and still have clinical fibromyalgia.

There is much disagreement and controversy among medical professionals and patients about categories and subsets of fibromyalgia or similar conditions. I'm not attempting to stir the waters with my version of the fibromyalgia spectrum, rather I'm trying to help you understand the fairly complicated nature of the condition and the different types I see. I find this model useful and practical in my everyday clinical practice. Remember one of my mottos: Keep things as simple as possible and make sure they make sense!

Chapter 10 — Survival Strategies

1) Find where your symptoms fit on the fibromyalgia spectrum.

2) Learn as much as you can about your subset so that you can determine which symptoms need attention.

3) Develop a treatment plan based on your findings.

4) Set appropriate goals and expectations for your subset.

5) Find ways to work "with" your fibromyalgia so that you can adapt your life-style to be more fibro-friendly.

SECTION III

TREATING FIBROMYALGIA

This section focuses on what I've learned about treating fibromyalgia. Many treatments are available and this section doesn't attempt to review every one possible, but rather, tries to give you the main one. General treatment strategies with specific types of programs are introduced. Specific and detailed treatments directed by the doctor are the main focus here. Personal "patient directed" treatment strategies that you can do are reviewed in the next section. Different doctors prefer different treatment approaches. I discuss my treatment styles and philosophies in this section and how I approach fibromyalgia patients.

Your goals with this section are to learn what can be done or what can be prescribed for your fibromyalgia. You should keep an open mind, and hopefully, you'll discover a few new ideas.

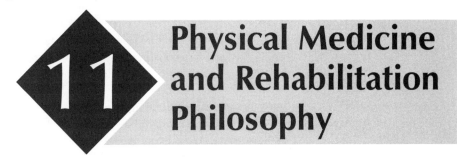

Physical Medicine and Rehabilitation Philosophy

Numerous medical professionals and specialists treat fibromyalgia. One specialty in particular, Physical Medicine and Rehabilitation, is especially skilled at diagnosing and treating such chronic conditions. A physician specializing in Physical Medicine and Rehabilitation is called a physiatrist. I am a board certified Physiatrist.

My field of medicine began in the 1930s to address musculoskeletal and neurological problems. Two historic events occurred to help shape and broaden this particular specialty. The first was the polio epidemic, which caused millions to suffer from acute pain and weakness and led to the physical medicine component of my specialty. Physical medicine modalities such as heat, electric stimulation, and water therapy along with exercises to stretch, strengthen, and condition became important treatment approaches for acute polio, and ultimately for any problem that caused pain.

The second historic event that helped shape the rehabilitation component of my specialty occurred after World War II. Improved medical technology and techniques on the field, plus the availability of penicillin led to increased survival among injured soldiers. Many soldiers with head injuries, spinal cord injuries, infections, and amputations survived. Consequently, the number of disabled soldiers also increased. Rehabilitation strategies were developed to help these disabled veterans improve functional and vocational skills, and ultimately to help them return to civilian society as productive workers. Thus, the rehabilitation component was more focused on optimizing functional abilities and included retraining and an interdisciplinary team approach.

Physiatrists treat a wide range of problems from musculoskeletal pain to brain injuries. The specialty serves all age groups and treats problems that touch upon all of the major systems in the body. The focus is on restoring function. A physiatrist diagnoses conditions that cause pain, weakness, and numbness, and may prescribe drugs, assistive devices, or a variety of therapies to improve this function.

Specific philosophies unique to physiatry include a team approach involving various medical professionals, identifying rehabilitation goals to improve function, and focusing on improving one's quality of life. The word "habile," from which rehabilitation is derived, is Latin for "to make able again." This word is an embodiment of our unique treatment philosophies.

This approach applies naturally to the diagnosis and treatment of fibromyalgia because fibromyalgia affects all aspects of our lives and makes it hard to function. The Physical Medicine and Rehabilitation strategy empowers the fibromyalgia person with abilities to improve the quality of life, even if the condition is still present.

Fibromyalgia Treatment Goals

It is a mistake to think of people with fibromyalgia as if we all have the same thing. Although we all have fibromyalgia, we certainly do not behave in the same manner, nor do we all respond the same to treatment. What works for one person may not work at all for another, because each of us is unique. We each need to be handled with special unique care, and each of us needs to identify our own specific treatment goals.

Specific fibromyalgia treatment goals that I identify for each individual include:

1) **Decreasing pain, even if pain is still present.** It would be great if everyone could go into remission and be pain-free, but this rarely happens. What usually happens is that the pain decreases, sometimes considerably, to a much lower and more stable level. Some people achieve remissions where they feel hardly any pain.

2) **Improving function.** Even if the person is unable to resume activities enjoyed prior to developing fibromyalgia, one can improve by learning to focus on current abilities. That is why I like the word "habile," because it focuses on abilities, the positive. Too often, we tend to focus on the negative, our inabilities, by concentrating on things that we used to do. Remember habile!

3) **Learning a successful program to self-manage the condition.** Each of us with fibromyalgia has to live with this condition every day, so we should try to find out what works and learn to do it ourselves. We can't sling our doctors and therapists over our backs, carry them with us throughout the day, and pull them out when needed because of increased pain. We must manage our pain as best we can by ourselves on a daily basis.

Specific philosophies unique to physiatry include a team approach involving various medical professionals, identifying rehabilitation goals to improve function, and focusing on improving one's quality of life.

As I've said earlier, one does not have to be a physiatrist to diagnose and treat people with fibromyalgia. Many doctors and specialists want to help, will be open-minded, and use the best of all available treatment options to enable each individual to **achieve the highest quality of life with the least amount of pain possible.** Your qualifications are the most important. You're the one with fibromyalgia, and you must want to do better!

Evaluating the Patient

When I see a patient for the first time, I perform a comprehensive Physical Medicine and Rehabilitation evaluation. This includes a complete history and physical examination. I gather information on pain and various symptoms and particularly on how functional abilities have been impaired. Careful palpation is included as part of my physical examination. I examine the 18 designated tender point regions in addition to the rest of the musculoskeletal system to identify all areas that are particularly painful. I search for abnormalities that could help determine a diagnosis (spasms, weakness, swelling, etc.). Any abnormalities are documented.

If the evaluation is consistent with fibromyalgia, I document this diagnosis. I note any diagnosis that may apply to the individual's pain, even if it is different from fibromyalgia. For example, there may be shoulder bursitis, rotator cuff tendinitis, spinal facet arthritis, lateral epicondylitis, hip sprain, or many other painful conditions. I don't simply put "fibromyalgia" as a diagnosis, but try to be as descriptive as possible. If a cause such as trauma or infection can be determined, I will note posttraumatic fibromyalgia or post-infection fibromyalgia. If the fibromyalgia is widespread, I will note generalized fibromyalgia. If it is more localized or regionalized, I will note regional fibromyalgia. If certain areas are particularly flared up, or if particular associated conditions such as myofascial pain syndrome, sleep disorder, and irritable bowel syndrome are present, I will note those as well.

The following patient is an example of how I might approach my evaluation and conclusion.

Mrs. Jones is a 36-year-old woman who reports pain throughout her body, particularly involving the muscles. She has a history of scoliosis. Her pains began in her early 30's and became generalized but fairly stable. In her late-teens she was involved in a couple of motor vehicle accidents where she had whiplash injuries. She received some therapies for these whiplash injuries, and said her pains completely resolved within a few months of treatment.

In her early 30s she began to develop aches and pains that became more generalized and ultimately led to a diagnosis of fibromyalgia. A month ago she took a job as a librarian and has noticed increased pain and fatigue since starting this job.

Her mother has been diagnosed with fibromyalgia. Mrs. Jones has two children, a 17-year-old son who has frequent headaches and a 20-year-old daughter who has scoliosis. Mrs. Jones' examination revealed numerous painful tender points including 14 of the 18 positive designated tender points, not the costochondral or medial knee areas bilaterally.

I would diagnose Mrs. Jones with generalized fibromyalgia. I note that there are various contributing factors to her fibromyalgia which include:

1) **Heredity**. Her mother has fibromyalgia and her two children may have prodromal symptoms.

2) **Scoliosis**. This condition increases the risk of fibromyalgia, presumably due to increasing strain on the back muscles and alteration of the biomechanics. This may be a form of cumulative trauma.

3) **Trauma**. This includes both the cumulative trauma from scoliosis and the trauma from the motor vehicle accidents. The accidents did not appear to cause the fibromyalgia immediately because the pains disappeared after treatment, but they may have created pain memory and increased vulnerability that made it easier for fibromyalgia to involve these injured areas at a later date.

Mrs. Jones' fibromyalgia represents a good example of how the exact cause may be unknown, but more than one factor are known to be involved. I may not know exactly which factor(s) caused the fibromyalgia, but I know the cause is probably one or more of the three factors that I described. I would put Mrs. Jones' fibromyalgia in subset 5, generalized fibromyalgia. The new physical activities required of her librarian job has caused a flare-up of her fibromyalgia.

Treatment Recommendations

I review my findings and diagnosis with each patient. I discuss fibromyalgia in detail and make treatment recommendations. Sometimes, I recommend that other specialists to be involved. For example, if I note my patient is clinically depressed, I may recommend a psychiatrist (specialist in depression) to specifically address the depression. I'll certainly treat the fibromyalgia but I'm not a depression specialist. My fibromyalgia treatment recommendations will try to decrease pain, improve range of motion, decrease spasms, improve function, increase knowledge, develop a successful home program, improve interpersonal skills and relationships, and optimize quality of life. The first treatment (and the most important, I believe) is education.

Chapter 11 — Survival Strategies

1) Identify treatment goals for yourself.

2) Understand that a goal of treatment is to decrease your pain. Eliminating all pain is not likely.

3) Accept that some activities will be beyond your limits, even though you could do them prior to developing fibromyalgia. You have a "different" life now, but nothing says it can't be better!

4) Learn to self-manage your fibromyalgia. The more control you have over your pain, the healthier you will be, both physically and mentally.

5) Understand what a physiatrist does and how this specialist may be most helpful in treating your fibromyalgia.

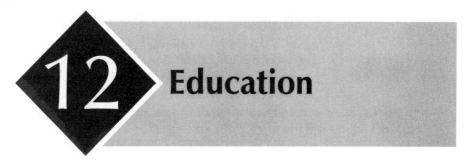

12 Education

As I said earlier, the single most important treatment is education. Learning about and understanding fibromyalgia is over half the battle. John Patrick has a memorable quote in which he said, "Pain makes man think. Thought makes man wise. Wisdom makes life endurable." Education is the first step to making your fibromyalgia more manageable.

Once your doctor has diagnosed your fibromyalgia, he or she will need to review some important points:

1) **It is a real condition.** You are validated with this diagnosis. This confirms once and for all that you are not crazy. You have a definite unique condition called fibromyalgia.

2) **Fibromyalgia is not life threatening.** You will not die from it. You may feel miserable and scared, but it is not fatal. Even if it's not life-threatening, it can be life-dreadening. You need to find ways to improve your quality of life with fibromyalgia.

3) **Fibromyalgia is not deforming or paralyzing.** It can cause joint pain and weakness, but it does not cause destruction of joints or paralysis like certain rheumatologic or neurologic conditions.

4) **Fibromyalgia does not turn into a life-threatening, deforming or paralyzing condition.** You will not get lupus or rheumatoid arthritis from your fibromyalgia. Some people have fibromyalgia in addition to these condition, but fibromyalgia doesn't turn into them. You may be stuck with fibromyalgia, however.

5) **Fibromyalgia is a treatable disorder.** It can improve. It can go into remission. It can be healed even if it can't be cured.

6) **It will not be easy having fibromyalgia** but everyone knows that good things never come easily! Fibromyalgia is a nuisance and can be debilitating. Not everyone achieves the hoped-for pain reduction or functional abilities. You have to work hard to keep fibromyalgia under control, and you have to continue to work hard to maintain a stable baseline.

I educate all of my patients on my treatment philosophy, which uses a multidisciplinary approach to achieve two general goals: 1) Find out what works. 2) Teach the person a successful home program. The patient needs to understand that she/he is an active member of the multidisciplinary team approach. There are numerous health professionals who treat fibromyalgia, and I explain my role as a team member, primarily the "coach," while the patient is the team "captain." I try to guide the patient to consistent "winning" strategies.

Realistic Goals

Part of the education process is establishing realistic goals. We live in a time when we expect perfection, and we expect results. We are used to custom-ordering and getting what we order. For example, we go into a restaurant and we say "I'd like my steak well done," "Put some lemon in my water," and "Where is the ketchup?" Or we go to a hair stylist and say, "That looks good, but take a little more off on the right." We expect our requests to get done, and done well!

> We need to set goals that are realistic. We may not be pain-free, but we can try to decrease the pain, make it more stable, or get it into a remission. Perhaps we cannot do sports like we did in high school; we can never do what we did in high school because we have gotten older. But we can learn to increase our activity level and quality of living in spite of having fibromyalgia.

So we go to the doctor and expect the same custom-order results. We say, "Doctor, I would like to be pain-free," or "I would like to play sports again like I did in high school."

I explain to the patient with fibromyalgia that we need to set goals that are realistic. We may not be pain-free, but we can try to decrease the pain, make it more stable, or get it into a remission. Perhaps we cannot do sports like we did in high school; we can never do what we did in high school because we have gotten older. But we can learn to increase our activity level and quality of living in spite of having fibromyalgia. Even if we can't do a particular sport, we can find other activities that are enjoyable.

By gently guiding patients towards realistic expectations, I try to ease the burden of perfection. It is okay to change our expectations to something that may be less than perfect, but much more easily accomplished.

Self-Responsibility

I encourage all patients with fibromyalgia to learn everything they can about the condition and how it affects their everyday life. I emphasize the importance of self-responsibility: learning to take control of fibromyalgia and striving to cope successfully with this condition each and every day. It is your responsibility to actively discover what works best for you. The more you know and understand, the less frightening or unbearable it becomes and the more "normal" you will feel again. Being self-responsible means that you recognize and accept fibromyalgia as part of you, and you learn how to adjust your life-style to best control your symptoms. Part of being self-responsible is increasing others' awareness, particularly your family, friends, and employers. We need to help others understand what we are going through.

Another key part of self-responsibility is following through with your treatment program. This takes daily work on your part. Your doctor and medical team can give you a lot of recommendations and ideas, but it is up to you to carry out the recommendations and find the right program and right balance for you and your everyday life. Medical professionals are here to help, but you have to live your own life.

Learning About Fibromyalgia

There are literally hundreds of books, brochures, newsletters, and articles to educate health professionals about fibromyalgia. I provide patients with a brochure on fibromyalgia and a handout listing various reference sources. I have been pleased to see an increasing number of fibromyalgia newsletters.

Various support groups and organizations have developed excellent and informative newsletters that include personal stories, research updates, and coping tips. I encourage my patients to read as much as they can and ask questions. When you follow-up with your doctor,

> There are a lot of people on the Internet who provide medical advice but have no medical license or medical background. This is often done to try to sell a particular product or solicit something from unsuspecting individuals. This can be dangerous because if an unsuspecting individual follows what is believed to be medical advice from a fraudulent person, that unsuspecting person could sustain injury or harm.

ask questions and work together to develop the best treatment program. Your doctor will also be able to learn from you, so share your knowledge and work together.

Internet

A wealth of fibromyalgia information is available on the Internet, and many patients take advantage of this remarkable resource. I advise people to be cautious when gathering information and advice on the Internet, and to be aware of potential pitfalls as well as benefits.

The benefits include a readily available "encyclopedia" on fibromyalgia and a good place to get basic overview information. There are also numerous fibromyalgia chat groups and support groups that can provide valuable support and bonding experiences. Many friendships have been established via these cyber support groups. Many reputable hospitals, universities, and organizations have Websites that provide reliable and helpful information on fibromyalgia.

The possible pitfalls of the Internet include the potential for overwhelming, complicated, and confusing information from a variety of sources. Invariably, if you talk to a hundred people, you will get a hundred different recommendations on how to best manage your fibromyalgia. A lot of good advice can be obtained from caring individuals, but the reality is that there are a lot of people on the Internet who provide medical advice but have no medical license or medical background. This is often done to try to sell a particular product or solicit something from unsuspecting individuals. This can be dangerous because if an unsuspecting individual follows what is believed to be medical advice from a fraudulent person, that unsuspecting person could sustain injury or harm.

I instruct people to be careful when interpreting information. The best strategy is to gather the information and share it with your knowledgeable medical professional and come up with a mutually agreeable treatment plan.

Support Group

A support group can be a valuable means of both education and treatment in fibromyalgia. Having the opportunity to share experiences with someone who has the same condition can be a powerful therapeutic tool. The Internet can be a place to meet people and participate in a support group. "Real life" support groups can provide a unique treatment dimension. A support group consists of individuals who share a common problem, fibromyalgia, and who are interested in meeting on a regular basis to share information and experiences (and doughnuts!). A successful support group can consist of as few as five members, but usually has between ten and twenty members. Of that group, there are individuals with newly diagnosed fibromyalgia who are in the early stages of accepting and coping with their condition and need guidance and support from more experienced members. Those with more experience can relate to the newer members, yet still learn new things themselves.

About nine years ago, many of my fibromyalgia patients expressed an interest in forming a group. With the help of a facilitator, we organized and have been meeting on a monthly basis ever since. My interests are both personal and professional; my involvement with the support group includes being both an active participant and a professional advisor. Our group has been fortunate to have wonderful people who are committed to helping each other.

Try to find a support group in your area. There are different kinds of groups, but the usual one would meet on a monthly basis for a couple of hours, with perhaps one hour being devoted to education and the second hour being devoted to support. Self-help groups that are run by patients can focus on more "personal" issues. Educational sessions could include having guest speakers on different topics involving fibromyalgia. One meeting a year, members could perform a literature review and discuss different aspects of fibromyalgia. Support can take the form of helping a member resolve a difficult situation; discussing issues such as anger, depression, and stress management; and sharing strategies.

I emphasize involving the patient's significant others in the education process. Fibromyalgia involves the spouse, family members, co-workers, and more. Education helps the patient's significant others to understand the condition and to provide support and encouragement.

Chapter 12 — Survival Strategies

1) Develop realistic expectations.

2) Learn everything possible about your condition and actively discover what works best for you.

3) Take responsibility for your condition.

4) Increase others' awareness about fibromyalgia, particularly your family, friends, and employers. You may be surprised to find support from others once they understand the condition.

5) Follow through with your treatment program.

6) Learn to live your life with fibromyalgia.

7) Remind yourself that one treatment or one supplement will probably not resolve your pain.

8) Participate in a support group.

Pledge for Fridge

Cut out at dotted line and tape to refrigerator

Fibromyalgia Patient Affirmation

1) I have a real condition called fibromyalgia.

2) My fibromyalgia is not life threatening and I am not going to die from fibromyalgia.

3) My condition is not deforming or paralyzing.

4) Fibromyalgia does not turn into a life threatening, deforming, or paralyzing disease.

5) I can do many things to "heal" my fibromyalgia even if it can't be cured right now.

6) It won't be easy having fibromyalgia but I will learn as much as I can about my condition.

7) I will use that knowledge to manage my condition and gain control of my life with fibromyalgia.

8) My goal is to achieve the best quality of life with the least amount of pain possible.

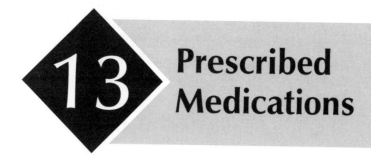

13 ◆ Prescribed Medications

Certain drugs reduce pain and improve overall feelings of well-being. No one type of medication works for everyone, and no one medication causes 100% improvement. You and your doctor need to experiment and work together to find out what is best for you. Pain relief, improved sleep, and improved mood are examples of goals that prescription medicines can help you reach.

As a group, those of us with fibromyalgia do not tolerate medicines well. We are very sensitive to medicines and often experience side effects such as nausea, drowsiness, or light-headedness. We may have side effects that the drug companies never realize could happen with their medicines! One person may tolerate a particular medicine, but the next person will get sick on it. I am particularly sensitive to medicines, and I always joke that the day they discover a pill to cure fibromyalgia, I'll take it and within seconds will get sick! Prescribed medicines can provide great benefits to many, however.

Categories of drugs used in the treatment of fibromyalgia include:

1) Analgesics

2) Anti-inflammatory drugs

3) Antidepressant medicines (tricyclics and selective serotonin reuptake inhibitors)

4) Muscle relaxants

5) Sleep modifiers

6) Anti-anxiety medicines

7) Other medicines used to treat chronic pain

We'll review each category briefly.

Analgesics

Analgesics are pain killers and can include over-the-counter medicines such as aspirin and acetaminophen, or prescription-strength pain pills like narcotics (opiates), codeine, Vicodin, Darvocet, Oxcontin and Percocet. Ultram is a pain reliever that differs from narcotics in its action on the central nervous system.

These medicines do not alter the fibromyalgia, but they can help take the edge off of pain. Narcotic medicines have potential for adverse side effects including drowsiness, difficulty with concentrating, and addiction, so they should be used carefully. Many people with fibromyalgia are sensitive to codeine medicines, which can cause nausea or an allergic reaction. Ultram can cause allergic reactions in people sensitive to codeine, and a small number of people taking Ultram have seizures (Ortho-McNeil pharmaceutical letter to healthcare professionals, March 20, 1986). As a pain specialist I will frequently prescribe analgesics, including narcotics for patients experiencing severe pain.

Anti-inflammatory Medicines

Anti-inflammatory medicines include aspirin, nonsteroidal anti-inflammatory medicine (NSAIDs for short) such as ibuprofen, Naprosyn, Lodine, Daypro, and the newer Cox-II inhibitors, and corticosteroids such as prednisone or dexamethasone. These medications are both anti-inflammatory and analgesic. Some of these medicines such as ibuprofen are available both over the counter and by prescription.

Cox-II inhibitors selectively block only the Cox-II enzymes, which control the production of chemicals that cause inflammation and pain; these chemicals are known as prostaglandins. Good prostaglandins that help the stomach lining, kidneys, and platelets are formed by the Cox-I enzyme system and are not affected by the Cox-II inhibitors.

Because fibromyalgia is not a true inflammation, these drugs may be less effective in reducing pain. However, these drugs can be helpful in reducing pain that flares up with excessive physical activity, tendinitis or bursitis. These medicines should be used only as needed. If the NSAIDs are helpful for overall fibromyalgia pain, they can be continued on a regular basis as long as there are no major side effects.

The major side effect of the anti-inflammatories is bleeding from gastrointestinal ulcers. This problem is more common the longer the medicine is taken. However, a new medication class is available, Cox-II inhibitors, which include Celebrex (Searle Pharmaceuticals), and Vioxx (Merck). This new form of NSAID selectively blocks only the Cox-II enzymes, which control the production of chemicals that cause inflammation and pain; these chemicals are known as prostaglandins. Good prostaglandins that help the stomach lining, kidneys, and platelets are formed by the Cox-I enzyme system and are not affected by the Cox-II inhibitors, thus avoiding gastrointestinal bleeding.

I prescribe various types of anti-inflammatories on a regular basis, and sometimes patients will respond very nicely to these medicines. To avoid risk of bleeding or other side effects, patients must not take over-the-counter anti-inflammatory medicines if they are taking them by prescription.

Antidepressant Medicines

The antidepressant medicines include tricyclics (for example, amitriptyline, nortriptyline, doxepin, and trazodone), and selective serotonin reuptake inhibitors (Prozac, Zoloft, Paxil, Effexor, Serzone, and Celexa). These medicines can treat pain and alter sleep and mood disturbances seen in fibromyalgia. The tricyclic medicines are effective, but frequent side effects include dry mouth and drowsiness. Sleep disturbances can be reduced by using low doses. Carefully controlled studies have shown that low doses of tricyclic antidepressants can benefit fibromyalgia patients (Karette *et al*, 1986, Goldenberg *et al*, 1986).

Because of the extreme sedation and morning hangover effect common with ami-triptyline, I've found that nortriptyline or trazodone have fewer side effects but give the same benefit. Even though the sedation side effect of the tricyclic medicine may have worn off by morning, the other benefits of the drugs (decreased pain, muscle relaxation, and improved mood) can continue throughout the day. Because the tricy-clic can provide more than one beneficial effect, I think these medicines are handy in fibromyalgia treatment. It is like using one pill to do the work of several.

The selective reuptake inhibitors work well in treating depression. They also block the breakdown of serotonin, the brain hormone that is low in persons with fibromy-algia and depression. Serotonin is important in the brain's regulation of pain and sleep. By selectively inhibiting the breakdown of serotonin, these medicines increase the serotonin concentration in the body and its beneficial effects.

These medicines have fewer side effects than the tricyclics, although Zoloft and Paxil can cause sexual dysfunction. Some of the newer medicines, Effexor and Serzone, for example, do not inhibit sexual function. Using a combination of a serotonin reuptake inhibitor during the day and a tricyclic at nighttime can be an effective com-bination medicinal approach (Goldenberg, 1996).

Muscle Relaxants

Muscle relaxants can decrease pain in people with fibromyalgia. Medicines in this family include Flexeril, Soma, Skelaxin, and Robaxin. The most common side effect is drowsiness, although Soma and Skelaxin cause less of it. I have found that muscle

relaxants do not really de-crease muscle spasms or truly "relax" muscles, be-cause the painful area still has palpable spasms. Rather, the medicine ap-pears to help by a central neurologic mechanism that reduces muscle pain. If drowsiness is a side ef-fect, this medicine should only be taken in the

The selective reuptake inhibitors work well in treating de-pression. They also block the breakdown of serotonin, the brain hormone that is low in persons with fibromyalgia and depression. Serotonin is important in the brain's regulation of pain and sleep. By selectively inhibiting the breakdown of serotonin, these medicines increase the serotonin concentra-tion in the body and its beneficial effects.

evening so it doesn't interfere with driving or concentration. Flexeril is a popular medicine for evening. Although it is a muscle relaxant, it is very similar to amitrip-tyline in structure and effect, hence the benefits reported.

Medicines in the antispasticity category can be used to treat muscle spasms. Two of these medicines, Zanaflex and Baclofen, have been shown to help reduce back muscle spasms and pain. Antispasticity medicines are primarily intended for people who have neurologic conditions causing involuntary muscle spasms (such as spinal cord inju-ries, multiple sclerosis, or strokes). However, they may have a role in patients with fibromyalgia who have numerous muscle spasms.

Sleep Modifiers

Various medicines including those already mentioned can treat insomnia (analge-sics, antidepressants, and muscle relaxants). True sleep modifiers include benzodiaz-epines like Restoril and the hypnotic non-benzodiazepines such as Ambien. The most common reported concern about using sleep modifiers, especially benzodiazepams, is the habit-forming potential. Ambien is reported to be less habit-forming but can cause rebound insomnia when it's stopped. Sonata is a newer sleep modifier that is not habit forming and doesn't cause rebound insomnia. Sometimes sleep modifiers are prescribed in short intervals only.

I have found that sleep modifiers improve deep sleep, and particularly improve the morning perception of a good night's sleep. This improved sleep can carry over into a better day. Sleep modifiers are short-acting medicines, so they work during the night and are usually eliminated from the body by morning, hence the low chance of a morning hangover. Some people report nightmares with these medicines, but usually these medicines are "silent," that is, one doesn't realize any medicine was taken, other than knowing that sleep was better. I've devoted a chapter (Chapter 26) to review the sleep problem so many of us have.

Anti-Anxieties

Anxiety is a common problem in fibromyalgia and contributes to pain, muscle tension, and irritability. It can make depression and insomnia worse. Various medicines including antidepressants and muscle relaxants treat anxiety. Benzodiazepines such as Klonopin, Ativan, and Xanax are commonly used medicines. These medicines also cause sedation and thus can improve sleep. Possible side effects include depression and decreased memory. Sometimes it is hard to determine whether symptoms are due to fibromyalgia or are side effects of medication.

No medicine will completely cure fibromyalgia or eliminate the symptoms, but it may help improve symptoms and comfort level, hopefully without side effects.

I have found Klonopin to be a particularly useful medicine in the evening especially when there are leg symptoms (pain, restless leg syndrome, jerking of the legs called myoclonus) that interfere with sleep. Low dose Klonopin therapy is one way to improve the balance of the inhibitory receptors (GABA) and excitatory receptors (MMDA) in the central nervous system. Most fibromyalgia patients have too much activity in the excitatory receptors (MMDA receptors), and Klonopin can increase the pain inhibitors' activity to achieve a more normal balance, improving sleep and reducing pain.

Other Medicines Used to Treat Chronic Pain

Other medicines can be used to treat pain. Some pain medicines were originally developed for a different purpose. For example, anti-seizure medicines known as neuroleptics (including Neurontin, Dilantin, Depakote, and Tegretol) were later found to be helpful in treating pain, particularly neuropathic pain. People with fibromyalgia who have a lot of burning or electric shock feelings in their hands and feet may improve from a trial of neuroleptic medicines.

Headaches are a common problem with fibromyalgia, and various headache medicines are available. In addition to the medicines described above, headache medicines include ergot alkaloids, sumatriptan, calcium channel blockers and beta blockers.

Other conditions associated with fibromyalgia such as irritable bowel syndrome can cause severe cramping pain and may require separately prescribed medications.

Medicines used to treat irritable bowel syndrome include Metamucil, Levsin, and Levbid.

In addition to the variety of medicines available for fibromyalgia treatment, a variety of doctor "strategies" are also available. Doctors who prescribe medicine will usually find, through trial and error, an effective or favorite strategy. There is no single right way to prescribe medicines for fibromyalgia, and more than one strategy may work for different people and different doctors. Over the years, I have discovered basic strategies that seem to work best for me when using prescription medicines.

Antibiotics can have a role in treating fibromyalgia. Dr. Garth Nicolson has isolated a microorganism, *Mycoplasma fermentens*, as a possible infectious cause of Gulf War Syndrome (remember, this may be a type of fibromyalgia). Some patients had less pain and fatigue after taking antibiotics (for example, doxycycline, Zithromax), presumably due to the eradication of the *Mycoplasma*. Antibiotics may also inhibit certain enzymes that cause inflammation (anti-inflammatory mechanisms) rather than by acting as an anti-infection mechanism.

I have had some patients who improved after a course of antibiotics and many who did not, so I'm not convinced that these drugs are helpful for the long term. Antibiotic use increases one's chance of getting a Candida yeast infection, which can increase fibromyalgia symptoms. Yeast antibiotics (Nystatin, Sporanox, Diflucan) may be in indicated in fibromyalgia if there is a Candida infection that is causing increased pain and other symptoms. Over time we may identify a specific subgroup of fibromyalgia patients who have antibiotic-responsive symptoms.

My Basic Strategies

1) **Educate about expectation with medication.** I tell patients that no medicine will completely cure fibromyalgia or eliminate the symptoms, but it may help improve symptoms and comfort level, hopefully without side effects. Let me give you an example of how educating about medicinal expectation is important.

   Say you came to me with pain, and I prescribed a medication. I tell you to take the medicine to see if it helps your pain. I don't clarify what to expect. You go home, try the medicine and come back. I ask you how the medicine worked, and you say, "It only took away half the pain, I'm still hurting, I need something else."

   Now take the same situation, same exact medicine, but when I give you the medicine I tell you, "This medicine is not going to eliminate all of the pain. It may help reduce your pain, but it will not make the pain disappear. Hopefully, you will find that at least you feel better than you did before, and there will not be any side effects to interfere with the success of the medicine. Give it a try, and let me know how it works." When you come back for the next visit, and I ask you how you did, you will say, "Great! This medicine took away half of my pain. I haven't felt this good in years!" If the patient is educated on what to expect, the medicine can be much more effective.

2) **Try to use the lowest effective dose of medicine** and wean off medicines whenever possible, especially if the patient is at a "stable baseline." Believe it or not, fibromyalgia can stabilize and require less medicine than before. I always

try to challenge the fibromyalgia by decreasing the medicine to the lowest effective dose that controls symptoms. Sometimes when decreasing the medicine, we are able to actually stop the medicine altogether, and to our pleasant surprise the symptoms do not return. This approach considerably reduces risk of side effects or developing tolerances to the medicines. If the symptoms flare up at a later time, the medicines can be resumed or increased.

3) **Discontinue any medicine that is not working.** Many times, patients come to me with a list of a dozen different medicines they are taking, and then report that none of them are helping. Yet they are continuing the medicines! I will instruct the patient to stop, or if needed, wean off the medicine. Sometimes a patient will stop a medicine and the symptoms increase, indicating that the medicine probably was helping. If this occurs, the patient can resume that particular medicine and monitor for improved symptoms.

Sometimes medicines help to maintain a stable baseline, and we don't realize how much they are working until we stop them. Other times, a medicine had helped in the past, but is no longer effective because the body has developed a tolerance to it, or perhaps a higher dose is needed. I avoid automatically adding any new medicine to the group of medicines that are not working. I often do the "add and subtract" strategy, where I add a new medicine to try, but at the same time, subtract one that does not appear to be working.

4) **Narcotic/opiates can be used sparingly and responsibly for pain control.** There are certainly risks for habituation, dependency, and addiction with the use of narcotic medications. In my experience, most patients are terrified of using narcotics on a regular basis for fear of becoming addicted. If patients use prescription narcotic medications responsibly and as prescribed for pain control, the risk for addiction or other serious side effects is very low. Patients must be instructed on the importance of using narcotics sparingly and responsibly exactly as prescribed, and agree to strictly adhere to these rules.

I rarely have problems with my patients misusing narcotic medications. From time to time, there are "red flags" that go up and must be addressed immediately. I have found that the responsible use of narcotic medications for pain control is much more beneficial than the occasional risk of side effects, but the physician has to monitor these prescriptions closely.

5) **Be flexible and keep it simple.** There are many different strategies, and sometimes we can try all of them and still not have much success. I have my favorites, but I am willing to try different things. I also try to keep it simple, because the more medicines added to the mix, the more the potential for adverse side effects, sensitivity, and interactions among the medicines.

Trigger Point Injections

Therapeutic injections are a different way to administer medicine for pain management. The most common form used for fibromyalgia is a trigger point injection. I recommend that trigger point injections be considered when a few areas, perhaps one to six, are causing most of the patient's severe pain. Trigger point injections are most effective if they are done in the points where the patient is experiencing the most pain, even though other trigger points may be painful on palpation.

A trigger point injection sends medicine into a painful soft tissue area, usually the muscle. I use a local anesthetic and sometimes a corticosteroid such as Dexamethasone or Celestone if I feel the combination will prolong the effect of the injection.

Painful areas are located and injected with a small diameter needle. The patient is instructed on the potential benefits and risks of the procedure. The benefits include significantly reducing the pain and spasm, confirming that the area injected was indeed the source of pain, and hopefully achieving a benefit that lasts for weeks. The risks include a temporary increase in pain, localized bleeding, and rarely, blood vessel damage, lung puncture, or a skin infection. The procedure is carried out in the doctor's office.

For an average trigger point injection, I generally use lidocaine. I've learned to get the needle in, inject quickly, and get the needle out. I do not "fan" or "pepper" the needle. I find this provides the minimum amount of needle trauma and helps achieve the quickest and most prolonged benefit from the injection. During the actual injection, a few seconds of increased pain confirms the right location. Then, the medicine works quickly to cause a numbing effect. After the injection, I perform stretching and soft tissue mobilization to decrease pain and relax spasms.

There is no way to determine how long a particular trigger point injection will last in a given person, as it can be anywhere from a few hours to a few months. I've found that the average trigger point injection lasts three to four weeks. Trigger point injections are not a permanent solution. Many times they reduce severe pain, and when they wear off, the pain is not as severe as it was before the shots. Trigger point injections can also help other treatments work more effectively. If injections are helpful, they can be done on a regular basis depending on the patient's needs and physician preferences.

Botox injections have been used to treat painful tender points. Botox is a purified chemical made from the same botulism compound which causes a potentially fatal food poisoning. When injected into a painful muscle area, Botox causes a disruption of the nerve-muscle junction around the injection site. This releases the muscle spasm by blocking the nerve signals to the muscle area, thereby reducing pain.

I have used Botox injections on a number of people who have tender points that are resistant to usual trigger point injections. About 50% to 60% will have improvements lasting several weeks to several months.

Other types of therapeutic injections have been tried in patients with fibromyalgia. These include epidural steroid injections, selective nerve root blocks, joint injections, and a technique called proliferative injections (prolotherapy). Prolotherapy has shown a lot of potential for treating resistant tender points (see Chapter 16).

> Trigger point injections reduce severe pain, and when they wear off, the pain is not as severe as it was before the shots. Trigger point injections can also help other treatments work more effectively. If injections are helpful, they can be done on a regular basis depending on the patient's needs and physician preferences.

As with prescribed oral medications, therapeutic injections can be considered on an individual basis as part of a multi-disciplinary treatment approach. I use a combination of prescription medicines and injections along with other treatment approaches. We need a lot of weapons to go after this "enemy" of our state of well-being!

Chapter 13 — Survival Strategies

1) Understand there is no magical pill that will get rid of all fibromyalgia symptoms.

2) Experiment with your doctor to determine which medicines can help "control" your symptoms.

3) Responsibly use analgesics and narcotics to take the edge off the pain. These medications will not relieve all your pain but may improve symptoms and comfort.

4) Educate yourself about expectations of medication.

5) Use the lowest effective dose of medicine; wean off whenever possible.

6) Be flexible with medications. Keep it simple.

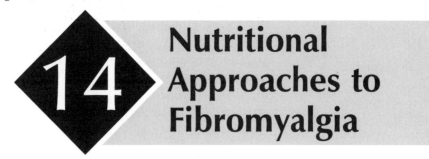

Nutritional Approaches to Fibromyalgia

Proper nutrition is important for maintaining health. Medicine has long recognized the importance of nutrition therapy and dietary modifications in diseases such as diabetes, heart disease, osteoporosis, gout, and hypertension. There has been increasing interest in the role that nutrition plays in managing fibromyalgia, and numerous studies have been published to describe nutritional aspects of pain management. Indeed, nutritional strategies can play an important role in the overall treatment of fibromyalgia.

Special Eating Problems Related to Fibromyalgia

Fibromyalgia causes problems with everyday living, so it is not surprising that it would interfere with eating. A variety of conditions can pose unique eating problems.

1) **Pain**. Pain has a way of making us forget about everything else, including hunger. Pain interferes with eating, cooking, and thinking about preparing food as well. Some people use food as a "reward" for being in pain (I'm in pain so I "deserve" ice cream!).

2) **Fatigue**. Next to pain, fatigue is the most common symptom of fibromyalgia, and it causes us to not think about eating or cooking at all. Extreme fatigue alters our eating pattern, so we tend to minimize any effort involved in preparing food and enjoying meals. Some people overeat to "try" to get energy.

3) **Depression**. Depression is common in conditions that cause chronic pain. Part of the depression picture can include under-eating, overeating, or eating disorders such as anorexia or bulimia.

4) **Irritable bowel syndrome**. This common condition causes episodes of constipation, diarrhea, abdominal cramping, pain and bloating. People with irritable bowel syndrome are usually sensitive to foods that are greasy, fatty, or bulky, as well as nuts and raw vegetables. Many patients with irritable bowel syndrome require an evaluation by a gastroenterologist. Foods that trigger an attack need to be avoided. Medications used to treat irritable bowel syndrome include those that decrease bowel spasms (called parasympatholytics) or increase the stool consistency (natural fiber medicines).

5) **Food sensitivities and allergies**. People with fibromyalgia have a lot food intolerances. Practically anything can aggravate our symptoms. I believe if we eliminated all foods that can cause allergies or irritate our symptoms, there would be nothing left to eat!

If food intolerances are present, the most common foods (sugar, wheat, dairy products, citrus fruits, eggs, and chocolate products) are usually the ones that create problems. Many of us are lactose intolerant, meaning that milk and milk products can cause gastric attacks, gas, cramping, or diarrhea. Others do not tolerate food additives or preservatives. Also, food smells may be nauseating to our overly sensitive nostrils. People with fibromyalgia can be more susceptible to chronic yeast overgrowth infections, especially with diets that are high in refined sugars and fermented foods. This can create additional gastrointestinal symptoms.

Avoiding foods that cause sensitivities or allergies is certainly the main emphasis in treating this problem. A trial elimination of offending foods may cause noticeable improvement in some fibromyalgia symptoms and pain level; these symptoms may reoccur if the offending foods are reintroduced into the diet. Allergy testing or specific allergy medicines may be necessary as well.

6) **Hypoglycemia.** People with fibromyalgia are more prone to developing hypoglycemia, or abnormally low blood sugar. This is probably due to our dysfunctional autonomic nervous system. Hypoglycemia can cause dizziness, lightheadedness, a feeling of passing out, extreme fatigue, and listlessness.

A hypoglycemia attack is usually brought on by eating foods rich in sugar — candy, pastries, cookies, and snack foods. After eating, the sugar gets quickly absorbed into the blood stream. This rapid increase in blood sugar tells the autonomic nervous system to release insulin. Insulin is a hormone that opens the "sugar gates" in the muscles. Thus insulin allows sugar to leave the blood and go into the muscle cells. In fibromyalgia, it appears that the insulin "overshoots," causing too much sugar to be taken out of the blood stream and put into the muscle, thus leaving too little sugar left in the blood stream (hypoglycemia).

In addition, the person begins to experience a carbohydrate craving as the blood glucose level drops too low. Within a few hours of eating a snack loaded with sugar, the person begins to crave more sugar, but eating another snack loaded with sugar repeats this cycle. Adding more carbohydrates simply encourages more hypoglycemia.

How does one avoid hypoglycemia? By eating meals or snacks that have a higher protein content, eating more natural sugars such as fruits and vegetables, and avoiding refined sugar. Protein controls the amount of glucose absorbed into the blood stream and the amount of insulin released, so it makes sense to increase the protein we eat. Later in this chapter, I will review a fibromyalgia diet.

7) **Temporomandibular joint dysfunction.** This condition commonly associated with fibromyalgia causes pain in the jaw and can lead to difficulty in opening the mouth and chewing. Chewy foods, sandwiches, and hard foods can pose special difficulties for someone with TMJ dysfunction. A dental specialist may need to be consulted, and specific treatments could include customized bite splints, crowns and bridges, or other TMJ restorative procedures. People with TMJ dysfunction may notice decreased jaw pain if they avoid hard and lumpy foods, take smaller bites, and chew the food slowly and completely.

Nutritional Problems with Fibromyalgia

In order to develop good nutritional strategies for coping with fibromyalgia, one needs to understand how fibromyalgia can interfere with proper nutrition. Various studies have yielded clues to underlying biochemical and hormonal abnormalities that can interfere with nutrition.

Biochemical studies show that fibromyalgia patients have low ATP (energy molecules) in their muscles due to a deficiency of the compounds that make ATP such as oxygen and magnesium (G.E. Abraham, J.D. Flechas, *General Nutritional Medicine,* 1992). Swedish investigators, Drs. Bengtson and Henrikson, have shown that a lower concentration of oxygen than expected is found in fibromyalgia muscle and Dr. T.J. Romano (1994) found magnesium is low in the muscle cells of fibromyalgia patients. Muscle mitochondria, the small organelles in cells that produce energy, have difficulty making ATP without enough oxygen and magnesium around. A lack of ATP contributes to fatigue and interferes with energy-requiring processes such as digestion and nutrient delivery.

Other studies have shown hormone deficiencies or imbalances (cortisol, thyroid, serotonin, growth hormone) in fibromyalgia. Insulin and other hormones are probably affected as well. Dr. Leslie J. Crofford (1998) has described hormonal abnormalities in fibromyalgia and how they interfere with physiologic communication between the brain and the body. Closely linked with hormones is the autonomic nervous system. The autonomic nerves are the small nerves vital in the coordination of the body's hormones, and thus they play a role in the regulation and delivery of nutrients to our cells. The hypoglycemic roller-coaster effect is a good example of the combination of hormonal imbalances and autonomic nervous system dysfunction leading to hypoglycemic symptoms.

Still another problem occurs with increased food sensitivities. If one is sensitive to a particular food, the body may not properly digest this food. This in turn may interfere with the ability to digest and absorb other nutrients and perform other necessary nutritional activities. In other words, the body cannot absorb needed nutrients.

An imbalance between friendly and unfriendly microorganisms can lead to digestive and nutritional problems (*e.g.,* diarrhea, bloating and hypoglycemia). "Friendly" *Lactobacillus* yeast and "unfriendly" *Candida* yeast both inhabit the intestinal tract and carry out vital tasks in the digestion of sugars and release of key enzymes and nutrients. *Candida* in small colonies are good for our body and necessary as part of our "normal" microorganisms.

As long as the *Candida* yeast are kept in check by the other yeast, all is well. But when certain conditions prevail, the *Candida* yeast can grow uncontrollably and become "unfriendly." These conditions include antibiotic usage, excessive sugar consumption, stress, estrogen usage, and often, fibromyalgia! An overgrowth of *Candida* will disrupt the smooth digestive and nutritional processes and create problems until the "normal" balance is restored.

Part of our treatment includes finding an ideal nutritional balance in spite of our body's nutritional dysfunctions. This helps our fibromyalgia symptoms to be more stabilized. There is no nutritional cure for fibromyalgia at the present time, but we can increase our nutritional awareness as it pertains to fibromyalgia, and make changes gradually and slowly (like — we should chew our food!).

The goals in nutritional therapy for fibromyalgia would be to improve nutrient absorption and entry into the cells, boosting the immune system, eliminating toxins from the body, creating optimal biochemical pathways, minimizing food sensitivity or adverse reactions, maintaining a healthy microorganism balance, and improving energy levels. I believe there are some basic principles in trying to accomplish these goals and optimizing nutrition for patients with fibromyalgia.

1) **Eat at least three meals a day to help maintain proper energy for daily needs.** Many people with fibromyalgia actually do better by eating six smaller meals a day, or by eating three smaller meals and two larger snacks. Those who are bothered by irritable bowel syndrome will often do better to eat smaller portions more frequently. Eat slowly, and take your time to chew foods well.

2) **Emphasize a diet that is higher in protein and lower in carbohydrates.** Americans eat well over half their daily calories in carbohydrates. Those who would avoid fats usually end up eating more carbohydrates and too little protein as "low fat" foods are usually high in carbohydrates and low in protein. I believe a diet high in carbohydrates and low in proteins aggravates fibromyalgia symptoms, especially fatigue, irritable bowel syndrome, and weight gain.

   If we "reverse" the usual diet, that is, eat a diet higher in protein and lower in carbohydrates, many of these symptoms can improve. Particularly reduce or eliminate refined sugars, potatoes, breads and pasta; and try for more natural fruits and vegetables. Emphasize lean meats, chicken, turkey, eggs, beans, and nuts. Avoid fried foods, but don't try to eliminate fat from the diet. Fat is a necessary part of our daily diet, although we might reduce the amount we eat. A natural fiber supplement could be considered.

   Eat proteins first. Proteins require hydrochloric acid for proper digestion, not carbohydrates. If we eat carbohydrates first, hydrochloric acid may not be activated, and proteins eaten may not be properly digested. Also avoid eating raw vegetables and fruits at the same meal; different digestive enzymes are required for each.

3) **Avoid nicotine, caffeine, and alcohol, as these all interfere with the body's ability to manufacture energy and carry out efficient biochemical reactions.** They act as drugs in our bodies. Artificial sweeteners such as aspartame which is marketed as Nutrasweet, Equal, and Spoonful have been shown to cause a variety of symptoms in some people. These symptoms can include pain, numbness, dizziness, headaches, and fatigue. Symptoms are thought to be caused by sensitivity to the aspartame or sensitivity to the by-product of the aspartame breakdown, formaldehyde. Formaldehyde is poisonous in higher concentrations. If you are sensitive to aspartame, avoid products that contain it. Watch your diet pop habit; it usually contains both Nutrasweet and caffeine.

   Most patients tell me their fibromyalgia feels better if they are able to quit smoking. Your doctor may be able to prescribe a patch or a medication to help you quit. Drink a cup of "real" coffee in the morning, and no caffeine after lunch. I've read that the chemicals used to remove caffeine from coffee can be hard on your body so watch the decaffeinated coffee, too! A universal medical recommendation is "use alcohol in moderation, and do not use alcohol with prescription medicines." Common sense needs to prevail when considering whether or not to use these products and how much to consume.

4) **Drink six to eight eight-ounce glasses of water a day.** Adequate fluids are needed to run the body's machinery and eliminate wastes. Also, people with fibromyalgia are more susceptible to dips in blood pressure which can cause

light-headedness or fainting. If too little water is consumed each day, one is more likely to have these hypotensive episodes, so make sure you are drinking lots of water.

5) **Consider a trial elimination of certain foods that may exacerbate fibromyalgia symptoms.** If you do not notice any improvement after a few weeks, there is probably no relationship between the fibromyalgia symptoms and those foods, so you can reintroduce them. If there are noticeable improvements during the trial elimination, then try reintroducing these foods to challenge the body. If the fibromyalgia symptoms increase, avoid these foods as much as possible. These elimination/reintroduction/challenge trials can be done with various "suspicious" food categories.

6) **Nutritional supplements.** Various nutritional supplements have been used to improve energy, detoxify, encourage weight loss, and optimize nutrient absorption. As with any other treatment, different nutritional supplements may work for some, but not for others. Various complementary medicines are discussed in Chapter 16. I recommend that patients take a good daily multivitamin. A magnesium and malic acid combination supplement can be helpful. A few studies have found this combination decreases pain in fibromyalgia patients (Abraham G.E. and Flechas J.D., 1992; Russell I.J. *et al*, 1994). Manganese, Vitamin B_1 and B_6, Vitamin C, and Coenzyme Q10 are additional nutrients that help feed the muscles to optimize their energy production. *Lactobacillus* supplements can help replenish the friendly microorganisms in the intestinal tract.

Numerous nutritional products are available, and I work with my patients in an open-minded and responsible manner about trying them. Educate yourself by reading up on various products. Ask your doctor, and base your decisions on your knowledge and experience and not on a product's good marketing strategy. Try one supplement at a time for one or two months. If you notice no improvement the product is not helping. If you think it might be helping but you're not sure, try it for another month and reevaluate its effect. Remember to work together with your doctor.

There are dozens — no, hundreds — of diet plans out there and I don't pretend I have all the answers about diet. I try to enhance patients' awareness of dietary possibilities and encourage them to experiment with their diets to see if their fibromyalgia symptoms can be improved. I have come up with a diet handout to assist patients and give them some specific guidelines:

Dr. Pellegrino's Fibromyalgia Diet

Factors Contributing to Weight Gain in Fibromyalgia

1) **Decreased metabolism.** Numerous deficiencies and dysfunctions of hormones can occur in fibromyalgia and cause a decrease in metabolism. These affected hormones include thyroid, growth hormone, and cortisol. Decreased metabolism results in slowing down of the body's machinery, making it difficult to burn calories.

2) **Dysautonomia.** The small nerves that control hormones, blood flow, heart rate, and blood pressure become dysfunctional and probably result in increased sensitivity to hypoglycemia and hyperinsulinism. Since insulin is the

main hormone that causes fat formation, any process that increases insulin sensitivity will increase weight gain.

3) **Medicines.** Side effects of medicines used to treat fibromyalgia can cause weight gain by decreasing metabolism, altering hormones, causing fluid retention, and increasing appetite. The most common offending medicines are the antidepressants, particularly the tricyclic antidepressants. Other substances such as estrogen and prednisone can contribute to weight gain.

4) **Decreased activity due to pain.** People with fibromyalgia hurt more and are not as active because activity increases pain. Thus, it is difficult to increase the energy expenditure or calorie burning related to exercise and activity.

Dieting Myths

Myth #1. Obesity is a result of eating too much fatty foods. **Fact:** Obesity is usually the result of eating too many carbohydrates and having metabolic changes occur. Insulin causes sugar to turn into fat, thus it contributes to weight gain especially in carbohydrate-rich diets.

Myth #2. You eat less on a low-fat diet. **Fact:** You actually eat less on a low-carbohydrate diet than on a low-fat diet. Foods higher in fat and protein suppress the appetite and satisfy hunger more than eating carbohydrates. In a low-fat diet, you eat more carbohydrates, have more hunger, and are more likely to consume more total calories overall.

Myth #3. You can't lose weight unless you eat fewer calories. **Fact:** You can actually lose weight by eating a higher number of calories if you eat the right food combinations. Diets that are heavy in carbohydrates can cause weight gain, but eating the same amount of calories, or even higher calories, on a diet heavier in proteins and fats and lower in carbohydrates can cause weight loss. The quality of food is important, not the quantity of the calories.

Myth #4. Most overweight people overeat. **Fact:** Actually, most overweight people do not overeat. They may have a craving for carbohydrates, and the carbohydrates are easily converted to fat, especially when a high secretion of insulin is occurring.

Rationale for a High Protein, Low Carbohydrate (HIPLOC) Diet

Specific problems related to fibromyalgia that may respond to dietary modifications include weight gain, fatigue, brain fog, hypoglycemia symptoms (irritability, anxiety, dizziness, carbohydrate craving), irritable bowel symptoms, yeast and parasite symptoms, (bloating, abdominal cramping, rectal itching), food intolerances, and food sensitivity.

Fibromyalgia patients may be hypersensitive to insulin. The increased insulin causes glucose to get "pushed into" the cells. Glycogen, which is the form in which glucose is stored in our cells, fills up the glycogen storage spaces, so the leftover glucose that is being pushed into the cells is converted into fat. The end result, sugar turns into fat.

The fibromyalgia diet changes the composition, not necessarily the quantity, of the diet. If you are overweight, the goal is to promote a steady weight loss, but improve energy. If you are already at your ideal body weight, the goal is to promote improved energy and feeling better all over. Appetite and hunger can be reduced naturally.

On a metabolic level, the high protein, low carbohydrate diet will induce ketosis. Ketosis is the act of breaking down fat and converting it to glucose. The ease of getting into ketosis, which is also known as lipolysis, is based on the ratio of fat to carbohydrate. The more fat there is in relation to carbohydrate, the more ketones. An overweight person is resistant to ketosis. With a decrease in dietary carbohydrate, the body will mobilize its own glucose for energy. First it uses up the stored glycogen, which takes a couple of days, then the body will start burning fat which forms glucose. It is this process which puts us into ketosis or lipolysis. Once in ketosis, the appetite is actually suppressed and the carbo cravings stop.

Goals of the HIPLOC Diet

Numerous high protein/low carbohydrate diets have been described. I have combined some of the features of different diets, especially Dr. Adkin's Diet and The Mayo Clinic Diet, to come up with a fibromyalgia diet. There are some key goals intended with this diet:

1) Promote steady weight loss (if overweight) to reach the ideal weight

2) Improve energy

3) Reduce appetite naturally and eliminate hunger

4) Develop a dietary life-styles change

5) Consistently improve overall fibromyalgia symptoms

6) Change the composition, not the quantity, of the diet

7) Allow yourself to periodically go off the diet to eat your favorite foods

Fibromyalgia Diet Plan (HIPLOC Diet)

Foods that should be reduced or eliminated:

1) Sugars (dessert, candy, cookies, most fruits, sugared drinks, yogurt, potato chips, even "Wow" brand)

2) Breads and starches (bagels, muffins, pancakes, waffles, noodles, pizza, breaded meats, pasta)

3) Certain vegetables (potatoes, sweet potatoes, corn, popcorn, cole slaw, peas, navy beans, black beans, kidney beans, rice)

Foods that are okay:

1) Meats (steak, hamburger, chicken, fish, lunch meat if it does not have sugars)

2) Most red and green vegetables

3) Certain fruits such as avocado, raspberries, and strawberries

4) Dairy products, cheese, cream, butter, skim milk

5) Any salad dressing, mayonnaise, or olive oil. Salad garnishes which include nuts, olives, bacon, grated cheese, mushrooms, and allowed vegetables

6) Artificial sweeteners and beverages with no sugar

Daily meals:

Breakfast

Two eggs, any style

Two slices of bacon, Canadian bacon, or two links/patties sausage

Lunch

Salad (with any dressing) and salad garnishes

Meat, any style, any amount

Eat until full

Dinner

Meat, any style, any amount

Vegetables cooked in butter or any seasoning, or salad as above

Eat until full

Bedtime Snack

Snack foods can include protein and fatty-rich foods (macadamia nuts, pecans, walnuts, Brazil nuts, cream cheese or fried pork rinds) or can have sugar-free gelatin dessert with cream or cottage cheese

One cup of raspberries or one cup of strawberries per day allowed and can be eaten as a snack or mixed with sugar-free gelatin or cream

Rules of the HIPLOC Diet

1) Don't skip meals, and at any meal you may eat until you are full. Follow the HIPLOC Diet.

2) Don't eat in-between meals except for an evening snack. You may have one 6-oz. glass of skim milk per day. The combination of foods should eliminate cravings; if you get cravings, eat protein, fat-rich foods.

3) Take nutritional supplements along with the diet: Multivitamin and mineral tablets, magnesium and malic acid combinations, and Colostrum may be recommended, along with others.

4) Exercise: Stretch on a daily basis. Try to perform a light conditioning exercise at least three times a week (more if able), such as walking at least one mile or some type of similar exercise for 20 to 30 minutes.

5) Stay on the diet twelve days, stop for two days, and then go on again. Repeat this cycle until ideal body weight is reached, then modify the diet to maintain stable weight. Modifications need to be individualized but may include increasing foods allowed and allowing more days off the diet.

6) Record initial weight, weigh once a week and keep a record. Record how you feel or if you have any problems or questions. You can lose an average of one to two pounds every two days with this diet; usually you will not lose weight for the first four days.

Who Can Benefit?

Everyone's nutritional balance is different, and there are no magical nutritional approaches to cure fibromyalgia. Rather, there are effective nutritional approaches that can be part of its successful treatment. Common sense needs to prevail. If you have a condition that can definitely be treated by nutritional modifications—overweight, irritable bowel syndrome, a yeast infection, lactose intolerance, or an eating disorder such as anorexia or bulimia – prescribed nutritional strategies may be medically required. I frequently work with a dietician and nutritionist to help fibromyalgia people make the changes.

You should notice more energy and less pain, better weight control, and more mental alertness, better sleep, and fewer fluctuation in symptoms. If your fibromyalgia bothers you less, you will feel better about yourself as a result of your nutritional life-style changes, and you will have improved your well-being.

Chapter 14 — Survival Strategies

Nutritional approaches

1) Observe how what you eat may be affecting your fibromyalgia.

2) Learn and understand how fibromyalgia can interfere with proper nutrition.

3) Evaluate your nutritional strengths and weaknesses.

4) Develop realistic strategies to deal with food problems.

5) Eat 3 – 6 meals per day.

6) Increase protein in your diet. Decrease carbohydrates.

7) Avoid nicotine, caffeine, and alcohol.

8) Increase fluid intake to 6 – 8 eight- ounce glasses per day.

9) Consider a trial elimination of some foods from your diet.

10) Evaluate your need for nutritional supplements, particularly a multivitamin and a magnesium and malic acid supplement.

11) Improve your nutrition plan. You should notice more energy, less pain, better weight control, more mental alertness, better sleep, fewer fluctuations in symptoms.

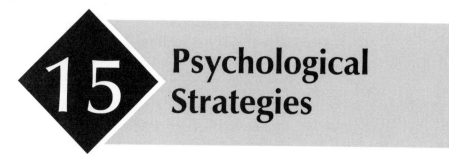

15 Psychological Strategies

Fibromyalgia affects your entire body. As a physician, I look at the whole person, not just a bunch of tender points. The body, mind, and soul are all affected by fibromyalgia, and all need to be treated together for healing. We need to consider the mental pain as well as the physical pain; one can't heal without the other.

In the past, fibromyalgia was mistakenly called "psychogenic rheumatism," which suggested that the condition was an imagined one. We know that is not the case, although people can benefit by working on the psychological aspects of this condition. Even if you don't understand at first how fibromyalgia really bothers you, or why therapy may help, you know that having a chronic illness is stressful and has affected your life in many ways:

1) You may have financial stresses because you can't work as much as before, and have less money.

2) You may feel you can't give enough to your significant other or your family because of pain and fatigue, and you feel worthless.

3) You may feel cheated and angry because chronic pain wasn't in your life plan.

4) You may be unable to accept fibromyalgia or view yourself as chronically "ill," yet you know you don't feel "healthy."

5) You don't want to reevaluate yourself; you want things to be the way they were before fibromyalgia.

If it is suggested that you work with a mental health professional to help manage your fibromyalgia, that is not the same as saying the pain is "all in your head, or that "you are crazy." Rather, it is a recognition that chronically painful fibromyalgia affects all of you, including your mental outlook. It is OK to get help for *all* of you.

Many people with fibromyalgia develop associated psychological problems. These include decreased self-esteem, depression, anxiety, strained interpersonal relationships and altered coping mechanisms. That is not the same as saying, however, that psychological problems are the cause of fibromyalgia. In fact, studies conclude that depression, stress, and anxiety do NOT cause fibromyalgia, and that people with fibromyalgia have no more psychological problems than other people with chronic medical problems or chronic pain. Nor do past psychiatric diagnoses determine the severity of fibromyalgia (Dr. Lawrence Bradley, 1997).

Chronic physical pain can lead to very real psychological reactions. It is normal to become fearful, frightened, frustrated, angry, anxious, and depressed because of chronic pain. If these feelings lead to decreased self-esteem or depression, psychological therapies need to be considered as part of your overall treatment program. A psychological therapist will not take away your fibromyalgia, but will help you sort things out and support you while you go through the process of accepting your condition. This is not an easy process, but worth the work! A therapist can help you find the "new" you, realistically. Psychological strategies can include a variety of approaches.

1) **Psychotherapy.** For fibromyalgia, this treatment is designed to evaluate mental aspects of a chronic illness through reeducation, reassurance, and support. Techniques such as psychoanalysis and hypnosis can be employed in psychotherapy. Psychologists and social workers usually perform this one-on-one intervention aimed at reinforcing your mental strategies, identifying and resolving conflicts, and achieving successful coping strategies. If a person with fibromyalgia is overcome with feelings of depression, anger, or has had negative childhood experiences or traumatic experiences, this technique may need to be considered.

To give an example, one of my patients reported to me she was feeling more depressed and having suicidal thoughts because of her severe fibromyalgia pain. I referred her to a psychiatrist who was knowledgeable about fibromyalgia. He helped my patient see that she was trying to be a "super woman." Her mother died when the patient was 11 years old, and the patient, who was the oldest child, always felt she needed to be the "mother" figure for her three younger siblings. Later in life, she submerged herself in her "mother" role, with her own family, with work, and with her church. Fibromyalgia came along and prevented this, and caused severe depression. My patient responded to this psychotherapy by realizing what was happening and redefining her role to allow herself to do less and focus on getting her fibromyalgia under control.

If it is suggested that you work with a mental health professional to help manage your fibromyalgia, that is not the same as saying the pain is "all in your head, or that "you are crazy." Rather, it is a recognition that chronically painful fibromyalgia affects all of you, including your mental outlook. It is OK to get help for *all* of you.

2) **Counseling.** This is professional "guidance" by using information gathered from the patient's history, interviews, and various tests. The counselor gives advice to the individual, couples or a group. A session of counseling is like talking to a friend, you feel comfortable and "safe." This counselor "friend" is an impartial, non-judgmental, but trustworthy professional who will listen to you and offer helpful suggestions. Fibromyalgia creates problems and stresses that not only affect the individual's sense of control or balance, but also can seriously affect the relationships with the significant other, family, and friends. Relationship difficulties including sexual dysfunction can occur and may benefit from psychological counseling. I recommend counselors who are knowledgeable in fibromyalgia. Sometimes patients may need some coaxing, but they are usually very pleased with the results.

3) **Pain and stress management.** This is a more specialized form of counseling which includes cognitive and behavioral therapies. These therapies try to help patients think about themselves and behave in a manner that is "positive" in spite of the chronic pain. Pain management techniques are used to identify problems such as feeling depressed, hopeless, or disabled as a result

of chronic pain. The treatment goals are to work on developing successful mental strategies, think more positively, and improve mental and physical outlooks and abilities. These techniques can teach the mind how to relax muscles and decrease pain, stress, and anxiety.

Guided imagery is a popular technique that uses therapist-guided mental images to relieve stress or relax muscles. The therapist may describe a setting and ask the patient to imagine being in this setting and performing imaginary steps to reach goals. For example, one therapist helped patients with burning pain by having them imagine they were using ice to cool it off. The well-known technique of counting sheep jumping over a fence to fall asleep is an example of using guided imagery. Specific programs can be played on cassette tapes to allow patients to practice this technique at home. About 60% of patients do very well with guided imagery.

4) **Biofeedback.** This is a specific technique for pain management in which individuals learn to control their body responses so as to achieve relaxation and pain relief. Numerous bodily functions are automatic, not controlled by our conscious selves: heart rate, pulse, digestion, blood pressure, brain waves, and muscle activity. These automatic functions are controlled by the autonomic nervous system. If one can recognize the autonomic nervous system signals, he can consciously create favorable autonomic nervous system responses like relaxing muscles or reducing stress.

Biofeedback devices monitor skin temperature, heart rate, muscle tension, electrical conductivity of the skin and/or brain wave activity. An individual with fibromyalgia will train with a biofeedback device under the direction of a qualified biofeedback counselor. These devices measure the body responses to stress or certain brain wave activities, and often give a signal — a noise, beep or visual reading — that the individual can recognize. These responses are automatic at first. The patient notices these random responses and consciously starts wondering, "What was I doing or thinking that caused this response?" The patient may then appreciate a pattern between what she/he is doing or thinking when the "desired" response occurs. Once the patient identifies this pattern-response relationship,

> Biofeedback devices measure the body responses to stress or certain brain wave activities, and often give a signal that the individual can recognize. These responses are automatic at first. The patient notices these random responses and consciously starts wondering, "What was I doing or thinking that caused this response?" Once the patient identifies this pattern-response relationship, she/he can practice CAUSING the response.

she/he can prac-tice CAUSING the response. The more this learned response is practiced, the better the biofeedback skills become. Thus, the person can learn to consciously achieve relaxation.

Dr. Stuart Donaldson has been doing research on EEG-driven stimulation as a way of controlling favorable brain waves in the treatment of fibromyalgia. The patient uses biofeedback information to recognize the "good" brain waves on the EEG and tries to consciously "think" good brain waves. The more good brain waves one can think, the less the fibro-fog. Any treatment that can give a person feedback can enable the individual to develop skills to control pain, improve concentration, and relax.

5) **Relaxation.** In addition to counseling, pain and stress management, and bio-feedback, many counselors teach relaxation using complementary or alternative strategies. Yoga, tai-chi, meditation, music therapy, dance therapy, and other types of therapy can be helpful.

6) **Support group.** Therapeutic support groups provide more group psychological therapy and can address specific issues that are common to patients with fibromyalgia — anger, grief, and loss of abilities. This may be more treatment-oriented than the regular support groups we previously discussed.

Whether it be one-on-one psychological intervention or group therapy, patients can develop better coping mechanisms and improve their outlook with psychological strategies. Psychologists, psychiatrists, counselors, social workers, clergy, and other qualified individuals can assist patients to cope with fibromyalgia and make the necessary life-styles adjustments. Patients learn to change their attitude can help make the change from "I can't because of my fibromyalgia," to "I can in spite of my fibromyalgia."

I never hesitate to recommend psychological intervention for someone who may need this help. If you think you may need this help, please make an appointment with someone right away. You may find a professional "good friend" who can help you in ways your other "good friends" can't.

Chapter 15 — Survival Strategies

1) Consider getting help from a professional therapist to help manage your fibromyalgia.

2) Realize the chronic pain of fibromyalgia affects all aspects of your life.

3) With a therapist, determine and set realistic goals.

4) Change your attitude about therapy. Make the mental aspects of your illness as important as the physical.

5) Asking for help doesn't mean "you are crazy", or it's "all in your head." You just want help reevaluating where you are in life and being OK with that.

6) Recognize early symptoms of depression, anxiety, and decreased self esteem. The earlier these are treated the better.

7) Seek treatment immediately if/when emotions reach crisis proportion.

16 ◆ Complementary Medicine

Complementary or alternative medicine has become more popular in the past few years. This type of medicine has been around for thousands of years, much longer than traditional or conventional medicine. Historically, the United States has embraced the conventional medicine approach, so complementary or alternative medicines have been viewed with skepticism. As patients and the public in general have become more aware of alternative medicine, its popularity has increased.

A study described in the Journal of *American Medical Association* (Eisenberg, D.M. *et al*, 1998) found that the total number of visits to alternative medicine practitioners rose by nearly 50% from 1990 to 1997. In 1997, the most popular alternative therapies were vitamins and herbal medicine, massage, energy healing, chiropractic, and homeopathy. In the United States, over 21 billion dollars was spent in 1997 on alternative medicine.

It is not surprising that people with fibromyalgia are interested in alternative medicine approaches. If there is one area in which conventional medicine often fails, it is in the management of conditions causing chronic pain. Conventional medicine emphasizes the diagnosis and pharmacologic treatment of various medical conditions based on scientific research. The main philosophy is to identify the cause of the disease and treat it with medicines or surgeries to eliminate the cause. Conventional medicine is wonderful in curing patients with bacterial infections by treating them with antibiotics, saving persons with diseased organs by transplants, treating diabetes by providing insulin replacement and saving an individual with acute appendicitis by performing an appendectomy. But if someone has chronic pain, does not respond to medications, is not a candidate for a surgical procedure, and has had numerous diagnostic tests that were normal, conventional medicine may be literally helpless.

Complementary or alternative medicine strategies emphasizes the interaction between the body and the mind. The main focus is on maintaining homeostasis, which is the body's natural ability to maintain a stable harmony and balance among its hormones, enzymes, muscles, and organs to prevent disease or to allow the body to heal itself. This type of medicine focuses on the whole individual instead of the individual symptoms, and seeks to optimize homeostasis by promoting healthy life-styles, appropriate exercise, restful sleep, proper nutrition, and self-responsibility.

Those who endorse complementary medicine will tell you that the body does not end with the skin. Instead, energy fields extend beyond the body that affect one's well-being. We can respond to energy therapies. And no, you do not have to be radioactive to emit an energy field, you just have to be alive!

Conventional medicine sets a high research standard for approving certain treatments. Scientific studies are valuable tools in proving effectiveness (or harmlessness) of certain treatments. If a particular drug treatment has been studied and shown to be scientifically effective, this drug may be helpful (and safe) for patients.

Sometimes, this scientific standard can be a double-edged sword. Most conditions that doctors treat do not have scientific studies that "prove" a particular treatment is effective. But that does not stop us from treating conditions, nor should it. Medical practitioners need to be open-minded. If we always waited for scientific proof, most diseases that exist today could not be treated. Complementary medicine has long

You are encouraged to be open-minded when it comes to complementary/alternative medicine strategies. Numerous treatments are available and many people have benefited from them. Like any other treatments, there can be side effects from or lack of response to complementary treatments, so you need to work with qualified, knowledgeable health professionals. Choose your care wisely and responsibly, and hopefully you will find many ways to control your fibromyalgia!

been stereotyped as "failing" to hold up to scientific standards of conventional medicine. Fortunately, an increased number of scientific studies are being published that support the effectiveness of many complementary medicine treatments. Complementary medicine may still need to "catch up" on its scientific credibility, but it already has a long and successful history in clinical applications. Just ask people with fibromyalgia!

Placebo Effect

I remember learning that the placebo effect was "bad." The placebo effect occurred when a person reported improvement in pain after being given a sugar pill instead of the actual drug. The placebo effect has to be accounted for in a research study. The placebo response needs to be cancelled out, so as not to mistakenly attribute all of the positive benefits to the drug being tested.

Placebo is derived from the Latin word that means "I will please." It is a positive human response to hopefulness and wanting to get better with a treatment. Even though the person wasn't given an actual drug, she/he felt measurably better simply because of HOPE. Studies show the placebo effect may happen up to 30% of the time with ANY treatment. This means three of ten people will feel better when given any type of treatment, with no obvious relationship to the actual treatment.

The placebo effect is a powerful physician "tool" that is not limited to a pill. Suggestions that a physician makes can have a dramatic effect on how a patient will respond to a particular treatment. In a study done by Drs. Staat and Hekmat (1998), the role of one's pain threshold in response to suggestion was examined.

Three groups of college students were to place their hands in a tank of ice water. Each group was instructed differently. The first group was told "neutral" things: don't think about anything, just keep your hand in the water until you need to remove it. The second group was told "positive" things: ice water can improve circulation, strengthen the heart, cleanse the skin cells, and other beneficial effects. The third group was told "negative" things: ice water can be dangerous by causing numbness, decrease in blood flow, tissue damage and hypertension. All three groups were told to keep their hands immersed until they couldn't tolerate the pain anymore.

Guess what happened? The "positive" group held their hands in longer and reported less anxiety. The "negative" group took their hands out much quicker and reported more anxiety. The "neutral" group was in between the other groups. This study demonstrated how the physician can affect the patient's response to treatment. Reassuring positive words are more likely to increase the therapeutic response — cause a positive placebo response. I have found much better responses to medications in my patients when I ex-

> Conventional medicine is wonderful in curing patients with bacterial infections by treating them with antibiotics, saving persons with diseased organs by transplants, treating diabetes by providing insulin replacement and saving an individual with acute appendicitis by performing an appendectomy. But if someone has chronic pain, does not respond to medications, is not a candidate for a surgical procedure, and has had numerous diagnostic tests that were normal, conventional medicine may be literally helpless.has had numerous

plain what to expect, tell them the medicines may help but won't take away all the pain, than if I just gave them the medicines and said, "Take this and let me know if it helps."

A number of years ago it dawned on me that the placebo response from hopefulness and one's desire to improve is EXACTLY what we are trying to accomplish in the treatment of chronic pain related to fibromyalgia. We want people to feel better, even if we can't explain how it happened. This approach would seem to be one of the major philosophies of complementary medicine, to improve the well-being of body and mind. With this realization, I've washed out all of the negative connotations I learned about placebos from conventional medicine and have become more open-minded. Now one of my philosophies is, welcome placebo! We WANT to achieve a positive placebo response.

My Specialty Blends Both Medicines

My specialty is actually a blend between conventional and complementary medicine strategies. By using a multidisciplinary approach, we blend the best of everything to help fibromyalgia. I was "conventionally" trained at The Ohio State University (both M.D. and Residency), but my training included learning and understanding physical medicine treatments, physical therapy, massage therapy, manipulation therapy, nutritional therapy, biofeedback, and many other areas that are considered "alternative" treatments. I also received training in diagnosis, testing, prescribing medications, and research, areas that are considered "traditional."

Over the years, the line between traditional and alternative medicine blurred. Acupuncture, physical therapy, and nutritional therapies are examples of alternative treatments that have become traditionally accepted. I think it is a pointless exercise to try to separate conventional and alternative medicines; we need to recognize that chronic pain requires the best of everything.

Many people are frustrated at the lack of improved conventional treatments for chronic pain, and if the physicians are not open-minded and flexible in their treatment approaches, these people will search elsewhere for relief. A knowledgeable physician treating pain should accept whatever works and not be limited to any particular treatment.

Many doctors specialize in complementary medicine and have undergone years of training to become experts in their field. However, many nonmedical people have ventured into alternative medicine treatments with little or no experience, training, or supervision. They promote themselves as so-called "experts" in managing pain. I advise patients to be open-minded, but to check credentials and training and make sure that the practitioner is licensed. If the answers to these licensing and credential questions are too "vague" or "mysterious," stay away from him or her.

This chapter is not meant to be a complete, comprehensive guide to all of the alternative medicine strategies available for chronic pain. There are many good reference books on alternative medicine. One good one is *Alternative Medicine, The Definitive Guide*, compiled by the Burton-Goldberg group. This chapter will highlight some specific approaches I have found useful in the overall treatment of fibromyalgia. Many others, which I have not included here, may be helpful.

Chiropractic Medicine

Chiropractic medicine can be effective in treating back problems, headaches, and other pain disorders including fibromyalgia. Dr. Daniel David Palmer founded the modern chiropractic system in 1895, and today chiropractic medicine is the most popular of alternative medicine fields. Chiropractic treatment can be effective in persons with fibromyalgia since patients have pain along the entire spine.

A key philosophy in chiropractic medicine is the holistic approach with an emphasis on the relationship between the spinal column, the nervous system, and the soft tissues of the body. Proper alignment of the spinal column is necessary to achieve homeostasis and optimal health by allowing unimpeded nerve flow and enhanced neurologic and soft tissue function. In other words, it is believed these treatments enable "clearer" nerve signals to travel through the spine to the brain. If an imbalance, dysequilibrium, or misalignment occurs in the vertebrae or soft tissues, nerve pressure can occur. This results in altered signals which eventually lead to impaired nerve function, disease, and pain.

Manipulations are forceful movements of body parts (*i.e.*, pelvis, shoulder) to bring about a greater range of movement and to relax muscles. Adjustments are the application of a sudden and precise force to a persistent point in the vertebra or muscle to properly align the tissue. The desired outcomes of properly aligned vertebrae and muscles are improved balance, better neurologic flow, better circulation, and ultimately, decreased pain and tension.

Many chiropractors use a device called an Activator to perform adjustments. This hand-held device has a spring loaded plunger mechanism which delivers focused pressure energy to a specific body part to achieve proper alignment. A chiropractor is trained in all types of adjustments and can determine which techniques would be most appropriate for a given individual. Chiropractic medicine also deals with preventive, nutritional, strengthening, and fitness measures in helping individuals achieve their highest state of well-being.

I believe the professional relationship and communication between chiropractic and medical physicians will continue to improve, and patients will benefit.

Applied Kinesiology

Specific muscles may be overactive causing a spasm, or underactive, causing weakness. These muscles can create dysfunction that causes pain and impairment. An applied kinesiologist uses procedures that strengthen weak muscles and relax tense muscles to help return injured or dysfunctional muscles to their normal state. Specific muscles are thought to be related to specific organs, and thus improving the muscle balance improves organ function. Since patients with fibromyalgia have muscle imbalances because portions of the muscles are overly tense and other portions are weak, applied kinesiology techniques can help. Many chiropractors and manual therapists have learned applied kinesiology skills.

Acupuncture

Acupuncture originated in China thousands of years ago and has been successful in pain relief, particularly as an alternative to conventional pain medications. Acupuncture is based on the theory that energy pathways called meridians are present in the body, and that they link the nervous system with the organs. Multiple acupuncture points within these meridian systems can be stimulated to improve the energy flow. These points are stimulated using special needles, electrical stimulation, or pressure.

Acupuncture stimulates the body's own natural pain killers, endorphins. It also affects neurotransmitters or hormones that transmit nerve impulses in a way that decreases the perception of pain. Many studies have shown the effectiveness of acupuncture as a substitute for surgical anesthesia and the temporary relief of pain.

A growing number of physicians have been trained in acupuncture and are practicing this technique in treating pain disorders. In November of 1997, the National Institutes of Health consensus panel on acupuncture issued a statement indicating that pain from musculoskeletal conditions could be successfully treated with acupuncture. Indeed, many patients with fibromyalgia have benefited from acupuncture treatments.

Magnetic Therapy

Magnetic therapy use magnets to decrease pain by improving energy and blood flow in the body. Therapeutic magnets work on the same principle as acupuncture, but without the needle. Magnetic fields surround us, generated by natural mechanisms such as the earth and weather changes. The fields can be man-made, caused by power lines and electrical devices. This theory maintains that these magnetic fields can affect the body's function in both positive and negative ways by influencing the body's metabolism and oxygen availability to cells.

Magnets have two poles, a positive and a negative. It is felt that the positive pole causes negative effects such as decreased metabolic function, especially with prolonged exposure. The negative pole is felt to cause beneficial effects by normalizing the body's metabolic and energy functioning. Magnetic therapy can be used in numerous ways, from magnetic strips applied to parts of the body to magnetic beds, pillows, and shoe inserts.

Some people believe that reduced exposure to the earth's natural geomagnetic fields can lead to a magnetic field deficiency syndrome. People who live in cities, in high rise buildings, or who have minimal contact with the "bare" earth would be at risk for magnetic field deficiency syndrome since asphalt, concrete, bricks, and metal block our exposure to the natural geomagnetic fields. This syndrome causes pain, headaches, insomnia, stiffness, and fatigue (sound like fibromyalgia?). It is felt that magnetic therapy can be used to correct this deficiency and help restore health in some of these people.

Magnetic fields are used in diagnostic testing procedures such as MRI (magnetic resonance imaging), magnetic encephalography and nerve conduction studies to safely and accurately measure structures and electrical activity. Magnetic field diagnostic techniques are already established in mainstream medicine, and therapeutic magnetic therapy is rising in popularity. It is considered a safe treatment, and many qualified health professionals are using magnets in their clinical practices.

Energy Therapy

Energy therapy is a practice of promoting healing by working on the body's energy fields. It is deeply rooted in the ancient practice of laying-on of the hands. If one assumes that human beings have energy fields that extend from their bodies and that energy flows to and from the body, then one can understand how energy therapy may be a helpful modality. Energy therapy can also be called therapeutic touch, although it is not necessary for the energy therapist to physically touch the patient.

Energy therapy has its roots in ancient Chinese medicine that was based on increasing and balancing the flow of Chi, which means "life force." Acupuncture, another ancient treatment development, is also based on altering the flow of Chi by identifying and treating specific acupuncture points in the body.

Energy therapists believe that some illnesses are related to blocked or uneven energy. Various stress-related problems such as headaches, irritable bowel syndrome, breathing difficulties and autonomic nervous system dysfunction may be caused by altered energy flow in the body. Energy therapy has been promoted as an effective way of reducing stress and pain and relieving various stress-related symptoms. Accelerated healing and boosting the immune system are the results promoted by energy therapy.

It is believed that energy can be transferred from one person to another, hence an energy practitioner can access an energy field and rebalance or re-pattern the energy of a symptomatic patient. The energy therapist usually accesses the energy field by moving the hands over the body from two to six inches away. The energy therapist reports that her hands sense cues from the patient's energy field such as a pull, tingling, pulsation or a temperature change. The therapist identifies these specific cues and tries to modulate and rebalance the energy field by moving the hands over the area towards the periphery of the field. Sometimes actual physical touch is needed in combination with non-contact "touch." The average treatment lasts 15 to 20 minutes, and each person responds differently. Patients have reported feeling sensations during the treatment such as tingling or warmth.

The goals of energy therapy are to reduce pain and stress-related symptoms. Certainly any treatment that can help achieve a relaxation response and reduce pain and stress is welcome in the fibromyalgia world.

Homeopathic Therapy

Homeopathic medicine had its origins over two hundred years ago with Dr. Samuel Hahnemann. It is a practice that approaches each individual disease as a consequence of an imbalance within the homeostasis. Each individual's condition is unique, and the homeopathic doctor learns as much as possible about the patient and then prescribes natural substances, called remedies, to treat him or her.

Homeopathic remedies are administered by mouth and should have no toxicities or side effects. Homeopathic ingredients are based on the principle that *like cures like*. It is thought that a small diluted dose will stimulate the body to control its symptoms by healing and restoring balance. If the substances were given in larger doses, they would usually cause the symptoms the patient is complaining of, not eliminate them. For example, ipecac is given to induce vomiting after a poison is ingested. However, homeopathic remedies use very diluted doses of ipecac to treat symptoms of nausea and vomiting. Think of remedies as vaccines which are small, harmless doses that stimulate a specific body reaction to actually protect the body against this substance.

If the person is given a homeopathic remedy for inflammation, this should gently stimulate the body to heal the inflammation and return the body to health and harmony, or homeostasis. Homeopathic remedies stimulate the body's own immune and defense system to initiate the healing process. The homeopathic practitioner approaches the individual's unique problems and prescribes individualized medicine based on the person's total symptoms, including physical, emotional and mental.

Conventional medicine has used homeopathic-like therapy. I have already given the example of vaccination to induce a protective immune response against the actual infection. Other examples include using radiation to treat people with cancer (radiation can cause cancer), using Ritalin for hyperactive children (Ritalin is an amphetamine-like drug which causes hyperactivity), and using digoxin for heart conditions (digitalis can actually cause heart abnormalities).

Homeopathic medicine is actually a sophisticated practice in which remedies are prescribed to help the body heal. It is gaining in popularity as more and more people are seeking alternative means for helping pain. A number of my patients have reported substantial benefits in reducing their pain through homeopathic means. If you are considering homeopathic medicine, I recommend you see only a licensed physician who is trained in homeopathic medicine to ensure optimal safety.

Prolotherapy

Prolotherapy is a simple, safe, and effective treatment for numerous painful conditions. The term "prolotherapy" was coined in the 1940s by George S. Hackett, M.D., a Canton, Ohio industrial surgeon who developed and later refined the modern technique. The "prolo" in prolotherapy is short for proliferate because the treatment actually induces growth, or proliferation, of tissue. It is a form of injection therapy directed at weakened ligaments and tendons. Typically, a dextrose (sugar) based anesthetic solution is injected into the injured ligament and tendon areas. These injections stimulate an injury–repair sequence. (Sounds painful...well it is a little bit...!) The chemical environment of a fresh injury is recreated in a controlled manner, and this activates the healing cascade.

Studies have shown that ligament and tendon size and strength can increase as much as 35 to 40% in areas treated by injections. It has been shown to be an effective treatment for chronic low back pain, and usually there is a 75% or greater success rate (less pain, less tenderness) in treatment of other types of chronic musculoskeletal pain including fibromyalgia.

Prolotherapy has been used successfully in posttraumatic fibromyalgia, particularly neck pain from unresolved whiplash injuries. Sprains and strain injuries that do not heal on their own can go on to develop chronic myofascial pain syndrome/fibromyalgia, and perhaps a major mechanism in this particular pain is persistent weakened ligaments and tendons which "destabilize" a region. Muscles tighten up to try to "stabilize" this region, causing painful spasms. Because prolotherapy actually creates new tissue in the injured structures, it may be considered a more permanent treatment in many instances, and indeed many patients have received long-term benefits (Dr. Vladimir Djuric, *Prolotherapy Treats Pain*, Chronic Pain Solutions, 1998).

Nutritional Therapy

As we discussed earlier (Chapter 14), there has been a lot of exciting research on the nutritional and biochemical aspects of fibromyalgia, and I think this area is the "hotbed" in fibromyalgia research and treatment. An explosion of nutritional products is available on the market. These over-the-counter supplements and health foods are not subjected to the same strict Food and Drug Administration (FDA) regulations as are prescription medicines. Remember, we discussed the scientific standards that apply to acceptance and use of prescription medicines.

The FDA is the scientific accrediting and regulating agency for prescription medicines. In some instances the FDA has warned consumers about potential side effects or contaminations of health food products that could cause medical complications. For example, there have been FDA warnings about the use of tryptophan contamination which has caused serious blood reactions (eosinophilia). Also, the FDA has warned about using dietary supplements that contain both ephedrine and caffeine, as this combination may cause heart attacks, heart arrhythmia, or hepatitis.

Many effective nutritional therapies have been used for hundreds and even thousands of years, resulting in a lot of accumulated clinical experience. That is not the same as saying scientific studies have confirmed the success, or that the FDA has approved the use of particular products. We have to remember that not everything we use to treat medical conditions has been studied or approved, and that does not mean we shouldn't use it. We need to be open-minded about nutritional approaches, but we also have to optimize safety and therapeutic efficacy by being responsible and knowledgeable about products that we use. An average consumer works closely with her/his doctor, nutritionist, pharmacist, or knowledgeable colleagues to learn about a product and make intelligent decisions. You should not try anything unless you know exactly what it contains and your doctor has approved its use.

A good quarterly newsletter, *Health Points*, published by To Your Health, Inc., Fountain Hills, Arizona, focuses on nutritional articles with information about ordering nutritional products. A recommended reading is *Prescription for Nutritional Healing* by James and Phillis Balch.

There are no magical nutritional approaches; rather nutritional approaches can be part of a successful treatment plan for fibromyalgia. Doctors who specialize in fibromyalgia treatment have found particular strategies that work well for their patients. For example, Dr. Jacob Teitelbaum has blended traditional and complementary strategies in his treatment of chronic fatigue syndrome and fibromyalgia which he describes in his book, *From Fatigued to Fantastic*. Dr. Paul St. Amand reports success in treating patients with guaifenesin and has published information regarding this strategy. Guaifenesin is a cough medicine that has found a "new" application in fibromyalgia treatment. Another cough medicine, dextromethorphan, can lead to reduced pain by decreasing pain signals. Maybe with additional research, we can find medicine that will stop both our pain and our coughing!

For my patients, I also use a variety of complementary/nutritional approaches. I've summarized my Top Ten approaches below.

Dr. P's Top 10 Nutritional Medicines

1) **Muscle nutritional supplements.** I recommend a combination magnesium/malic acid supplement for the muscles. I have found about 70% of people will have decreased pain, improved energy, a more stable baseline, or a combination of the above with these supplements. These supplements can be combined with Vitamins B_1, B_6, C and/or manganese.

2) **Colostrum.** Colostrum has been promoted as an immune system booster and a supplement that promotes healing. It has helped nearly 75% of my fibromyalgia patients improve their energy levels and concentration abilities, as well as helping to control the pain. Dr. Bennett (1998) found that people with fibromyalgia have decreased growth hormone level as measured with IGF-1 (Insulin-like growth factor, a derivative of growth hormone). He also found that daily growth hormone injections not only increased the IGF level in these patients but also resulted in significant improvement in the treatment group versus the placebo group. Growth hormone injections are expensive, averaging about $1500 a month and are not routinely covered by insurance, hence limiting the widespread application for fibromyalgia treatment.

   Colostrum has a high concentration of growth hormone, IGF and immunoglobulins. Bovine (beef) colostrum is essentially identical to human IGF-1. Bovine colostrum given orally has been found to raise the serum IGF-1 levels in humans.

3) **A good multivitamin and mineral supplement.** People can take other products that contain vitamins and minerals, but I recommend that they still take a daily multivitamin and mineral supplement.

4) **Topical muscle medicines.** These can decrease muscle pain in the areas applied. The three I use most commonly are Biofreeze, which gives a cool sensation; Tiger Balm, which gives a hot sensation; and lidocaine patches, which numb the skin.

5) **Vitamin B_{12}.** Many people with fibromyalgia have a relatively low B_{12} level. A "relatively low" B_{12} level could contribute to fatigue, numbness, and decreased biochemical pathways, particularly in the nerves and red blood cells.

   If patients have relatively low vitamin B_{12} levels and are bothered by extreme fatigue, I frequently prescribe a B_{12} injection protocol. One milligram of B_{12} is injected intramuscularly once a week for six weeks or more. B_{12} replacement improves erythropoiesis (red blood cell manufacturing), and improves the pathways in nerves, fatty cells, DNA synthesis, and folate metabolism. I do not find that pain levels decrease significantly with B_{12} injections, but the energy levels improve. B_{12} can be taken sublingually and be absorbed directly through the blood vessels in the mouth, but it is not absorbed well from the stomach.

6) **Natural anti-inflammatories.** Many people with fibromyalgia also have degenerative or arthritic problems that are contributing to the overall pain. Natural anti-inflammatories not only help reduce inflammation (which is great in people who do not tolerate NSAIDs), but are also building blocks to repair and regenerate cartilage and ligaments. Glucosamine sulfate and chondroitin are two popular ones in this category. I have used MSM (Methyl Sulfonyl Methane) as well, which can help reduce fibromyalgia pain and reduce inflammation from other conditions. MSM is a sulphur derivative which can help improve hormone and protein function.

7) **Natural serotonin supplements.** The two that are commonly used are 5-HTP and St. John's Wort. I don't use them together. 5-HTP is 5-hydroxy L-tryptophan which is a modified amino acid that the body uses to manufacture serotonin. In addition to helping the body produce serotonin, 5-HTP can be an appetite suppressant and a sleep inducer. Impurities were discovered in some pills which caused a condition known as eosinophilia/myalgia syndrome, which can be life-threatening. The impurities, not the 5-HTP, caused this condition. I use reputable brands with companies that have a proven track record, and have not had any problems with contaminated supplements. Dosing of 5-HPT is 50 mg at bedtime on an empty stomach to start, and can increase to 100 mg three times a day under the direction of your doctor.

St. John's Wort has been used as a natural antidepressant. One should not use St. John's Wort with a prescription antidepressant, and I don't like to use 5-HTP and St. John's Wort together because I don't want patients to have too much serotonin effect or adverse reactions (sweating, rapid heart rate, anxiety). Some reports have shown that combining natural serotonin medicines with prescription ones can cause problems in a few patients. Typical dosing of St. John's Wort's is 300 mg up to twice a day.

Sam E (pronounced Sammy) is a natural medicine used in Europe for over 20 years to treat mild to moderate depression. Recently it is being promoted for use in the U.S. It stands for S-Adenosyl-L-methionine, and it helps make the body's mood enhancing chemicals. Usual dosing is 200 to 400 mg twice a day on an empty stomach, whatever your doctor recommends. Side effects can include upset stomach and headaches.

8) **Natural sleep modifiers.** 5-HTP and St. John's Wort can be sleep modifiers. I also use melatonin, Kava Kava, and valerian root as natural sleep modifiers and natural stress relievers.

9) **Immune boosters.** Colostrum, Vitamin C, zinc, echinacea, cinnamon, garlic, goldenseal, or a combination can help boost the immune function. Those who are prone to frequent colds are candidates for an immune booster, particularly Vitamin C and zinc. Antioxidants are helpful in fighting free radicals, supporting the cellular function, and improving the immune function. Common antioxidants include Vitamins A and E, grape seed extract, and lipoic acid. Licorice root and Ginseng can help improve the adrenal gland function and boost our stress and immune response.

10) **"Others."** I use many others depending on a given situation. For example, Feverfew is commonly prescribed for migraine headaches. Nystatin is a natural antibiotic that can help treat yeast infections. Coenzyme Q10 is a muscle

nutritional supplement that can help boost energy production. *Lactobacillus* supplements can help restore friendly microorganism balance in those with chronic *Candida* yeast overgrowth.

You are encouraged to be open-minded when it comes to complementary/alternative medicine strategies. Numerous treatments are available and many people have benefited from them. Like any other treatments, there can be side effects from or lack of response to complementary treatments, so you need to work with qualified, knowledgeable health professionals. Choose your care wisely and responsibly, and hopefully you will find many ways to control your fibromyalgia!

Chapter 16 — Survival Strategies

1) Explore alternative medicine approaches.

2) Understand the importance of improving the mind-body connection. Choose alternative therapies that embrace this philosophy.

3) Consider working with an M.D. who specializes in Physical Medicine and Rehabilitation. This will give you a comprehensive treatment approach that combines conventional and complementary medicine.

4) Evaluate and choose alternative medicine treatments responsibly — check credentials of practitioners.

5) Share all information with your doctor.

6) Educate yourself about nutritional products so you can make knowledgeable choices.

7) Be consumer savvy.

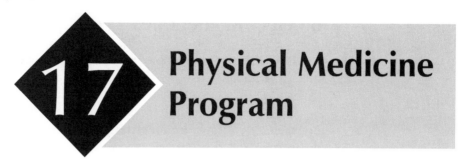

Physical Medicine Program

A physical medicine program is an important part in the overall treatment of fibromyalgia. A physical medicine program includes such modalities as heat, cold, massage, electric stimulation, or whirlpool. Manual exercises, stretching, strengthening, conditioning, aerobics, and aquatics can also be helpful. Not everyone with fibromyalgia needs a physical medicine program, but most of my patients have benefited from one. Different therapies work better for different persons, and doctors need to determine what is best for that individual.

Different health professionals who might be involved include physical therapists, massotherapists, chiropractors, and exercise physiologists. Any therapy program should be safe, relatively easy to do, affordable, and have a good chance of success. A successful therapy program should be one that the patient can learn to carry out by him/herself. Chapter 22 will address how to develop an individualized home program. This chapter focuses on initial prescribed therapies that can help get you started. As with any treatment prescription, the patient's therapy response and any changes or modifications should be monitored by a physician familiar with fibromyalgia syndrome.

Let's consider a number of available physical medicine treatments.

Therapeutic Modalities

Therapeutic modalities (physical medicine treatments) include thermal agents and bioelectric therapy. Thermal agents include cryotherapy, or cold therapy, and superficial and deep heat. Cryotherapy is often used for acute soft tissue injuries to decrease edema and spasm. In fibromyalgia, cryotherapy can reduce pain and muscle tightness. Therapeutic heat consists of both superficial heat (hot packs, warm water therapy, and paraffin bath), and deep heat (ultrasound, diathermy, microwave). Superficial and deep heating modalities can help decrease pain and improve flexibility of the soft tissues. About 20 minutes of a thermal application (heat or cold) is the usual treatment time. Sometimes heat and cold are alternated (called a contrast bath). This can help those with neuropathy-type pain.

Heat therapy is more popular with fibromyalgia, particularly moist heat. Cold treatments can be just as effective if the person can tolerate the first five minutes of COLD. After the first five minutes, numbness and desensitization of the skin allows full tolerance for the remaining 15 minutes of treatment. The deep muscle cooling effect of the cold modality can insulate the tissues and slow the blood flow, neurologic signals, and metabolism to give a longer-acting effect than heat. If an exercise program is also being performed, a combination of heat and cold can be used for the best effect. Heat modalities can be used before exercise to assist in the warm-up process, and cold modalities can be used immediately after exercising to help minimize swelling and pain and to assist in the cool-down process.

Bioelectric Therapies

Electric stimulation, sometimes called bioelectric therapy, can also provide relief. Electrical current delivered to the muscles ranges from a mini-electric current that is barely felt, to a stronger electrical current that causes the muscles to contract. Types of bioelectric therapy include transcutaneous electrical nerve stimulation (TENS), functional electric stimulation, interferential therapy, and iontophoresis. Each type works differently; your doctor may prescribe one or more types as part of your program. Drs. Melzack and Wall performed a landmark study in 1965 on the gate control theory of pain (see Chapter 8), and this led to the development of numerous electrical therapy modalities. The mechanisms of the bioelectric modalities include: 1) blocking the pain with "soothing" electrical sensation, 2) facilitating the entry of nutrients into the cells and waste products out of the cells, and 3) biochemical/neurologic reeducation to improve the body's efficiency at a cellular level. Bioelectric modalities are usually well tolerated, and with repeated treatments, the patient can tolerate higher intensities and get even more therapeutic effect, particularly when treating more acute pain and muscle spasms.

Manipulation and Adjustments

Manipulations and adjustments can be performed by trained osteopathic physicians, chiropractic physicians, and manual therapists. These techniques can mobilize joints, improve range of motion and relaxation, and reduce muscle pain, all of which can benefit patients with fibromyalgia. Manipulations are forceful movements of body parts such as the neck to bring about a greater range of motion and relaxation. Adjustments are the application of a sudden and precise force to a specific point in the vertebrae or muscle to properly align the body. The desired outcome of properly aligned vertebrae and muscle is improved circulation and neurologic signals and reduced pain.

Massage Therapy/Manual Therapy

Massage therapy can decrease pain by relaxing muscles, improving circulation and oxygenation, removing waste buildup in the muscles, increasing muscle flexibility, and reeducating muscles. Various massage techniques include:

1) **Stroking,** which is the gliding of palms and fingers firmly over the muscles in a slow rhythmic motion.

2) **Kneading,** when the muscles are grabbed between fingers and thumb and slightly lifted and squeezed in a slow rhythmic sequence.

3) **Friction massage** penetrates deep into the muscles and uses slow circular motions with the tips of the fingers or thumb.

Massage therapy is administered by a qualified therapist, and treatments usually last for about 60 minutes. This therapy is often combined with other therapies, but my patients love this treatment and consider it their favorite. There are different types of specialized massage.

1) **Swedish massage.** This is the traditional massage that involves stroking, kneading, and friction massage.

2) **Myofascial release.** This technique was developed by physical therapist John Barnes. It is designed to loosen up the fascia (or connective tissue) and allow the muscles to relax and improve blood flow.

3) **Trigger point therapy.** This technique involves sustained pressure applied to pain trigger points/tender points (no needles here!). This sustained pressure helps break up and desensitize the trigger points.

4) **Craniosacral therapy.** This gentle technique was developed mainly by Dr. John Upledger. It enhances the flow of the cerebrolspinal fluid which bathes the brain and spinal cord (craniosacral system). This therapy is promoted to reduce stress and enhance the body's natural healing mechanisms, hopefully reducing pain.

5) **Strain/counterstrain.** This technique uses opposing forces on muscles and connective tissue to relieve restrictions and tightness and cause the muscle fibers to lengthen. When properly performed, it will cause relaxation/lengthening of the muscles and improvement in spasms and mobility.

I often prescribe some type of massage or manual therapy as part of the overall treatment program. Techniques are individualized to the patient. As treatment progresses, more advanced and deeper techniques can be used as the patient begins to improve and tolerate treatments better. The massage therapist needs to be knowledgeable and experienced in treating fibromyalgia to use the best of many techniques for any given individual situation.

Self-massage is a simple procedure that patients can be taught. A spouse or significant other can also learn how to perform therapeutic massage. We offer couples massage classes. One criteria for the classes is that the patient with fibromyalgia has to agree to give the significant other a massage every once in a while, too!

Exercise Therapy

Exercises are beneficial in the long run for everyone and everything! Many people with fibromyalgia reject exercise outright because it's simply too painful. But everyone can find some type of exercise program that is tolerated and helpful, even if it's stretching only. I usually wait until the acute pain begins to subside before introducing exercises, then gradually progress them as tolerated. Patients often experience increased pain after exertion due to a combination of tight muscles and being less aerobically fit overall (Bennett R.M. *et al*, 1989). Fibromyalgia patients who attempt an exercise program often experience an increase in muscle pain which may discourage them from continuing to work on improving their level of fitness. I have found that staying with a prescribed supervised exercise program will gradually coax the patient's muscles to a greater fitness level with more flexibility and functional ability. Different types of exercises include:

Sometimes heat and cold are alternated (called a contrast bath). This can help those with neuropathy-type pain.

1) **Range of motion exercises.** Each joint is moved through its normal range. These exercises help maintain normal joint movements and decrease stiffness.

2) **Stretching and flexibility exercises.** This combines range of motion with a gentle yet firm stretching of the muscles and joints. The shoulders, neck, hips, and back muscles tend to be particularly stiff and painful, so they need to have regular stretching and flexibility exercises.

3) **Strengthening exercises.** These increase muscle strength. Isometric exercises (the person tightens the muscle, but does not move the joint) can be helpful if the joints are painful, because it makes the muscle stronger with little joint movement. Isokinetic or isotonic exercises (the muscles tighten using a weight or some type of resistance, and the joints move through the motion) are also effective because they allow for better blood flow and oxygenation. Two popular exercises that combine stretching and strengthening include therabands (long rubber bands) and a Swiss ball (an oversized inflated ball) used in different ways to stretch and strengthen muscles.

Specialized exercises to strengthen back muscles include McKenzie exercises and Williams flexion exercises. McKenzie exercises are a popular and effective way to strengthen back muscles, particularly the extensor muscles that arch the back. Many of my fibromyalgia patients have learned these exercises from trained therapists and have found them helpful in reducing back pain and improving posture and strength.

4) **Aerobic exercises.** These enhance the condition of the heart and lungs as well as strengthening and conditioning muscles. Common aerobic exercises include walking, biking, jogging, aerobics, and swimming (if the water is close to 90° F).

Prescribed Physical Medicine Program

A typical prescribed therapy program may start with therapies three times a week for ten to twelve treatments. The goals of such a program may be to decrease the pain by at least 50% over a month, and to gradually increase tolerance to activity. I want the patient to make progress from the pain management phase to the exercise phase, and ultimately to a successful home program. Progress is documented in four ways:

a) Pain Analog Scale (See diagram next page).

Everyone can find some type of exercise program that is tolerated and helpful, even if it's stretching only. I usually wait until the acute pain begins to subside before introducing exercises, then gradually progress them as tolerated.

NAME: _____ DATE: _____

REFERRED BY: _____

ONSET OF SYMPTOMS – DATE: _____

WERE YOU INJURED (ACCIDENT, FALL, BLOW, OTHER)? _____

CHIEF COMPLAINT: _____

SECONDARY COMPLAINT: _____

ON A SCALE OF 0 (NO PAIN) TO 10 (WORST PAIN) RATE YOUR PAIN:

TODAY: _____ WORSE DAY: _____ BEST DAY: _____

WHAT MAKES YOUR PAIN BETTER: _____

WHAT MAKES YOUR PAIN WORSE: _____

IS YOUR SLEEP AFFECTED: _____

MARK WITH THE COLORED PENS TO DESCRIBE YOUR SYMPTOMS:
ACHES = YELLOW   BURNING = BLUE
PINS & NEEDLES = GREEN NUMBNESS = BLACK
STABBING = RED

MEDICAL PROBLEMS:
_____
_____
_____
_____

RIGHT   LEFT   RIGHT

MEDICATIONS:
_____
_____
_____
_____
_____

ALLERGIES:
_____

OCCUPATION:
_____

DO YOU SMOKE: _____

This allows grading of the pain from 0 (no pain) to 10 (worst pain). Many patients rank their pain higher than a 10! This scale is particularly useful and valid for a given individual to note pain before, during, and after treatments to see if the treatments helped (*i.e.*, pain decreases).

b) Tender point examination or "mapping" results (shows fewer painful areas)

c) Range of motion (improves)

d) Functional accomplishments (patient able to do more)

Pain Management Program

This phase is designed to decrease pain and get control over a pain flare-up. It involves education, prescribing medicines and nutritional supplements, and specific Physical Medicine programs. I use multiple treatments at the same time because they have a better chance of reducing pain more quickly rather than trying one thing at a time, waiting to see if it works, then try the next thing if the first treatment didn't help. I want you to feel better FAST! If you should have decreased pain from the different treatments , but can't tell exactly what works, so what?! What a nice problem to have, feeling better but not sure what's working! We can figure out what is helping after you are feeling better. Most people can tell what helps, even if more than one treatment is helping.

Depending on the location of pain and the number of "worse" areas, I may try trigger point injections. Using either a local anesthetic only or a combination of a local anesthetic and cortisone, I may inject from one to six areas at a time. Other types of injections may be necessary including selective joint injections, nerve blocks, epidurals, or prolotherapy.

Prolotherapy has been highly effective in my practice. My associate, Dr. Djuric, has been trained in prolotherapy, and has treated many patients with fibromyalgia. A number of them have gotten permanent improvements with this treatment. The fibromyalgia isn't cured, but certain painful areas settle down and remain in remission. The conditions that have gotten the best results include: persistent spine pain from unresolved whiplash injuries, plantar fasciitis, lateral epicondylitis (tennis elbow pain), knee pain from persistent ligament/tendon strain, and occipital headaches.

With prolotherapy most patients achieve over 50% improvement in particular areas. Usually a series of proliferate injections are required, anywhere from two to six, but one can usually tell after the first injection if it is going to help.

The first part of my therapy program focuses on pain management. The patient works with me and other team members (therapists, primary care specialists, chiropractor, counselor, and other medical professionals) to decrease the acute pain as much as possible using different therapy or injection strategies. Hopefully, the pain stays settled down. If it does, the patient is ready to begin a progressive exercise program.

Exercise: Reactivation and Retraining

I shift the emphasis from pain management to reactivation and retraining. Now I want patients to increase their physical activity and fitness levels and develop a successful home program. This phase is usually started around the third week of treatment. Pain management modalities are winding down, and there is a progressive increase in stretching and range of motion exercises. Manual therapy/massotherapy is often continued. Pain management therapies may be renewed as needed, and the patient may continue to work with various team members.

I emphasize postural exercises (see Fibronomics, Chapter 20), stretching and flexibility exercises of all major muscle groups, and focus on a warm-up period that consists of stretching only. For some people, stretching may be the only exercise that they can do.

I also try to develop what I call a "light conditioning" program. Such a program can include walking, water aerobics, using an exercise bicycle, or performing low-impact aerobic exercises. This exercise program is introduced and gradually progressed as tolerated with the goal of achieving a stable baseline and developing a successful home program. I instruct patients to do a regular exercise program at least three times a week. I emphasize proper posture and body mechanics

It's better to have fit painful muscles than deconditioned painful muscles. In other words, you can improve your function even if the pain doesn't decrease.

to minimize strain on the muscles and joints. I always tell patients that it's better to have fit painful muscles than deconditioned painful muscles. In other words, you can improve your function even if the pain doesn't decrease.

I frequently prescribe water exercises. Aquatic exercises are beneficial even for someone who cannot swim. In water, most of the body weight is buoyed, so the gravity stress on the muscles and joints is reduced. The water needs to be kept at a comfortable temperature, usually around 90° F. Range of motion, flexibility, strengthening, and aerobic exercises can all be done in the pool, and can initially be supervised by a trained professional until individuals feel comfortable with following through on their own.

Sometimes the progressive stretching and exercise increases pain, even if the acute pain has subsided from the initial therapy program. Manual therapy/massage usually helps, but if this is not controlling the pain, additional pain management techniques can be reintroduced (heat, cold, injections). Ultimately, becoming knowledgeable about fibromyalgia and learning what works for you will allow you to find a regular program of proper body mechanics, stretching, and exercises that helps.

Home Program: Reintegration

In this phase, the patient is reintegrating into the "real world," armed with knowledge and self-management strategies. Patients use these techniques and life-style changes to live their everyday lives, work their jobs, and be themselves in spite of fibromyalgia. Patients will continue their program of medications, nutritional supplements, stretches and exercises, and hopefully will be able to maintain a stable baseline. I do not automatically follow up with people at this stage unless there is a new problem or a flare-up, but my patients know they are welcome to call me or see me at any time. If there is a new problem or a flare-up, we review together the need for any new treatments or changes in their program.

Regular prescribed treatments may be required. For example, a patient may continue with periodic manual therapies or massage therapies, or have periodic trigger point injections in addition to continuing prescribed or nutritional medicine. The ideal goal, however, is to have the patient be able to control her or his symptoms through a self-responsible and independent home program. The medical professionals are available if needed, and hopefully they will not be needed on a frequent basis.

As part of the home program, the patient may join a support group. I offer a fibromyalgia course that can be taken at any phase of treatment, and encompasses the overall understanding and management of fibromyalgia. Chris Marschinke, R.N. who co-developed the course with me, teaches the course in my office. The course consists of six weekly sessions, 2 ½ hours each week. It includes workbooks, lecture slides, and handouts. A different topic is covered each week and the last week includes a question and answer session with me, and a class graduation ceremony!

This comprehensive Physical Medicine and Rehabilitation approach in the treatment of fibromyalgia can help individuals achieve a realistic stable baseline. A stable baseline is not the same as no pain, rather it is a level where, while there may still be pain, it is not preventing the patient from performing desired activities. The baseline level is different for everyone, but each person can eventually learn what her or his baseline state will be. Actually, we all must learn this; our fibromyalgia doesn't give us much of a choice! At a stable baseline, the spontaneous pain is decreased. We still have painful tender points if poked at, but we can usually get through the day without getting poked!

What Kind of Results Do I Get?

I do not cure people of their fibromyalgia. Everyone who sees me does not get better. Sometimes people feel worse after they see me! But I try. A lot of factors are involved in determining how people do, including insurance issues, compliance issues, and severity of the fibromyalgia.

There are four categories of fibromyalgia patients that I see in my private office setting. They are:

1) The newly diagnosed fibromyalgia patient with no previous treatment (about 25% of my total fibromyalgia patients).

2) The previously diagnosed fibromyalgia patient who is referred for additional recommendations or follow-up of initial treatment approaches (about 25% of my total fibromyalgia patients).

3) The fibromyalgia patient who is experiencing a flare-up (about 40% of my total fibromyalgia patients).

4) The chronic fibromyalgia patient whose symptoms have been resistant to multiple treatment approaches (about 10% of my total fibromyalgia patients).

Results I Get for Each Category

I monitor the outcomes of treatment programs for my fibromyalgia patients. Certainly reduced pain is a major goal but sometimes a person can report improvement even if the pain remains the same. That person may be able to be more functional in spite of the pain, or is able to do more activities without increasing the pain. A key way that I monitor outcome is by using a pain outcome chart to determine a patient's pain level over time with treatment.

I reviewed 300 charts of patients treated for fibromyalgia in the first four months of 1999. By monitoring the patient's reported pain level over treatment, the following outcome results were noted:

1) In the newly diagnosed fibromyalgia patient (106 patients), 85% achieved 50% or more reduction of their pain level over an average of 10 therapy treatments; 15% achieved less than 50% (and of those, 5% reported less than a 10% reduction of their pain).

2) In the previously diagnosed fibromyalgia patient who was referred for additional treatment (73 patients), 80% achieved a 50% reduction or more of their pain level. Twenty percent achieved a pain reduction of less than 50%.

3) In the fibromyalgia patient experiencing a flare-up requiring treatment (109 patients), 85% returned to their previous stable baseline, and 15% improved but were still higher than their previous stable baseline.

4) In the chronic fibromyalgia patient who has been resistant to multiple previous treatments and who tried a treatment approach under my direction (12 patients), 20% achieved a 50% or greater reduction of their pain level; 80% achieved less than 50% pain reduction (and of those, 15% reported no change at all in their pain level). Newly diagnosed patients seem to get better results whereas those with chronic "resistant" fibromyalgia respond less favorably.

These results are general guidelines based on an average of 10 treatments. Each patient's treatments are individualized. Some patients may require additional therapies and get additional improvement. Other patients may flare-up shortly after their treatment program and experience a rise in their pain level again. I certainly want everyone to improve, but not everyone does. The goal is to try to help as many people as much as possible.

Here are some examples of patients' pain outcomes as indicated on the pain outcome chart in the following diagram. Each pain outcome chart demonstrates a different example of a treatment response in fibromyalgia patients. The patient names are fictitious, but the pain outcome charts are derived from real patients. On the chart, the "●'s" represents pain level before treatment and "✖'s" represent pain level immediately after treatment. The treatment sessions occur over time and, in general, ten treatments represent approximately a one-month time period.

Diagram 1: Improvement. Sally's pain outcome chart demonstrates an improvement in the overall pain. This is the most common type of pain outcome and shows a consistent response to the treatments and lowering of the pain scores. In this particular example, the pain decreased from 10 out of 10 to 3 out of 10, a 70% improvement.

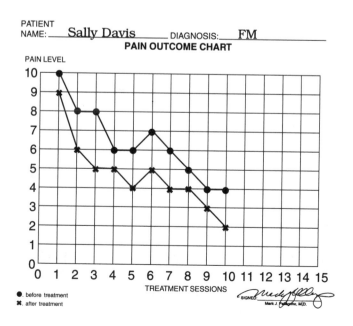

Diagram 2: Resistant Fibromyalgia. Sue's pain outcome chart shows very little response to treatment and a persistent high level of pain that stays around a 10. This is very little improvement in the pain immediately after the treatment.

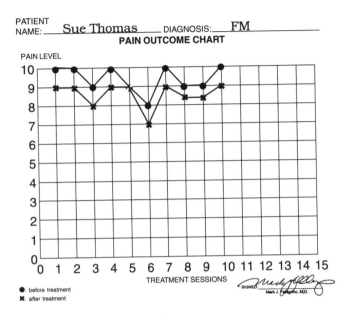

Diagram 3: Unstable Fibromyalgia. Mary's pain outcome chart indicates the pain levels bouncing up and down and variable responses to treatments. This pattern is actually *no pattern* and characterizes unstable fibromyalgia.

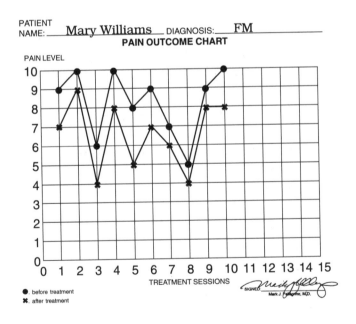

Diagram 4: Flare-up. Jane's pain outcome chart shows an initial good response to therapy with improvement of the pain scores. However, between the fifth and sixth treatments, there is a sharp increase in pain which causes a peak to occur on the graph. In Jane's case, she planted a garden which caused her flare-up. In spite of the flare-up, she continued to improve over time with additional treatments, and in the end her pain decreased from 10 out of 10 during her flare-up to 3 out of 10.

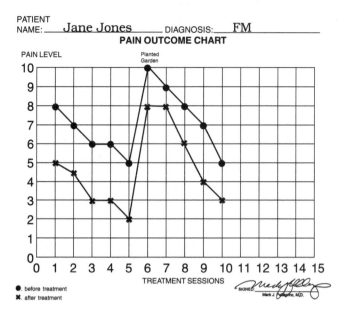

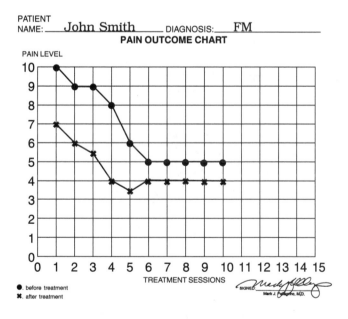

Diagram 5: Stable Baseline. This chart shows that John's pain improved, but around the fifth treatment his improvement stabilized and plateaued, and he remained at a stable baseline even with a few additional treatments. Overall, his pain improved from a 10 to a 4, a 60% improvement.

The fibromyalgia patient is a unique individual who has specific problems and needs. There is no generic patient. The physician should approach each patient on an individual basis using the types of strategies I described above. Each patient requires an individualized program, and hopefully everyone will get some improvement.

Summary

As complicated as fibromyalgia treatments can be, I still adhere to the philosophy of trying to keep treatments as simple as possible. If medicines aren't helping, they need to be stopped. If they help, use the lowest effective dose. If certain therapies help, teach the patient how to do them on her/his own. Sometimes the best treatment is simply trying to point the patient in the right direction, and watching the patient take control of the fibromyalgia!

Chapter 17 — Survival Strategies

1) Consider being treated by a Physical Medicine and Rehabilitation doctor.

2) Experiment with modalities such as heat, cold, massage.

3) Consider some type of massage therapy.

4) Remember that any new treatment may cause a "temporary" increase in pain.

5) Increase any exercise or treatment gradually.

6) Work with therapists who are knowledgable and enjoy working with fibros.

7) Don't give up!

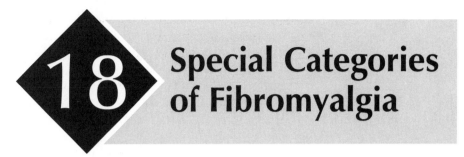

18 Special Categories of Fibromyalgia

Some categories of people with fibromyalgia have special features that are different from the traditional fibromyalgia patient. Different evaluation and treatment strategies may be necessary for these special categories.

1) Children with fibromyalgia

2) Men with fibromyalgia

3) Resistant fibromyalgia

4) Chronic pain syndrome associated with fibromyalgia

Children with Fibromyalgia

I see a number of children in my practice who have fibromyalgia. The youngest I have seen was a boy aged three.

A child who has a parent or sibling with fibromyalgia or connective tissue disease is at risk. If this child at risk is involved in a competitive sport that stresses the muscles — tennis, dancing, gymnastics — risk is increased. Children can get post-traumatic fibromyalgia, especially those who have a hereditary vulnerability. A number of young female patients in my practice have been involved with dancing, gymnastics, or baton twirling for many years. Hours of practice and competition have been involved. Symptoms of pain appear and ultimately fibromyalgia develops.

Other risk factors in children include the presence of scoliosis (curvature of the spine) or forward posturing (rounded shoulders). Postural changes cause more strain on the back muscles which, over time, can lead to traumatic changes that trigger fibromyalgia. Girls are more likely to have scoliosis than boys (genetic risk). I see many youngsters who have intermittent back strains related to postural changes, and some have gone on to develop "full blown" fibromyalgia. There is no way to predict who will develop clinical fibromyalgia in those who are at risk, especially in those who are completely symptom free.

In children, girls still outnumber boys, but the gap is smaller, about 60% girls and 40% boys in a survey of children with fibromyalgia in my practice. This is consistent with the research reported by Dr. Buskila. Causes of fibromyalgia in children are similar to the causes in adults: genetics, trauma (either a major trauma such as a fall or car accident or cumulative type trauma as with certain competitive sports), infections such as mononucleosis or other viral infections, or secondary to another condition. Primary fibromyalgia is more common.

In children, there may be generalized widespread pain, but usually there are some common initial symptoms, or ones that may be part of the prodromal state that can ultimately turn into fibromyalgia. These symptoms include:

1) Leg pains (may be called growing pains): This appears to be a form of restless leg syndrome in children.

> The main treatment may simply be a matter of reassuring the child and parent that there is no serious medical condition, but rather there is some evidence of fibromyalgia which can be handled with education, and tailoring an activity program to include stretches and specific exercises, nutritional approaches, and long-term monitoring.

2) Fatigue. Episodic bouts with extreme fatigue may occur.

3) Sleep problems. Both falling asleep and frequent awakening may occur.

4) Headaches. Frequent migraine headaches or tension headaches may occur with neck and shoulder pain or in the absence of any other pain. Allergies and dry eyes may be present and contributing to the headaches.

5) Abdominal pain. Frequent stomachaches and stomach pain, possibly accompanied by nausea. This may be early irritable bowel syndrome.

6) Cognitive difficulties. This can include difficulty with concentration and attention in school, difficulty focusing on a topic, difficulty with reading and reading comprehension, and complaints about vision. Often, school teachers will notice these difficulties first and mention them to the parents.

Certain aggravating factors may cause fibromyalgia to flare up in kids. I find that many kids will experience increased pain or more widespread pain during growth spurts. Perhaps fibromyalgia is thrown out of balance, so to speak, as growth is occurring more rapidly than the fibromyalgia can adjust, hence the increased pain. Girls may notice increased pain when their menstrual cycles start, and they have exaggerated premenstrual symptoms from the very beginning. Children are not free from stresses, whether it be at school or at home, particularly if there is marital discord among the parents. All of these factors can contribute to flare-ups of fibromyalgia in children.

Many times when I see these children with various symptoms or associated conditions, I find they have numerous painful tender points and ropey muscles with localized spasms. The diagnosis of fibromyalgia may be made.

Minimal Invasiveness

I will approach children with fibromyalgia a little differently than adults. I want to make sure there is no underlying problem other than fibromyalgia that could be causing symptoms. Usually I will obtain some lab work including blood counts, sedimentation rate, and possibly thyroid studies. If cognitive difficulties are a problem, I will consider neuropsychological testing to specifically test memory, auditory comprehension, reading comprehension, and other integrative skills of the brain.

My treatment philosophy with kids is mainly "let kids be kids." Children are active, they tend to sleep more, they can be moody. Sometimes parents' concerns are based more on the parents' experience with fibromyalgia and fear that the child may be going through the same thing. I address these concerns and try to offer encouragement. I believe that minimal invasiveness is required. The main treatment may simply be a matter of reassuring the child and parent that there is no serious medical condition, but rather there is some evidence of fibromyalgia which can be handled with education, and tailoring an activity program to include stretches and specific exercises, nutritional approaches, and long-term monitoring.

If there is a functional impairment as a result of fibromyalgia, if the child is missing school or important school activities, or unable to participate in sports because of pain and fatigue, I will treat more aggressively. Treatments could include specific, prescribed medicines such as Klonopin, nortriptyline, or a mild pain medication. I may prescribe a therapy program to try to find out what works and to develop a successful home program.

School modifications such as the following may be necessary on a temporary or ongoing basis.

1) Rescheduling student classes so the student may be able to arrive later and leave earlier and have a study hall/rest time in the middle of the day.

2) Physical adaptation such as using a back pack or luggage cart, avoiding steps and using the elevator, having another locker on another floor to decrease the need to carry a lot of books at any given time.

3) Excuse from school gym for the time being.

Sometimes it is necessary to temporarily remove the child from school and use a home tutor. If the process of getting to and from school is extremely difficult because of pain and fatigue, this may be a reluctant but necessary option.

I review the physical risks with each individual. If we determine that a certain athletic activity or a competition is the culprit in causing and aggravating fibromyalgia, I advise the child athlete on ways to modify or avoid the offending activities altogether. Several of my female patients were interested in a dancing major in college, but they developed fibromyalgia along the way that was made worse by repetitive dancing. I advised them on changing their major to one that is more realistic and did not involve activities that aggravate the fibromyalgia. Dancing could still be pursued as recreation, but fibromyalgia would probably not allow it as a career.

If gymnastics, tennis, or any other competitive sport activity appears to be a major factor in the cause of fibromyalgia and of flare-ups, I will tell the young athlete to think about a different competitive sport. First, they will back off on the activity, get the fibromyalgia under the best control possible, and then see what happens when the activity is resumed. If the fibromyalgia flares up quickly, it is a good indicator that the continued activity will not be tolerated well. We need to look at this honestly and realistically.

I find that kids are more resilient and adaptable to change than adults. Their youth gives them a better chance at controlling the fibromyalgia and maintaining a stable baseline or remission. I remind the parents not to project their fears onto their child, because each child is unique and the fibromyalgia has a unique identity as well. Even if the mother is having a difficult time with her fibromyalgia, the child can reach a stage where his/her fibromyalgia is hardly a bother. Most of the children I've seen have done better over time, and I am hopeful that they will continue to do well.

Men with Fibromyalgia

Men get fibromyalgia, too. In adults, women outnumber men by at least six to one, but if 5% of the population has fibromyalgia, nearly 15% of those are men. Men seem to comprise a large number of the "undiagnosed fibromyalgia" category. If we go out and look for fibromyalgia, we will find it in men who have never gone to the doctor. In people younger than 18, the ratio of girls to boys is three to two, so young men commonly get it, too.

Men have some "unique" characteristics with their fibromyalgia.

1) The two main risk factors are heredity and trauma. When comparing the population of men and women with post-traumatic fibromyalgia, men account for about 30% of this group, so the ratio of women to men is seven to three. Men with a parent or parents with fibromyalgia are more at risk.

2) Men are less likely to seek medical attention for pain problems. Men who finally present to the doctor and are diagnosed with fibromyalgia usually have a more severe form. Women are more likely to seek medical attention sooner, and thus are more likely to be diagnosed earlier with milder stages of fibromyalgia than men.

There is nothing unique on the men's exam for fibromyalgia when compared to women; they have painful tender points, localized spasms and trigger points,. Their tests give the same results (except their estrogen levels are much lower!). They can benefit from the available treatments; I don't find any unique medications or treatments that work better for men than women.

Men have specific issues and concerns regarding their fibromyalgia that are similar to those of women. Some of these issues include:

1) **Self-image.** Often, it is difficult for a man to see a doctor to discuss chronic pain. Many men have the stereotypic notion that they should be able to handle pain and should not complain. The mere fact that they have reached a point where they have to see a doctor can be perceived as both a failure on their part and an indication of just how severe the pain has become.

2) **Job and Financial Issues.** Men who have difficulty performing their jobs because of pain may experience a lot of fear and anxiety about whether they will be able to continue their livelihoods. Men take a lot of pride in their abilities to use their bodies to perform jobs in skillful manners, bring in income, and pay the bills. The thought of losing this, or the actual loss, can be very difficult for men.

3) **Disability.** Men often need to pursue disability because their fibromyalgia prevents them from working. It is usually not possible or practical to simply find another job. Many job skills require physical abilities, and if fibromyalgia interferes, job skills cannot be performed. This creates a paradox where a man can no longer be proud of his abilities, but rather, is forced to highlight his inabilities and failures.

4) Interpersonal and Intimacy Problems. Many men report erectile dysfunction or loss of libido because of pain and emotional issues that accompany a chronic pain disorder. Interpersonal relationships may be strained. Many men admit that pain causes a lot of frustrations that may be physically expressed — anger, yelling, irritability, throwing things, and feeling like they are ready to beat up someone at the slightest provocation.

These specific male issues need to be addressed as part of the overall fibromyalgia treatment. It can be challenging for men to get out of the disabled or victim mode once they have entered it. I try to use encouragement and to teach mental management strategies. Additional professional counseling may be needed. Education is crucial, and involving the spouse or significant other in a supportive role can help keep a man's goals and initiatives in focus. Life-style and vocational changes are part of coping with the fibromyalgia.

David Squires of *To Your Health* in Arizona is a great example of a man who has overcome severe fibromyalgia to reshape his life and accomplish successful life-style changes. Even with his condition, he has a positive approach to life and work. He runs his own business and devotes many hours to helping others with fibromyalgia. David has been active in support groups and is particularly interested in getting men with fibromyalgia to seek help and support.

Affected men represent the "silent minority" in fibromyalgia. They often suffer silently, though. Men should feel comfortable expressing their pain and concerns and, ultimately, learn to cope better with fibromyalgia.

I have the pleasure of knowing David and working with him at two support group workshops FOR MEN ONLY! It is apparent from these workshops that men have unique issues and concerns in dealing with fibromyalgia, and that many have a difficult time. Since men are the minority, it is difficult for them to gather in numbers for a support group. Usually the men at fibromyalgia support groups are spouses of a woman with fibromyalgia. No one is present who can truly connect with the severe daily pain from a man's perspective. Also, support group facilitators are usually women, and men can feel uncomfortable being surrounded by women, although they certainly can benefit from support groups even if all the other members are female.

Affected men represent the "silent minority" in fibromyalgia. As a male professional with fibromyalgia, I can relate to the men and appreciate that men hurt and have their lives disrupted. They often suffer silently, though. Our challenge is to reach out to this segment and help them connect. Men should feel comfortable expressing their pain and concerns and, ultimately, learn to cope better with fibromyalgia.

Resistant Fibromyalgia

This category represents those with fibromyalgia who do not respond to any treatment or get worse. They may have had brief responses to treatment, but nothing has made a long-term difference. The baseline pain remains very high and flares up frequently. There are various reasons why pain levels stay high and flare up easily.

Trauma. A new trauma may be superimposed on a previously stable fibromyalgia. This new trauma can cause permanent escalation of the baseline level of pain and involve new areas not previously painful. New traumas can occur with a single event such as a work injury or a car accident, or it may result from cumulative trauma such as repetitive activity from a job.

Worsening Due To Another Condition. Worsening can also be related to another condition that is progressive such as arthritis or neurologic diseases. Anyone who has fibromyalgia secondary to another condition (subset 8) or existing with another condition (subset 7) can be at the mercy of the other condition. If the other condition progresses over time, the fibromyalgia can worsen as well. Fibromyalgia is notorious for being easily aggravated with only mild increases of disease activity of another condition.

Fibromyalgia "Mutates." Like a virus, fibromyalgia can "mutate" to resist treatment, particularly in unstable fibromyalgia. There may have been a window of improvement with a particular treatment, but the fibromyalgia always finds a way to break through and cause increased pain. Needless to say, this is very frustrating and people become discouraged. I have several patients who felt so great with a particular product that they began selling the product (nutritional supplements, magnets). But, the improvements did not last. Over time, the fibromyalgia pain gradually took a renewed hold on them, and they had a hard time running their businesses, causing further pain.

As a physician, it is difficult to address the issue of resistant fibromyalgia, and it needs to be handled with compassion and hope. I try to emphasize that their pain is not their fault or caused by something they are doing wrong.

It is hard enough for the patients to accept fibromyalgia, but they have to try to accept a persistently higher level of pain that is resistant to treatment. There are no easy answers. Sometimes I have to say, "I don't know" when asked what the future will hold. I emphasize the importance of continuing with a regular program in spite of pain. We try different things, and if new treatment strategies are reported or discovered, we are open-minded in trying these.

I rotate treatments. Sometimes an initial treatment works and then stops working. Then we will try another treatment that may work and rotate back to the first treatment at a later time. The more therapeutic options that are available, the more opportunities to find successful programs that can be rotated.

Individual job situations need to be addressed. Preserving the job or some modified version of it is a high priority, but at times the person with fibromyalgia is disabled. My goal is to keep the person active and gainfully employed for the longest time possible.

Chronic Pain Syndrome Associated with Fibromyalgia

Some individuals develop a condition known as chronic pain syndrome. This is defined as a state of overwhelming chronic pain that interferes with the person's physical, emotional, and psychological functional abilities and causes depression in everyday life's activity. This condition is more overwhelming than fibromyalgia alone. Drs. Keefe and Block (1982) described characteristics of a person with chronic pain syndrome. They include:

Significant subjective and functional limitations out of proportion to the objective physical exam findings. TRANSLATION: Patients will report they are unable to do certain activities, but the doctor would expect they could do these activities based on the physical exam. For example, patients may say they cannot put on shoes even though they demonstrate the abilities to bend their back and move their arms in a manner required for that activity.

Dependency and addictive behaviors. This includes the use of excessive narcotic or opioid medications, increased alcohol or nicotine consumption, and an increased dependency on others to assist them in everyday activities.

Well-defined pain behaviors. Examples of pain behaviors include slow, deliberate movements, walking with an inconsistent limp, exaggerated flinching upon palpation, frequent facial grimacing and sighing, and frequent indications of "I can't" when asked to perform a certain movement or physical task.

Most people who have severe pain from fibromyalgia do not develop chronic pain syndrome. However, it does commonly develop from fibromyalgia. In my experience, about 2% of people with fibromyalgia develop chronic pain syndrome. These patients will give a history of terrible pain which continues to get worse, although everything has been tried. The patient may report that he or she spends most of the day in bed, and often complains of feeling depressed, frustrated, and anxious, and describes himself/herself as disabled. Typically, the physical examination is difficult because of pain behaviors. There is difficulty examining the muscles, because light palpation results in significant pain responses. Neurologic testing, particularly muscle strength testing and muscle sensory testing, may be impossible because the patient is not able to cooperate reliably.

The Person Has True Pain. The person with chronic pain syndrome has true pain. A psychological reaction to the pain has occurred, however, resulting in the syndrome described above. In this situation, both fibromyalgia and chronic pain syndrome are present even though it is usually difficult to isolate specific painful tender points because the patient complains of diffuse pain wherever touched.

Treatment of chronic pain syndrome, in my experience, is very difficult. It's hard to achieve consistent high success rates with treatments. This difficulty stems from the fact that in chronic pain syndrome, fibromyalgia is no longer the main condition causing symptoms. Rather, the chronic pain and pain behaviors become the primary conditions. Chronic pain syndrome is a separate disease entity that requires its own separate treatment. It is a very complex condition and the patient is actually more resistant to treatment.

A comprehensive multidisciplinary approach with knowledgeable personnel is once again necessary. The evaluation process includes core personnel of the chronic pain management team, that is, physician, psychologist, physical therapist, occupational therapist, social service counselor, rehabilitation nurse, vocational counselor, pharmacist, and dietician. The treatment emphasizes modifying and reducing medications, behavior management of pain by modifying pain behaviors and how pain interferes with one's life, addressing psychosocial and vocational issues, and increasing physical activity and vocational abilities. This type of intensive multidisciplinary evaluation and treatment with emphasis on behavior modification is probably the best.

When the Pain Doesn't Settle Down

Unfortunately there are a number of patients who have had multiple treatments but continue to be bothered by significant pain. The pain is disabling for them, and they are not able to carry out their daily activities or job functions. They have fluctuations of pain above and below their baseline, or have frequent flare-ups, but at their baseline level, they continue to have severe disabling pain.

What causes one's pain level to be worse? There may be ongoing trauma or stresses that worsens the fibromyalgia or another condition such as a progressive arthritis. The individual may be resistant to treatment because of well-ingrained disability and pain behaviors. The person expects to hurt and not get better. The patient may remember what it was like to have less pain, and this "remembered standard" is what is expected of successful treatment. If this standard is not reached, the perception is that the treatment is failing. There may be increased anger, frustration, anxiety, and depression contributing to the increased pain. Sometimes the person is just unlucky and has a more severe, resistant form of fibromyalgia. Even in patients who have not been compliant with the recommended treatment program, I do not confront them, but give them their options and respect the choices and decisions they wish to make regarding their fibromyalgia.

I'll also review any additional treatment considerations for the patient whose severe pain has not settled down. New medicines or medicine combinations, chronic pain and stress management programs, other medical professionals, supportive counseling, reassurance, or addressing work or disability issues are various treatment considerations. At times, people with fibromyalgia become disabled. In surveys, people with fibromyalgia rank their condition as more disabling than individuals with rheumatoid arthritis, heart disease, lung disease, and other chronic disorders.

Pursuing disability should be a last resort, in my opinion, and should be a decision mutually arrived at by patient and doctor. My experience is that fewer than 5% of fibromylagia patients receive a permanent disability award. Patients do not want to become disabled from fibromyalgia or any condition. They all want to be better. If everything has been tried and the

I rotate treatments. Sometimes an initial treatment works and then stops working. Then we will try another treatment that may work and rotate back to the first treatment at a later time. The more therapeutic options that are available, the more opportunities to find successful programs that can be rotated.

patients are still doing poorly and not functioning well, the disability route may need to be considered. I will write a disability report, but that is not a guarantee that disability will be awarded. The ultimate decision rests with "organizations" who review the applications and determine if the "criteria" are met. Sometimes it seems as if the "criteria" are as complicated as fibromyalgia itself!

Long-term follow-up studies on patients with fibromyalgia who have been rendered disabled or awarded a legal settlement have shown that the majority of them continue to be bothered by fibromyalgia and seek medical treatment for this condition. There is no question that the debilitating effect of fibromyalgia persists even if the jobs are stopped, stresses are relieved, life-style are altered, or disability is awarded.

However, I find that the majority of people with fibromyalgia do not reach the severe disabling stage, and I believe we can further decrease the number of those who do by aggressively identifying and treating fibromyalgia as early as possible.

Chapter 18 — Survival Strategies

1) Recognize that there are numerous treatments for fibromyalgia. Different approaches and styles can be successful. There is no "right" way to universally treat fibromyalgia.

2) Set goals in your treatment plan. The first should be to start tolerating a "gradual" increase in activity, then progress to the increasing of your activity and fitness levels. Begin developing a successful home program. Conclude with the ability to control symptoms through a self-responsible and independent home program with the goal of achieving a realistic stable baseline level.

3) Realize that a percentage of patients cannot get a stable baseline level and become disabled. This is a small percentage. Use all of your energies to overcome the situation by aggressively identifying and seeking treatment as early as possible.

Special Categories of Fibromyalgia   Inside Fibromyalgia with Mark J. Pellegrino, M.D.

150

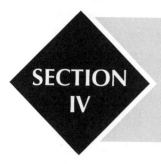

SECTION IV

SELF-DIRECTED STRATEGIES FOR MANAGING FIBROMYALGIA

This section emphasizes what you can do (need to do!) to manage your fibromyalgia. The last section reviewed prescribed treatments or doctor-recommended strategies. We medical people want to help point you in the right direction, but you have to work hard yourself to keep fibromyalgia under control. This section focuses on patient directed strategies.

Some information in this section is a "revisit" of previous discussions, except now I want you to appreciate how important you, the patient, are in directing your own care and managing your fibromyalgia, your way!

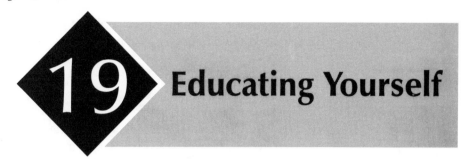

19 ▸ Educating Yourself

You need to take an active role in becoming an informed fibromyalgia patient. The more you understand your diagnosis, the more qualified you become, and the easier it is for you to make a decision regarding your condition. You can also learn what specific questions to ask your healthcare professionals.

Information therapy is a term for supplying patients with health information, enabling them to make informed decisions about their health and care, participate in their own well-being, and thus decrease the use of healthcare resources (Donna J. Mitchell, 1994). By increasing your knowledge, you will increase your confidence in your abilities to responsibly manage fibromyalgia.

It is hard for today's physicians to keep up with all of the medical literature. We read current journals, make information requests to libraries for articles, read books, take advantage of online technology, and more, all in our spare time! Physicians also learn from you, the patients. You ask us questions that we may not know the answers to, so we find the answers for you. You bring us articles and current information, and we review them and learn additional strategies.

I have a special inside informant with fibromyalgia who helps me gather information, Ann Evans. Ann works in a library and is an information expert. In addition to being knowledgeable in gathering information from all sources, she prepares a detailed information handout on fibromyalgia resources available in my area.

So I asked Ann, "How do you educate yourself about fibromyalgia?" She said the simplest answer to that question is, "Start by asking questions." (Isn't she smart!?) "The best places to start would be libraries, the Internet, and support groups." Let's review these places.

Libraries

Libraries are a great resource for people with fibromyalgia. Personally, I think I've spent a third of my life at various libraries at The Ohio State University. There are many types of libraries that have a wealth of information via books, magazine articles, videos, and computer technology. Types of libraries include public libraries, academic libraries, medical libraries/health sciences libraries, hospital libraries, or patient/consumer health libraries. Find a library that can accommodate your specific needs, that include a physically accessible building, well-trained staff, technology assistance, and guidance to specialized resources.

Ask for help! Try to find library workers who have a special interest in medical research. These people are good contacts for fibromyalgia networking. If you want a specific article or book, try to have the most complete information possible regarding the title, author, journal name, publishing company, date of publication, etc. The library worker can help you search databases using key words.

Remember to write down the information while you are reviewing the material. Don't trust yourself to remember this a month later. Keep your information organized so you can easily track down the necessary information when you need it. Library research can be confusing and overwhelming, but research will be easier once you understand the system. Remember, learning is supposed to be fun.

Remember to write down the information while you are reviewing the material. Don't trust yourself to remember this a month later (or even an hour later! Or in my case...what were we talking about?). Keep your information organized so you can easily track down the necessary information when you need it. Library research can be confusing and overwhelming, but research will be easier once you understand the system and identify a knowledgeable library worker. Remember, learning is supposed to be fun.

And also remember, libraries are big, so don't get lost. Wear bright clothing so it can easily be spotted by the night cleaning crew!

Internet

Internet resources on fibromyalgia provide an endless opportunity. Information on fibromyalgia as well as discussion groups are available, so the Internet can be both educational and supportive. Numerous websites are available for information both from medical university centers and from patient support and consumer standpoints.

The Medline is an example of an Internet site that provides accurate, up-to-date medical research information. Most articles referenced in Medline are written by and for health professionals, but they can prove extremely helpful for consumers. Medline searches can be done by subject, author, journal title, and text word, and there are citations from nearly 4,000 biomedical journals from around the globe.

To access the Medline, at no cost, 24 hours a day, 7 days a week, all that is required is a computer with Internet access. First, users should go to the National Library of Medicine home page (www.nlm.nih.gov) and click on the "Free Medline." The resulting screens will guide you to citations of articles from medical journals. Library staff who are trained to use the Internet can assist you in finding information on healthcare issues. You can know what your doctors know!

Support Group

Attending a support group is not just for emotional support, but also for information exchange. Special types of support groups/fibromyalgia courses are available that provide a formal presentation of fibromyalgia information by a trained medical professional combined with support opportunities.

Support groups are a great place to share the information. I have made my office facilities available for regular support group meetings, and we have a big bulletin board with fibromyalgia information about seminars, books, articles, and other pertinent information posted and available for regular review by interested people with fibromyalgia.

There are various Internet fibromyalgia support groups, so you don't ever have to leave your house. This may be a good option for patients with limited outdoor mobility or who may be more comfortable remaining "anonymous."

Beware of Misinformation

Not all information is medically accurate or helpful, especially Internet information. You need to be careful how you use it. Let's face it, as a group, we are more vulnerable to misinformation. Because of our severe, chronic pain, we may be more desperate for help, feel overwhelmed, have difficulty concentrating and processing information, may be more emotional and easily influenced, and be more easily convinced to try new products. Unfortunately, there are companies out there waiting to take advantage of us. They try to entice us with products that they claim will help us; help us spend our money, that is!

Here are 13 things to watch for to avoid being unlucky.

1) **It sounds too good to be true**. Like the old adage in investments, if it sounds too good to be true, it probably is. Trust your fibromyalgia knowledge, and don't let your hope override good common sense.

2) **It will cure fibromyalgia**. There is no cure for fibromyalgia at this time. There are a lot of treatments for fibromyalgia, but if the proposed treatment uses the word "cure," stay away from it.

3) **The product involves multilevel marketing**. The main reason to avoid these is that they are expensive. You have to pay five other people's profits when you purchase your product.

4) **The product involves a secret technique or formula**. If the promoter fails to disclose specific information about the product or how it works, stay away from it. I know a massotherapist who promoted a unique technique that gave great results but would not disclose the technique; you have to pay $2,000 to join this "special program." It turns out that the techniques used are commonly used by massotherapists.

To access the Medline, at no cost, 24 hours a day, 7 days a week, all that is required is a computer with Internet access. First, users should go to the National Library of Medicine home page (www.nlm.nih.gov) and click on the "Free Medline." The resulting screens will guide you to citations of articles from medical journals.

5) **The product is supported by personal testimonies only.** Consider this typical story for a product:

Poor Michael used to be so active, but then he developed fibromyalgia and couldn't even get out of bed. Then one day, he discovered *Fibro-Be-Gone* and began taking it. Within one week, his fibromyalgia symptoms were all gone. Now he is running three miles a day, skiing on weekends, and working full-time as the owner of a company that sells Fibro-Be-Gone.

This type of sensational advertising based on personal testimony is designed only to sell you a product. Maybe a particular product worked for a particular person, but everyone is a unique individual who responds differently to treatments.

6) **Questionable medical qualifications**. Many times, the supposed "medical professional" has no actual medical credentials. On the Internet, anyone can be a medical professional. Individuals can mislead you by putting M.D. after their name. There is no law that prohibits someone from putting initials, including M.D., D.O., or D.C., after their name. The M.D. can mean macarena dancer.

> Because of our severe, chronic pain, we may be more desperate for help, feel overwhelmed, have difficulty concentrating and processing information, may be more emotional and easily influenced, and be more easily convinced to try new products. Unfortunately, there are companies out there waiting to take advantage of us. They try to entice us with products that they claim will help us; help us spend our money, that is!

To avoid becoming a victim of fraud or misrepresentation, ask about credentials and do research. If the person says he or she is a medical doctor but won't disclose what medical school was attended or give any specific information about medical training, then this person is probably a fraud.

7) **Medical recommendations are made by non-medical professionals**. Unfortunately, many non-physicians try to make medical diagnoses and medical treatment recommendations to people with medical conditions such as fibromyalgia. This is illegal. If the person giving the advice is misrepresenting himself/herself as a licensed physician, this is fraud. The privilege of making medical diagnoses and treatment recommendations should be reserved for those who dedicated many years of their life to obtain medical knowledge and training and who maintain current medical license. If you follow fraudulent medical advice, you could be injured. According to the American Medical Association and the Federal Trade Commission, there is little investigation or enforcement of Internet fraud regarding falsely impersonating a medical doctor or giving medical advice without a medical license. Check qualifications before you deem a source credible, no matter how good this person sounds. Call the AMA, the State Medical Board, or the local medical society office if you have a question about a doctor's qualifications.

8) **The promoter has a vested financial interest in the product**. I recently received a flyer in the mail that said, "A very special workshop is about to take place in your area." The flyer then described a doctor who was experiencing great results with fibromyalgia patients using a new product. It reported, "In just 11 weeks, he has increased his monthly revenue by $4,000, and is enjoying his practice like never before."

The promoter of this product was trying to entice me to pay for the workshop, become a distributor, and try to encourage my patients to use this product. The promoters benefit financially from this arrangement, thus they have a vested financial interest. How can you trust the promoters of this product to be unbiased when giving you information about the products?

9) **The promoter of the product has a painful condition — fibromyalgia.** Beware of the person who knows exactly how you feel because he/she has the condition, and has just the product for you to get rid of the condition.

10) **High pressure marketing system.** What better way to get our money than to use fancy sales pitches, brightly colored literature, catchy slogans, and so forth and so on. If you feel that you are being presented with a heavy marketing pitch, you are. Don't buy things because you feel pressured into doing so.

11) **A video tape or audio cassette tape comes with the marketing kit.** I've learned to stay away from products that have any type of tape that comes with the marketing kit!

12) **The product is unavailable anywhere else.** Two problems with this. If it is not available anywhere else, they usually charge an arm and a leg for it. Also, if it is not available anywhere else, maybe it is not really a good product. If you can't compare this product with something else, stay away from it.

13) **Your doctor won't know anything about this product.** This is a double whammy. Not only does the promoter try to convince you that your physician is misinformed, but tries to qualify themselves as knowledgeable people who will inform you instead of your doctor. Don't get suckered in by this technique.

I'm not saying that no product can be helpful if one of the 13 red flags above is raised. Nor am I saying that someone who has fibromyalgia can't give you helpful advice or recommend products. I know many caring credible business people who sell products or services for people with fibromyalgia. I am simply telling you to be cautious, and don't act upon your emotions or a pressure market sell. If a red flag goes up, STOP, and agree that you are going to take the pressure off yourself and defer any decision until a later time after you have done some research. Spur of the moment decisions are costly ones, so make your decision LATER.

I have some strong feelings about those who prey on people with fibromyalgia. I can be diplomatic, though, and say simply that it is your responsibility to avoid being an unsuspecting victim.

Work with Your Doctor

Your goal is to interact with your physician to become as informed as possible, and to feel as well as possible. Some physicians are more comfortable with knowledgeable patients than others. (This may be an understatement!)

Try to approach your physician in a way that does not seem confrontational. If you walk into your doctor's office with a list of 50 questions and a stack of ten articles, you may overwhelm a doctor who has 15 minutes scheduled to see you. Ask your most important questions and work together on strategies for increasing your knowledge.

Learning is an ongoing process. You can't learn everything about fibromyalgia in a day. My body of medical knowledge didn't stop when I finished my residency. I need to continue to learn by experience, by reviewing literature, and by interacting with you. You are doing the same. Together, we become even smarter!

Chapter 19 — Survival Strategies

1) Take an active role in becoming an informed patient.

2) Start by asking questions.

3) Take advantage of libraries, the Internet, and support groups. See what they have to offer.

4) Review the 13 strategies for avoiding being unlucky. They will help to develop good consumer skills.

5) Check credentials of your health care provider.

6) As a consumer:

   Be cautious

   Don't act upon your emotions or sales pressure

   If a red flag goes up stop, and take the time to think it over.

7) Accept the responsibility to be an educated consumer to avoid being an unsuspecting victim.

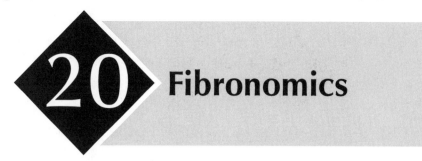

20 Fibronomics

With fibromyalgia, we have to pay extra attention to our bodies so our pain doesn't flare up so often. I believe the first step in any exercise or home program is observing proper posture and body mechanics. We can make time to stretch and exercise, but observing proper posture and body mechanics needs to be continuous and automatic.

All of us have experience with trying to achieve proper posture. We may remember Grandma reminding us to "sit up straight." I still remember the grade school nuns telling me, "Don't slouch!" It was as if somehow sitting properly at all times would prevent our spines from bending and curving or freezing in some abnormal position.

We learned how to lift heavy objects using our legs and not bending over at the waist to prevent back injury. As we became more sophisticated, we learned ways to maneuver our bodies to avoid causing injuries or pain, yet still complete the functional task at hand.

Ergonomics is a scientific study of posture and body mechanics and its relationship to various tasks. Ergonomics specifically involves designing equipment for work to fit the capabilities of the human body in order to minimize the risk of injury. Examples of ergonomic applications include tools that minimize

The four rules to fibronomics are:

1) Arms stay home.

2) Unload the back.

3) Support always welcome.

4) Be naturally shifty.

strain on the wrist, keyboards that are curved and slanted to fit the hand better, and secretarial chairs with armrests and back support. A key goal in ergonomics is to achieve a natural position for the human body where there is minimal or no strain on the joints and soft tissues.

The natural standing position of the human body is when the head is relaxed and slightly bent forward, the arms are loosely hanging down the sides with the elbows bent to a 90 degree angle, the wrists straight, fingers relaxed and slightly curled in, the back in a natural lordotic curve, the knees slightly bent, and the feet about 12 inches apart.

If an unnatural or awkward position occurs, more strain is placed on the joints and soft tissues. Examples of unnatural positions include: Head turned to the side or looking up, arms outstretched or overhead, elbows away from the body, wrists bent, palms up, body leaning forward and bending.

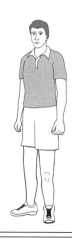

One cannot maintain natural body positions all day long. On the other hand, if we put a lot of strain on our tissues by repeated unnatural positions, we are at risk for injury or pain. A strategy: promote proper posture to prevent painful people!

With fibromyalgia, we have to develop a different concept of what is considered proper posture. All of the stuff that Grandmother told us just doesn't work. When we try to sit up straight for a long time, we hurt more. Slouching is actually comfortable. And, let's face it, we are not trying for modeling careers. We just want to be

> Activities that increase the load on the back are bending forward, prolonged standing, bending at the waist to pick up an object, or arching the back. All of these will increase the potential for mechanical imbalance and pain in our fibromyalgia muscles. We need to learn how to unload the back.

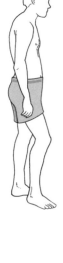

comfortable. Many of us who have had fibromyalgia for years develop a characteristic fibromyalgia posture that results from countless hours in a comfortable but less than perfect posture (see figure).

A different set of rules apply to fibromyalgia posture. We need to reprogram our minds and muscles and fit these fibromyalgia posture and body mechanic rules. We need to learn: Fibronomics.

Fibronomics is defined as *the art of properly manipulating our fibromyalgia bodies in the environment to enable completion of a function or activity with minimal pain.* Fibronomics can be applied to everything we do in life, no matter how simple it is. There are four easy rules to fibronomics, and once these are learned and applied, our bodies will automatically follow them.

The Four Rules to Fibronomics are:

1) Arms stay home.

2) Unload the back.

3) Support always welcome.

4) Be naturally shifty.

Rule #1: Arms Stay Home

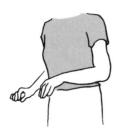

Fibromyalgia muscles in the neck, shoulders and upper back area do not like activity that involves reaching or overhead use of the arms. Isometric contractions occur when muscles stay continuously contracted. This causes decreased blood flow, decreased muscle oxygen, and increased pain. Any time the arms are away from the body, the trapezial, scapular, shoulder and upper back muscles all go into sustained isometric contractions, which usually causes increased pain after only a few seconds. Many will notice immediate increased pain or feelings of weakness in the arms when we reach. Sometimes we are so focused on what we are doing that we may not notice the early pain signals arising from our neck, shoulders, and upper back until it is too late.

The favorite position of our arms is at the sides with our elbows touching our sides and bent at a 90 degree angle (see figure). Our arms stay home (with the rest of the body) and do not reach away while performing a particular task. We should try to maintain this position as much as possible, so we need to move our whole body, not just our arms when we want to confront each specific task.

Examples of using Rule #1: Arms stay home.

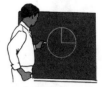

1) Problem: Reaching up to write on chalkboard.

Solution: Move body closer to board and write only in the mid to low portions of the board, not at the top of the board.

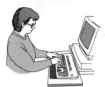

2) Problem: Reaching forward to type on a keyboard.

Solution: Raise chair, lower the keyboard by installing a drop keyboard mechanism into the desk, move chair as close to keyboard as possible. You might also place keyboard on lap. Enlarge the screen so you can see better.

3) Problem: Washing windows by reaching.

Solution: Get closer to the wall, use a long-handled tool such as a squeegee.

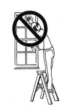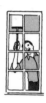

4) Problem: Prolonged driving with arms at the ten o'clock and two o'clock wheel position.

Solution: Move seat closer to steering wheel, place hands in four o'clock and eight o'clock positions.

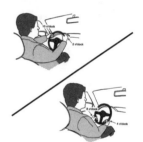

Rule #2: Unload the Back

The back actually includes the entire spine, pelvic, and hip areas with particular emphasis on the lower back and sacroiliac region. Many back and pelvic muscles interact with each other to maintain proper alignment. Anything that causes a shift in this alignment can create mechanical imbalance and or a misalignment. Pain occurs, whether it be from bones, ligaments, nerves or muscles. Activities that increase the load on the back are bending forward, prolonged standing, bending at the waist to pick up an object, or arching the back. All of these will increase the potential for mechanical imbalance and pain in our fibromyalgia muscles. We need to learn how to unload the back.

Ways that we unload the back include:

- Avoid bending forward at the waist; maintain a natural lordotic (arched) curvature of the spine.

- Cross our legs or put our feet up on a foot rest when we are seated.

- Lying in a fetal position on our sides with a pillow between our knees.

- Avoid bending over and picking up heavy objects; bend your knees and lift with your legs, keeping your back straight.

- Wear sensible shoes, no heels!

Examples of using Rule #2: Unload the back.

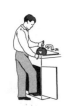

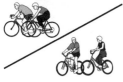

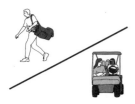

1) Problem: Leaning forward at the kitchen sink.

Solution: Keep back straight, open cupboard door under sink and lift leg into cupboard. Use long-handled sponges.

2) Problem: Riding sports bike bent forward.

Solution: Avoid rams horn style handle bars. Use a wider comfortable seat that places the back in a more natural position.

3) Problem: Leaning forward at the waist over a counter to sign papers.

Solution: Spread legs to lower body but maintain good back posture, then sign papers without bending forward.

4) Problem: Carrying heavy golf clubs puts strain on the back.

Solution: Play nine holes instead of eighteen, ride a cart or use a pull-cart, or use a caddy.

5) Problem: Applying make-up by tilting head back and looking into a wall mirror puts strain on the neck.

Solution: Look down into a magnifying mirror.

6) Problem: Bending and lifting at work causes low back pain.

Solution: Here are four techniques for lifting:

Modified Diagonal Lift:

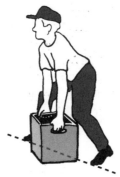

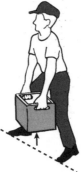

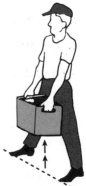

The modified diagonal lift is used for lifting heavy items which are one or two feet off the floor. Establish a wide stance with one foot in front of the other. Placing yourself slightly over the item, bend at the hips and at the knees. With the head and shoulders up, straighten the knees and hips to lift the object off the ground.

One Knee Lift:

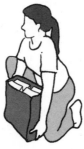

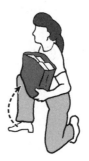

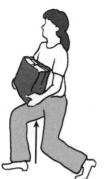
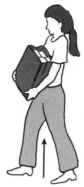

Place one foot beside the front portion of the object to be lifted; drop slowly to other knee. Grip the object firmly at near and far corners with head and shoulders up and lower back arched, then lift or roll the object onto top of thigh. Maintaining same posture, stand with object cradled. (Avoid this lift if you have knee problems.)

The Golfer's Lift:

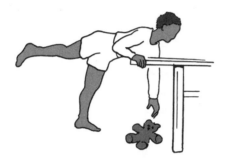

This lift can be used by people with knee problems, decreased leg strength, or when they must lift where there is a barrier in front of the item (such as a railing or deep storage container). Place one hand on table or other fixed object to support the upper body; arch the back, bend at the hips, and raise one leg behind yourself. By raising one leg, the upper body weight is counterbalanced and bending forward from the low back is reduced. To pick up item, the individual should look up, push off with free hand, and lower the raised leg.

Straight Leg Lift:

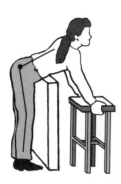
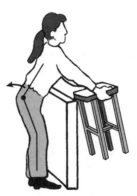

This lift is used when knees and hips cannot be bent. Position body as close to the object as possible. If you are reaching over something into a lower work area, press your legs forward against the object over which you are reaching. While bending slowly at hips (not the waist), you should firmly grasp item and bring it closer if necessary. With the low back arched and head up, complete the lift by rotating hips backward to a full standing position.

Rule #3: Support Always Welcome

We should take advantage of existing environmental structures to relieve some of the force on our bodies. Our muscles work hard everyday to support us and get us from one place to another. We expect that our muscles will get tired, and usually when they get tired, they hurt more. It is okay to use extra support to relieve our muscles whenever we can. Our muscles won't deteriorate or atrophy if we are responsibly using additional support.

Examples of using Rule #3: Support always welcome.

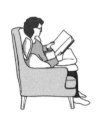

1) Problem: Our arms become tired and hurt.

Solution: Use armrests, pillows, or furniture (table, desk, or countertop) to rest arms. Cross arms or rest on head, lap, or body. Hold one arm with the other. Put arms in pockets, muffs, or slings.

2) Problem: Our back is tired and hurts.

Solution: Sit in a chair, particularly one with a good seat and back. Lean against a wall or other object. Use a footstool or pillow for additional support. Use a brace or a belt.

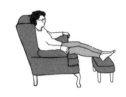

3) Problem: Our neck is tired and hurts.

Solution: Use pillows to support the head and neck. Hold the head in your hands. Wear a soft cervical collar when driving/riding on long trips or bumpy roads.

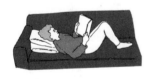

4) Problem: Our whole body feels tired and hurts.

Solution: Lay down. Use various pillows and cushions. Sit in a recliner.

Rule #4: Be Naturally Shifty

This rule emphasizes maintaining natural or neutral body and joint positions, and periodically moving the muscles. If we keep our muscles in one position for too long, we tend to get painful tightening and spasms. To counteract this, keep moving the muscles regularly. Some people have more tolerance than others, but we all have our limit, and if we spend too much time in one particular position, we will experience increased pain. We must learn to automatically alternate between positions such as sitting, standing, and walking. This strategy will enable various muscle groups to relax and stretch regularly.

Examples of Rule #4: Be naturally shifty.

1) Problem: Sitting up straight hurts.

Solution: Slouch at times, alternate this with sitting up straight.

2) Problem: Standing in line hurts.

Solution: Shift weight from side to side, walk around in your place.

3) Problem: Sitting in a hard chair for a long time causes the back and legs to hurt.

Solution: Be fidgety, shift around in the chair, move the legs, frequently stand up and stretch. Take a cushion with you!

Applied Fibronomics!

Use fibronomics to examine everything you do. First, determine why an activity may be causing pain by identifying the fibronomic rules that are violated. Sometimes the activity may be obvious, other times it may be subtle, but think about the rules and analyze every single thing that you do no matter how automatic it is. Correct these violations and practice these new strategies until they become automatic additions to your body mechanics. At first, you must consciously think about these violations and take steps to correct them. After a while, your subconscious takes over and the techniques will become automatic.

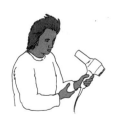

The following are some more examples of daily problems where proper application of fibronomics can be helpful.

Example 1—Problem: Sitting in bleachers at a sporting event causes significantly increased back pain.

Fibronomics rules are violated by prolonged sitting without alternating positions and unsupported sitting, which increases the load on the back.

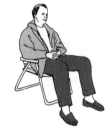

Solutions: Bring a folding chair with you to the bleachers and use it, allowing the back to be supported. Take frequent standing and walking breaks, averaging at least a minute of standing/walking for every 15 minutes sitting.

Example 2—Problem: The clock collection is posing a problem since winding up clocks once a week causes increased neck and shoulder pain and causes arm fatigue. (Isn't clock collection common in people with fibromyalgia!?)

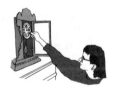

Fibronomics rules are violated by reaching your arms out to try to wind the clock. This increases isometric contractions in the neck, shoulders and back (causes timely PAIN!).

Solutions: Stand on a stool to lower the arms to a more natural position. Move closer to the clocks so the arms stay in, then wind, taking no more than 10 winds before stopping to drop the arms to the side for a few seconds; then resume the winding. Arms stay home when whining—I mean winding!

Example 3—Problem: Getting the hair ready in the morning can cause a lot of pain, yet we have to look presentable for the day.

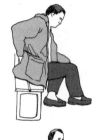

Fibronomics rules are violated by arms reaching up over our head, leaning forward over the sink puts an increased load on the back, and not taking advantage of any available support.

Solutions: Use the other arm to hold the arm used to fix the hair or hold the blow dryer. Hold hair dryer lower (arms more at sides) and direct air upwards. Bend head down so it is closer to the air. Obtain a folding director's chair to sit on in the bathroom and perform morning duties in a more favorable position. Consider a new hairstyle that is more fibro-friendly. Remember, you look beautiful just as you are!

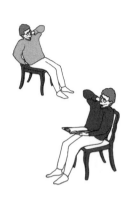

Example 4—Problem: Reading and studying causes considerable increased neck pain and headache.

Fibronomics rules are violated by the sustained positioning of the head and neck which causes painful tightening, and the lack of neck support while maintaining the studying position. When studying, we are so focused on the material that we don't notice the early clues our neck, head and shoulders may be giving about increased pain . . . until it's too late!

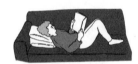

Solutions: Alternate positions every thirty minutes from sitting at a desk to lying in bed with a pillow propped behind the head. Set a timer to remind you when it's time to change positions. Use a pillow or book holder to prop up the book and allow you to more comfortably adjust your head position. Lean back in the chair so head and neck are more supported. Lay on the bed with neck and head supported with a pillow, bend knees, and put the book on your lap.

Example 5—Problem: Sitting in a chair is painful to the lower back, and when standing up after sitting in a chair for a while, spasms and stiffness in the back make it difficult to get out of a chair and stand up straight.

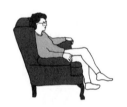

Fibronomics rules are violated by prolonged sitting without alternating positions, and lack of adequate support for the back due to poor chair design, which increases strain on the back.

Solutions: Crossing the legs is an excellent way to unload the back and pelvis. Remember to alternate the legs crossed. Use a footstool to rest both legs and raise the knees.

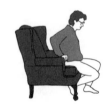

Sit in a good chair that has a sturdy back and arms to maintain proper body alignment; use a lumbar cushion or pillow to support the natural low back curvature.

When getting out of a chair, use the "back pedal technique." First, scoot forward to the front edge of the chair. Then plant one foot behind the chair as far as possible. With the arms pushing off the armrests, stand up while maintaining a natural back position without bending forward.

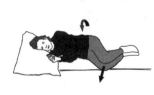

Example 6—Problem: Getting out of bed or off the couch causes severe back pain.

Fibronomics rules are violated because the back is under extreme stress when a "sit-up" is performed to get up. Also, the upper body is trying to lift up unsupported before the legs swing over.

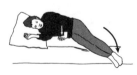

Solution: Transfer out of bed using a log roll technique. First, roll your body, log roll style, onto your side, then curl up your legs so your knees come forward and over the edge of the bed. Use the arm opposite the side on the bed to push on the surface near your waist level at the same time you swing your legs off of the edge to allow a quick yet smooth sitting up motion. This avoids undue stress on the back.

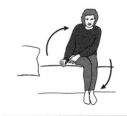

Wear a Mental Seat Belt

I pay particular attention to fibronomics in my everyday activities. In fact, I tend to be a little paranoid at all times. I don't want to do anything that will cause my fibromyalgia to flare up, so I try to be extra cautious to make sure I am following proper fibronomics!

We wear a car seat belt as a protective device to prevent injury in case of an accident. I say we should wear a mental seat belt at all times to help prevent a fibromyalgia flare-up and remind us not to be careless. Not only do we need to follow proper fibronomics, but we have to remind ourselves that every situation is a flare-up waiting to happen. One of the most common causes of flare-up is a body injury, so we need to avoid any potential harm or injury to our body as part of controlling our fibromyalgia.

Here are some examples of how I wear a mental seat belt at all times.

Whenever I'm going up or down steps, I always hold onto the rail. I've gone up and down steps a million times, and I know what it is to slip and fall. My last great stair wipeout occurred in college. I slipped on the top step on the way down, and slid or bounced down ten steps. My books went flying. I knocked books out of the hands of two girls walking up the steps. Luckily, only my ego was bruised.

By holding onto a rail at all times when I am on the steps, I not only remind myself not to fall, but I am physically preventing myself from falling should I lose my balance.

Whenever I am walking on icy ground, I assume I will fall and break a bone. No matter how close my car is or how much I'm in a hurry, I always walk slowly and carefully on ice. I make sure that my balance is stable at all times, and I avoid lifting one foot too far off of the ground when taking steps to minimize the chance of losing my balance.

Whenever I am picking up something off of the floor, I pretend it weighs 100 pounds. We usually don't hurt ourselves when we bend over to pick up something heavy because we know the object is heavy and take extra care in following proper posture. We get into trouble when we bend over quickly and twist to pick up something small like a little piece of paper. More often than not, this is the way we sprain our backs. I pretend that the little piece of paper weighs 100 pounds to remind myself to follow proper body mechanics and pick up the paper slowly so as not to catch my back off guard.

Fibronomics rules are violated by prolonged sitting without alternating positions, and lack of adequate support for the back due to poor chair design, which increases strain on the back.

Solutions: Crossing the legs is an excellent way to unload the back and pelvis. Remember to alternate the legs crossed. Use a footstool to rest both legs and raise the knees.

Whenever I feel a sneeze coming on, I make certain I assume the proper sneezing position: arms tucked tightly to the sides and bent, head and back slightly bent forward in a braced position, and knees slightly bent. I've had too many flare-ups in the past from "unprotected" sneezes. Now I am paranoid — and careful with my sneezes.

Remember to wear your mental seat belt at all times. It is a fibro law! Be especially careful on steps; wet, icy, slippery surfaces; or gravel, grass, hilly, bumpy surfaces. Be careful when you are carrying packages, and — all of the time! Remember to use your fibronomics.

We should wear a mental seat belt at all times to help prevent a fibromyalgia flare-up and remind us not to be careless. Not only do we need to follow proper fibronomics, but we have to remind ourselves that every situation is a flare-up waiting to happen. One of the most common causes of flare-up is a body injury, so we need to avoid any potential harm or injury to our body as part of controlling our fibromyalgia.

Chapter 20 — Survival Strategies

Fibronomics

1) Learn to follow proper posture and body mechanics at all times; this will help relieve pain.

2) Work to achieve a natural position for your body (ergonomics) so that there is minimal or no strain on the joints and soft tissues.

3) Use fibronomics to reprogram your mind to learn more fibro-friendly posture and body mechanics.

4) Apply fibronomics to "everything" you do in life, no matter how simple.

5) Wear a "mental seat belt" at all times.

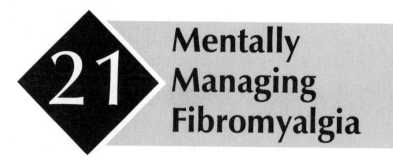

Mentally Managing Fibromyalgia

Physically, fibromyalgia bothers our bodies with pain and other problems. Mentally, it causes depression, mental fatigue, poor concentration, anxiety, fibro-fog, and more. The mind can have a powerful healing effect on the body, so we need to keep our minds healthy and use them to help the healing process. Hope is the most important tool in a loaded mental toolbox.

A lot has been written on how to reduce stress, relax, and think positively. If I were to line up every article, book or advertisement on these subjects...well, it makes me stressed, tense, and frustrated to even think about how long it would take!

Mental strategies can reduce the ill effects of stress on our bodies. Notice I said "reduce the effects of stress," not reduce stress itself. Stress is a major factor in fibromyalgia. A catastrophic stress may have caused it, and any stress can certainly aggravate it. Life is stressful, so we can never get rid of stress. I like to say that the last time we were stress-free was when we were in the womb.

We can learn how to reduce stress and minimize its effect on fibromyalgia. Everyone with fibromyalgia can benefit from mental techniques to manage their physical problems. There is no one right way; many ways can work. It takes motivation, practice, and perseverance to learn a new mental management strategy. It is hard!

Through the years each of us has evolved highly specialized thought processes to view ourselves and our world. For example, we always think of ourselves as young and healthy forever! Then all of a sudden, fibromyalgia comes along. Now these rules and processes are no longer effective. We are then asked to change our life-style, not only physically, but mentally. This is not an impossible task, but it involves a willingness to take that first step and to make a commitment to change our life-style. It is natural to be scared or even terrified of this process because we are not sure what to expect. But with encouragement, patients with fibromyalgia are truly impressive in their ability to change their thinking and achieve a positive mental outlook.

How can one make mental life-style changes? I approach this in a series of small steps that are integrated into a big leap to a successful new mental approach: to change the way you think about life with fibromyalgia. You have to take baby steps before you can jump. I have devised a mental strategy which I call the Five Repairs.

Five REpairs

1) REcognize and REdefine
2) REalistic REtraining
3) REliable RElationships
4) RElax and REfresh
5) REspect and REsponsibility

Each pair of "REs" is intimately related and addresses a different aspect of the mental approach to fibromyalgia. The ultimate goal is to be able to integrate all five into a positive mental strategy that works.

REcognize and REdefine

Fibromyalgia makes it easy to think negatively. Before we can correct this tendency we need to recognize the ways in which we think negatively.

Here are some examples:

- We over-generalize. One small incident seems like a catastrophe. For example, if we forget something, we think we are getting Alzheimer's disease.

- We anticipate bad things. If someone invites us to a party, the first thing we think of is that the party will cause a flare-up in our pain.

- We blame ourselves for everything. We believe it is our fault that we have fibromyalgia or that we have flare-ups.

- We label ourselves negatively. We think that because we are having a lot of pain, we must be bad or useless people.

- We expect things to get worse. If we talk to someone older than us who has fibromyalgia and is having extreme pain and disability, we expect that we will end up in the same way when we get older.

Continuous negative thinking about ourselves and our situation will ultimately lead to other negative emotions such as anger, frustration, hopelessness, and feelings of guilt and depression.

We also tend to be perfectionists and overachieving individuals, and this can lead to negative consequences when trying to cope with fibromyalgia. Our perfectionist nature can create "negative" traits which include:

- Inability to handle criticism
- Fear of failure
- Fear of rejection
- Feeling of inadequacy
- Anxiety
- Lack of control

By being overachievers, we also risk developing negative behaviors which include:

- Always searching for a fibromyalgia cure
- Doctor shopping for that magical treatment
- Inability to delegate tasks to others
- Feelings of being overwhelmed
- Procrastination

- Impatience

- Extreme guilt when unable to accomplish what we used to be able to do.

Once we've recognized this, we can change our thinking patterns. Fibromyalgia forces us to redefine our physical ability. Since we can no longer do what we used to, we must seek a new physical life-style that our fibromyalgia will tolerate. We also have to redefine our thought processes. We must now think of ourselves as persons with chronic pain, and from that perspective, try to imagine how we can feel better about ourselves.

To redefine, we ask ourselves, "What goals do we wish for ourselves?" and "How do we want to see ourselves?" and "What can we do?" A part of redefining our thinking is to redefine what it means to feel good. When we are so focused on feeling bad all the time, it is hard to look for things about ourselves that make us feel good.

You know how a picture can look bad to you at first, but when you move it to a different light it looks better? We must picture ourselves in a more positive light. We were not singled out to have this painful disorder for something we did or did not do, so we must stop blaming ourselves. Redefine ourselves as good, normal people who just happen to have fibromyalgia, and work on believing it. Focus on your strength and expect to live a good quality life in spite of having fibromyalgia.

For our tendency to be perfectionists and overachieving, we should try to redefine those qualities and see the positive. Examples of positive outcomes from our perfectionist tendency include:

- Organization and efficiency

- Industriousness

- Responsibility

- Trustworthiness

- Reliability

- Punctuality

Being overachievers can also have positive consequences:

- Innovative thinking that allows us to create new strategies

- Active participation in our care and decisions regarding fibromyalgia

- Proactive approach by reading everything we can about fibromyalgia and
    therefore acquiring knowledge

- Flexibility in learning to budget our energy and breaking big tasks into
    smaller tasks

Ultimately, we need to accept that fibromyalgia is a chronic illness. We need to take inventory of all the thoughts we have and the ways we feel about ourselves because of fibromyalgia. We then sort through this inventory to determine what we want to throw out, modify, or change — what we want to redefine. The next step in the process is realistic retraining.

REalistic REtraining

At this step, we ask the question, "How will we change our thinking to accomplish our redefined goals?" With fibromyalgia, it is not realistic to expect to be pain free. However, it is realistic to achieve a low baseline level of pain where we feel we are able to enjoy our lives as fully as possible. Sometimes we may even achieve a remission.

Retraining our thinking is not an easy or quick process. It took us a long time to reach where we are in our thinking process, so it will take time to change our thinking as well. A "quick fix" is not a good strategy since it only captures our initial enthusiasm and motivation as some of the fad diets do. We need a slow but long-lasting lifestyle change that has a higher chance of being successful for a longer duration.

A lot of people have been trained to think in black and white; it is either one way or the other. If we are then forced to start exploring the gray areas, it can create a lot of tension and even confusion in some people. We need to allow ourselves to look into and explore these gray areas. You may be surprised at the new mental strategies you can learn in that territory. Or at least you will be surprised at how many different shades of gray exist!

The individual with fibromyalgia who makes the effort has a much better chance of a positive outcome than the person who does nothing to start the adjustment or acceptance process. Some of the studies done on fibromyalgia patients over time have found some fascinating comparisons. Individuals who took an aggressive role in seeking strategies to control their fibromyalgia are less bothered by their condition as they get older. Those who took a passive role or were never given the opportunity to become an active participant in the management of the disorder fared much worse.

Set Mental Limits

Like setting physical limits, you need to set mental limits and learn to accept them. You must allow yourself to be forgetful at times without convincing yourself that you have a memory disease. You can be critical of your performance, but don't punish yourself personally and feel that you are worthless or unable to do anything. You can worry about certain activities causing a flare-up, but you have to set a limit on this, too. You can't let it cause you to avoid any type of activity.

Train yourself to change "I shouldn't" to "I'll try." That way, instead of completely avoiding a certain activity, you force yourself to try to find ways of doing it. This is a way of thinking positively, yet still respecting your mental limits. Saying "I'll try" also forces you to think of strategies and mentally rehearse them as a positive and constructive approach to your perceived limitations with fibromyalgia.

If you can train your mind to look for that opening and rehearse a way to get through it, the physical aspect will follow much easier. Here's an example: A minister with fibromyalgia experienced a severe flare-up following the flu. Because of increased pain and fatigue, she is no longer able to perform her hour-long Sunday service that includes a 20-minute sermon. At first she thinks that she shouldn't even try to complete a service because of too much preparation required, the prolonged standing, and the hand gestures that she uses while giving her sermon. Her initial thought is to avoid the Sunday service altogether until her flare-up resolves and she is able to perform all of her usual duties.

However, it's uncertain when her flare-up will resolve, and because of the importance of her church involvement, she takes a new approach. She reexamines every motion she makes during her sermon and tries to find ways to participate. Her mental plan is to first perform only the sermon, the vital part of the service. She would do this from a seated position, minimizing the hand gestures, and shorten the service from 20 to 10 minutes. From this she envisions being present during the whole service but being seated in a chair. Over the course of several Sundays, she would gradually increase her own participation in the service as she could tolerate it. She mentally rehearses these strategies and constructs her plan, then physically carries it out. She finds out that she is still able to be an active participant in spite of her fibromyalgia flare-up.

The retraining process does not work 100% when you first try it, and a successful behavior is never 100% perfect. Before we learned to walk, we first had to balance, learn to stand, learn to take slow, deliberate and unsteady steps, and practice this pattern until it became easier and automatic. Finally we developed walking skills that became part of our subconscious physical ability. We had to fall down many times before we became proficient at walking and even though we can walk well now, we still fall down occasionally. Our walking skills were achieved by a series of small, successful steps that were inefficient at first, but with practice, gradually became a successful and efficient system. This is how our mental retraining process works.

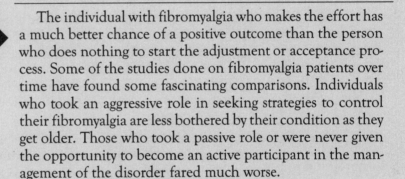

The individual with fibromyalgia who makes the effort has a much better chance of a positive outcome than the person who does nothing to start the adjustment or acceptance process. Some of the studies done on fibromyalgia patients over time have found some fascinating comparisons. Individuals who took an aggressive role in seeking strategies to control their fibromyalgia are less bothered by their condition as they get older. Those who took a passive role or were never given the opportunity to become an active participant in the management of the disorder fared much worse.

Mental retraining strategies can make physical performance easier. But doing physical things can also help us feel better mentally. If we make an effort to physically look good (dressing nicely, keeping our hair neatly styled, basic good grooming), we will feel better about ourselves, and thus receive a mental boost. We must also retrain our thoughts to achieve a proper diet, ideal body weight, and a regular exercise program.

REliable RElationships

This REpair step involves others in your life. Relationships mean family, spouses, significant others, friends, and co-workers. Your fibromyalgia affects not only you, but all those around you. Relationships change because of fibromyalgia, oftentimes for the worse. It is your responsibility to make your relationships positive in spite of fibromyalgia.

Even though you are in constant pain, your goal is to treat the ones you care about with compassion and kindness. This isn't easy if you hurt and feel downright mean and miserable. You might find yourself being short tempered and unpleasant with the ones you care about. Then you can feel guilty. You are allowed to feel miserable and be mean and short tempered. You can have these feelings or moods and still be a good person! You simply recognize that these are negative consequences of your chronic pain and you are going to work hard on overcoming them even if you aren't perfect at it.

You may also shut out the family and caring ones because of your pain. Sometimes you shut out the world, and you'll notice the pain more, because the world around you has become so small that there is nothing else in it except you and your pain. Don't shut out your relationships. Keep them in your world, even if fibromyalgia is crowding it.

Many times, families and significant others do not know how to respond to you and your fibromyalgia. If you do not communicate your problems, your family will not be aware of them. They may play a guessing game to figure out how you are feeling at any particular time.

You may also shut out the family and caring ones because of your pain. Sometimes you shut out the world, and you'll notice the pain more, because the world around you has become so small that there is nothing else in it except you and your pain. Don't shut out your relationships. Keep them in your world, even if fibromyalgia is crowding it.

Educate

Some families react to a chronic problem by denying its existence (just as you do sometimes). They think that your fibromyalgia will simply go away someday and you will be back to your "normal" self. You need to educate them about fibromyalgia. Give them literature to read. Let them know the types of things that aggravate your pain, what you are doing to help control your symptoms, and what works for you. Tell them that your fibromyalgia is not a tumor and will not cause deformities or paralysis and that you will not die from it. Hopefully, they will appreciate your teaching attempts.

In relationships, everyone brings his or her own unique perspective. Each person's perspective has been shaped by his or her individual past experiences, traumas, attitudes, limitations, and accomplishments. Everyone has "baggage." Most of our baggage, however, just happens to be from our physical experiences with fibromyalgia. Just as we would not reject someone for something in their past, we would not expect someone else to reject us just because we have fibromyalgia and a "past" associated with this problem. If we give others a chance, they can accept us.

At times you will think that no one is making any attempt to understand your problem, and at times they will think that you are simply using fibromyalgia as an excuse to avoid your responsibilities. A successful family support system recognizes the extremes that occur occasionally, but maintains a stable balance of understanding, acceptance and support that does not falter when these occasional bad times occur. Family life (indeed, any relationship) is difficult even in normal situations. Adding a chronic illness makes everything even more challenging.

Communication

How can individuals work together to form positive and reliable relationships? Open communication with your family and others you trust is important. They also have frustrations, needs and feelings about the fibromyalgia. Share your feelings with them, find out about their feelings, and work together to understand and accept your physical and mental limitations. Work on positively redefining relationships.

It helps if your family reads about fibromyalgia and maybe even attends your support group. When you attend the group, pay particular attention to what spouses and significant others share with the group. They are your best source of information on how healthy people look at and deal with fibromyalgia. Then you can ask your spouse or significant other if they have the same complaints. If so, work to make changes. You will learn to see your illness by others' perspectives. This may open a totally new line of communication.

Have frequent family conferences that function as your own family support group. Find out how everyone is feeling and how family members can help each other out. If you find the problem is too big to handle on your own, you may wish to seek professional help.

An area of concern to many patients with fibromyalgia is sex and intimacy. Chronic pain and illness definitely impact this aspect of relationships. There are particular fears and anxieties on whether individuals will be able to find an accepting life partner or continue to have satisfying and fulfilling relationships once chronic pain and fibromyalgia have intervened. This concern is discussed more in a later chapter.

Delegate

It is difficult to ask others for help. Feelings of low self-esteem, fear of losing our independence, and concern that we will be bothering this person by asking for help inhibit us. However, if fibromyalgia prevents us from doing things, we must learn to ask for help and delegate responsibility for various tasks to others. Practice on your family first.

Team chores can be performed by different family members with designated tasks. Everyone works together while performing his or her task. You do your part, also, and you can count "supervising" as a chore!

One patient compared this process to a corporation. If you are the CEO of the family, you have the ultimate role of making sure your whole family unit is functioning. However, you can set up your organization so problem solving and simple task completion can be done at different levels. Even though you are overseeing everything, you don't need to be approached directly for every task or problem. With your influence, these tasks are already handled automatically.

It is okay to ask for help from others outside of your family. We need to allow ourselves to approach reliable and trusted individuals to ask for help when we need it. Instead of "bothering" these people, we will probably discover that they will gladly help us. Family, friends and co-workers can become trusted people who are willing to help us when we ask. One patient said that whenever she is feeling her lowest, she always calls her most positive friend and can count on her to boost her spirits. We all need to find these positive people that can help pick us up when we are feeling down. We, in turn, will gladly help these people when asked.

Support Groups

Support groups are an excellent way to form reliable relationships. Sharing with others who know exactly how you feel has incredible power. Many of my patients are active in fibromyalgia support groups, both live and virtual. Other groups can be helpful and therapeutic even if they do not involve fibromyalgia. Card clubs, cooking groups, book clubs, and church groups are other therapeutic groups. Volunteering is an excellent way to stop thinking about our own problems and feel good about helping others deal with theirs.

RElax and REfresh

Perhaps one of the hardest things for people with fibromyalgia to do is to relax. With fibromyalgia we always seem to have tense bodies and minds. One woman described her tense mind as though she is "constantly running a marathon in her brain." We have a more hypersensitive autonomic nervous system, especially the sympathetic nervous system which is responsible for the "fight or flight" response.

Support groups are an excellent way to form reliable relationships. Sharing with others who know exactly how you feel has incredible power. Many of my patients are active in fibromyalgia support groups, both live and virtual. Other groups can be helpful and therapeutic even if they do not involve fibromyalgia. Card clubs, cooking groups, book clubs, and church groups are other therapeutic groups. Volunteering is an excellent way to stop thinking about our own problems and feel good about helping others deal with theirs.

The fight or flight response is normally triggered when we are in a threatening situation. Certain hormones, especially adrenaline, are released in large quantities to ready the body's protective mechanism, and we become tense, focused, and primed to either fight or run. It is not often, though, that a tiger jumps out of a bush in a parking lot and starts running after us, nor do we usually find ourselves standing in the middle of a railroad track facing an oncoming train. Yet, thanks to fibromyalgia, we manage to maintain such a continuous state of anxiety and tension.

The relaxation response is the opposite of the fight or flight response. It occurs when natural physiologic mechanisms cause muscles to loosen up, blood flow to improve, heart rate to slow down, and the mind to become calm. Our body's parasympathetic nervous system mediates this response, which is eliminated or distorted when the body is in a constant state of tension and anxiety. Thus, the chances of finding the relaxation response in fibromyalgia are about as good as finding an area that does not hurt! If we have lost the ability to subconsciously achieve the relaxation response, we need to consciously retrain our bodies to relax.

If there ever was something easier said than done, it has to be telling someone with fibromyalgia to relax. It is so difficult to relax that whenever someone tells me to do it, I actually get more tense. Saying the word "relax" elicits a fight or flight response! When trying to teach yourself a relaxation technique, keep in mind that there are literally dozens of techniques, and, as I have said before, there is no one way that works best for everyone, but there is probably a way that will work for anyone. For me, I like to read and watch video movies. Whether one is meditating, participating in a sporting event, praying, or performing Tai Chi, a type of relaxation exercise is happening. You, too, can learn to master the art of relaxation.

Comfortable Environment

The first rule of relaxation is to create a comfortable environment. This means picking a quiet spot and making sure that there is nothing to disturb you. Find a comfortable chair where you can stay in the same position for 20 minutes without increased pain. To get comfortable, wear loose, nonrestrictive clothing, place your body in a neutral position, then close your eyes.

Deep Breathing

The next step in the relaxation response is deep breathing. Once you have reached a comfortable position and told your muscles to relax, you should become aware of how you are breathing, and if you are breathing properly. Your stomach should expand when you breathe in through your nose and contract as you slowly breathe out through your mouth.

Take slow deep breaths through your nose, taking in as much air as your lungs will hold to the count of 3. When exhaling, breathe out slowly through a slightly opened mouth to the count of 6. Placing your hands on your stomach will give you tactile feedback that your stomach is properly moving out and in as it is supposed to with deep breathing. Repeat this cycle for 10 to 15 minutes, then sit quietly for 5 minutes with eyes either open or closed, continuing to think only calm thoughts.

Do not be disappointed if you don't achieve a deep trance or hypnotic state. This rarely happens. Breathing deeply can make you feel dizzy or light-headed at first. Try to stay relaxed as you feel yourself about to pass out! This exercise should be done at least once a day, but can be done several times a day if necessary.

This relaxation exercise can be an important part of your fibromyalgia management, once you practice and master this technique. There are other types of relaxation exercises, many that involve mental imagery. Daydreaming, fantasizing, and recalling pleasant memories are examples of mental imagery that can help to relax. These techniques can be done while you are performing other activities and with your eyes open. Many people can use mental imagery to induce a form of self-hypnosis which helps achieve successful relaxation.

> Take slow deep breaths through your nose, taking in as much air as your lungs will hold to the count of 3. When exhaling, breathe out slowly through a slightly opened mouth to the count of 6. Placing your hands on your stomach will give you tactile feedback that your stomach is properly moving out and in as it is supposed to with deep breathing. Repeat this cycle for 10 to 15 minutes, then sit quietly for 5 minutes with eyes either open or closed, continuing to think only calm thoughts.

Guided imagery can help. One fibromyalgia patient did a 4-week guided imagery study on volunteers with fibromyalgia. She was completing her training as a counselor and did this project as part of her schooling. She interviewed each participant and made a guided imagery cassette tape that instructed each person what to imagine. The tape was played daily. Nearly all reported better relaxation and improved sleep.

Biofeedback can also help. This technique is taught by trained psychologists or counselors, and involves muscle monitors and skin temperature measuring devices. Depending on the instructors, over half of people have success with relaxation techniques. Success means the ability to learn to relax and carry over this same response into your everyday life.

Ways to Relax

The following are ways people can relax and cope with fibromyalgia.

a. **A regular exercise program.** This is a powerful stimulator of the body's relaxation response. Exercise to relax, sounds like an oxymoron, doesn't it?

b. **Religion and prayer.** Many people are comforted by their beliefs and convictions.

c. **Enjoyable hobbies.**

d. **Volunteering to help others.**

e. **A hot bath.** This is a great way to both physically relax the muscles, and mentally relax the mind.

f. **Writing.** Keep a daily journal or diary — write a fibromyalgia survivor book!

g. **Music.** A universal stress antidote.

h. **Taking drives** on a rural freeway or country road during the day. (Avoid construction or slow semitrailers in front of you!)

i. **Playing video games,** particularly the hand-held type.

j. **Spend 15 minutes a day looking at three-dimensional pictures.** This is actually a great exercise to divert your thoughts and relax your mind and body.

Relaxation is not something that just happens. It is something that you first practice, and in time accomplish. Then you must plan your relaxation response on a daily basis. Set aside time and protect it. This is not the time to take a nap, but an opportunity to manage your fibromyalgia.

Handling Fibro-Fog

Chronic stress contributes to mental fatigue. We have difficulty with our attention spans and our ability to recall information. Achieving a relaxation response helps to counteract episodes of fibro-fog. Many times, we think our best thoughts and remember the most when we are laying down, relaxing, and trying to get to sleep.

Write notes frequently and organize the notes. When I write material for my book, I go through a routine. I jot down ideas and notes on pieces of paper and collect these papers. Then I start to organize these notes in an outline format. I think of details and let my thought processes evolve over days and weeks, while continuing to write notes and organize these notes. From there I can write the first versions of each chapter, revising and categorizing along the way. We need to take our time mentally, because the more pressure we put on ourselves the harder it is for us to focus and concentrate.

I always try to follow a specific routine. For example, my car keys can only be in three places, my pocket, on top of my desk, or on the kitchen counter. If I come home from work, I've trained myself to put them in those places. If I throw the keys on the bed, for example, I must consciously tell myself to stop everything and take the keys to the proper location. I used to think, "I'll remember where they are," but a few seconds later the memory was completely gone, and later on, I would spend many minutes searching for my keys which I had left on the bed.

You need to consciously train yourself to follow a routine with easily misplaced items. Strive for consistency. Once you have trained yourself, it will become automatic for you. Plus, it will save you a lot of time and frustration. If you misplace something, you will ultimately find it. Don't be too hard on yourself. Simply recognize that this is part of your fibromyalgia.

Being generally forgetful is part of fibromyalgia. Some people can do well with memory association tricks such as trying to associate a person's name or an object with a familiar object or something important. I find that the most reliable way is to write things down and knowing where to look for this written information. Writing things down forces you to focus on what you want to remember. You reinforce this memory by writing it down, and you can relax your mind better because you know where to look for this information when you need it. You give yourself "permission" to forget. Find out what your best memory technique is and use it. Fibromyalgia will certainly give you many opportunities to do so.

I may strive for a routine, but I am always forgetting things. I try not to get mad at myself when this happens and just simply work around what I'm forgetting. Sometimes I can't remember a particular medical word or phrase for a particular physical exam finding. When this happens, I forget about remembering the word and simply describe the abnormal finding. For example, I might not remember the term "Spurling's Sign," so I will say the person had radicular paresthesias when the head was fully rotated, laterally flexed, and extended, and a downward compression was applied to the top of the head. Sure, it would be a lot easier and less wordy to say the patient had a positive Spurling's Sign, but that would be too, uh, what is the word I'm looking for, umm, logical or easy!

Just to show you that this happens all the time, I decided to keep a memory diary for one day in April of 1999. I have summarized my memory diary for the day as follows:

Dr. P's Memory Diary

In the morning I was using a red pen to make some corrections. I set the red pen down, made a copy of my changes and could not find the red pen to resume my work. Eventually I found it on the shelf by the copy machine.

I wrote the wrong date five times on various prescriptions and notes throughout the day. This occurred in spite of wearing a watch with the date on it.

I told a particular patient, "Nice to meet you," even though I had met the patient before. After I examined the patient and was finishing up, I said again, "Nice meeting you," and caught myself and said "...again!"

I wrote down that a patient was a mall carrier instead of mail carrier. I spelled pain p-a-i-n-e, and wrote that spasms were caused by waltzing instead of spasms caused by walking. Instead of writing "dry eyes and numb face," I wrote "dumb face." I have no clue why I wrote these things, and please don't ask me to psychoanalyze myself!

After seeing patients, I got ready for track practice (I am a coach). I set my keys down, got dressed and forgot where my keys were. And I'm always bragging that I don't lose my keys. I was out of my ordinary routine, however, and misplaced the keys and had to find them.

Later in the evening I realized I didn't have an important paper with notes on it. I had worked on it earlier in the evening and thought it was on my desk, but no, it wasn't. I spent 30 minutes (yes, I did!) looking through my briefcase, my car, my desk, and various piles of paper in the office. I couldn't find the paper, so I assumed I had left it at the sports facility. I went to bed and one minute after I laid down, I thought maybe I had mixed the piece of paper up with my bills, so I got up and checked the basket with the bills in it and there was the paper!

How's that for a typical day!

> Try not to avoid doing something for fear of a flare-up. Rather, do whatever you can in spite of your fibromyalgia and its pain. You remember how you used to be before fibromyalgia, but now it is time to re-set your mental thermostat to a level that accommodates some baseline pain.

REspect and REsponsibility

The final step in repairing your mental approach to fibromyalgia is Respect and Responsibility. Having a painful syndrome is difficult because every day you hurt. I know this from personal and professional experience. We must understand and respect that fibromyalgia indeed does cause life-style altering pain, and that we will continue to have pain. Set a goal to achieve a minimal baseline level of pain. Try not to avoid doing something for fear of a flare-up. Rather, do whatever you can in spite of your fibromyalgia and its pain. You remember how you used to be before fibromyalgia, but now it is time to reset your mental thermostat to a level that accommodates some baseline pain.

The issue of control and fibromyalgia comes up frequently. While we have no control over whether or not we have fibromyalgia, we can learn to appreciate and respect the control we do have once we have the condition. We are able to control our posture, our response to stress, our activities, our home program, etc. We focus on respecting what we can control so we can decrease the risk of a fibromyalgia flare-up. In spite of doing everything right, we may still experience fibromyalgia flare-ups. However, by controlling what we can, we can reduce their number and frequency.

Good Pain Versus Bad Pain

I use the concept of good pain vs. bad pain as part of the control issue related to fibromyalgia. If we have chosen certain activities, we can deal with the consequences of increased pain because it is expected. If we like to wash the car one warm Sunday, then we can do it and accept the increased pain on Monday. After all, we did something we wanted to do. On the other hand, if we choose not to wash the car on Sunday and still wake up Monday with unexpected and severe pain, we consider this bad pain, or pain that we have no control over. It is better to make responsible choices in spite of having fibromyalgia than to use the condition as an excuse to evade responsibility.

> If we have chosen certain activities, we can deal with the consequences of increased pain.
>
> It is better to make responsible choices in spite of having fibromyalgia than to use the condition as an excuse to evade responsibility.

Find Balance

You need to seek a balance between detaching ourselves from fibromyalgia and integrating it into your everyday lives. Control what you can, learn what you can.

We tend to detach ourselves from our fibromyalgia by trying to ignore it or pretending we don't have it. When the pain level is lower, we may rationalize that there is no need to follow through with our home program since we "don't have a problem." Yet on the other hand, fibromyalgia goes with us wherever we go. It is always there to remind us that it is part of us. I am an optimist and believe that everyone can eventually find that balance, but he or she has to work very hard at it. The ultimate prize in mental coping is acceptance of fibromyalgia.

Chapter 21 — Survival Strategies

1) Learn the "effects of stress" to minimize how it bothers fibromyalgia.

2) Learn a new mental management strategy.

3) Reduce or eliminate negative thoughts to increase self-esteem and feelings of self worth.

4) Redefine your physical abilities.

5) Seek a new physical life-style with fibromyalgia.

6) Picture yourself in a more positive light.

7) Stop blaming yourself for having fibromyalgia.

8) Focus on your strengths.

9) Expect to live a good quality life in spite of having fibromyalgia.

10) Realize you will never be pain free. This is no longer a realistic expectation.

11) Achieving a low baseline of pain is our new goal.

12) Start a slow but long-lasting process of retraining your thinking.

13) Learn to ask for help.

14) Delegate tasks to others.

15) Remind yourself it is okay to ask for help.

16) Helping others, helps you!

17) Regain your ability to achieve relaxation.

18) Control what you can, learn what you can.

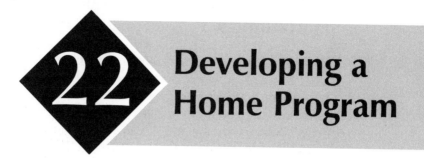

22 Developing a Home Program

Now that we have reviewed mental strategies, we need to include physical strategies for developing a successful home program. This is a difficult, yet necessary, challenge to help us cope with fibromyalgia. A home program can be time consuming, but it can also reduce the severe pain.

Our muscles are painful, tight, and easily fatigued, and when we attempt to exercise them, they often respond by increasing pain. Negative painful experiences may lead to decreased motivation, decreased activity, or exercise phobias. A cycle of increased muscle tightness, spasms, and pain starts again, and we seem to sink deeper and deeper into a painful unconditioned state. We want to accept responsibility for improving our activity level, and we need to choose wisely.

Basic Goals for a Home Exercise Program:

- **It is practical.** Buying a fifteen-piece indoor gym set for which we have to build an additional room isn't practical.

- **It should improve muscle endurance and fitness.** Even if it hurts, it is better to have fit and painful muscles than unconditioned and painful muscles!

- **The program can be easily modified.** If we have a flare-up, we should still be able to do the program, just less of it, or work on other parts of the body that are not painful.

- **The program should help maintain a stable baseline.** This is our prize goal, to reduce pain and keep it stable.

Our home exercise program is our responsibility and we have to be organized and consistent with it. Various medical professionals can help develop a home program: your doctor, physical therapist, massotherapist, fitness trainer, aquatics instructor, and aerobics instructor. As I have said over and over (and over!), no one program works best for everyone, but everyone should be able to find something that works. Each home program should include the following.

1. Fibronomics

2. Modalities

3. Stretching

4. Massage

5. Light conditioning

Fibronomics

Proper postures and fibronomics are the basic building blocks of a home program. There is a proper way of doing everything in our daily lives, whether we are at home, at work, or anyplace else. Once we practice these techniques, they will become automatic and ingrained in our subconscious so we don't have to think about them all the time. These techniques are discussed in Chapter 20.

Modalities

Modalities include heat, cold, electric stimulation, and water therapy. They can be applied at home to help relieve pain. Heat is the easiest home modality to apply and usually works the best. Heat can be a recurrent theme throughout the day: a heated mattress pad, an electric blanket, a hot morning shower, a heating pad during the day, heat-producing muscle creams before exercise, hot, jetted Jacuzzi after exercise, a hot tub in the evening. Since many fibromyalgia patients complain of cold skin and cold extremities, heat is a natural modality to warm the skin, improve the blood flow, relax muscles, and decrease pain.

Some people complain that a jetted Jacuzzi or whirlpool aggravates the tender points, due to the direct pressure. Other people describe it as a soothing massage effect. You need to determine if this approach would work for you prior to investing in a jetted Jacuzzi bathtub. A hot tub is a good investment for many people, since it not only allows deep therapeutic heat to relax the muscles, but it is mentally relaxing as well. If that is not feasible, taking a bath in water as hot as can be tolerated and soaking up to the top of your neck for 30 minutes can be an excellent substitute.

Hot showers are a great way to start off your stiff, painful morning. If you have a couple of tender areas that are particularly bothersome, a continuous hot shower stream on these areas can reduce the pain. If you are experiencing a flare-up, you can take extra showers during the day; or soak in the hot tub or a hot bath. You can never overheat your muscles by performing too many heat treatments during the day. Use heat more frequently during flare-ups, and once a stable baseline is achieved again, the usual program can be resumed.

Many people who use electric blankets will still complain of coldness coming from their mattress and sheets. I advise them to use an electric blanket only after having first acquired a heated mattress pad. Heat from below is better for skin and muscles than heat on top because the weight of our bodies pushing down on the heated surface increases the body surface area in contact with the heat, and improves heat conduction to the body. Plus, heat rises, so one wants heat rising from below to meet the body and not rising off the bed.

Some people like cold treatment, especially for muscle spasms. If you can stand the first five to ten minutes of an ice application, then a full twenty to thirty-minute treatment may provide considerable pain relief, muscle relaxation, and longer duration than heat.

Some people like cold treatment, especially for muscle spasms. If you can stand the first five to ten minutes of an ice application, then a full twenty to thirty-minute treatment may provide considerable pain relief, muscle relaxation, and longer duration than heat. However, very few people can tolerate the cold sensation against skin (including me) and opt instead for heat treatments. If heat is not effective, however, I always advise trying cold treatment, such as an ice pack or ice massage, to see if this modality is helpful. One patient told me she used a refrigerated gel pack for 10 minutes, then used the ice pack on that "cool" area and the ice pack didn't bother her skin.

Many people have found a TENS unit to be helpful. This is device that emits an electrical buzz that blocks the pain, and can be worn and used for different painful regions of the body. If this particular modality is helpful to an individual, he or she will continue to use it in spite of the hassles that are involved (putting the pads and wires in place, carrying the unit around, adjusting the controls, etc.).

Stretching

Stretching is a vital part of a fibromyalgia person's home program, and we need to stretch frequently during the day. Because muscles are so tight, they are more vulnerable to strains, so it is especially important that we counteract this tightness by stretching. I have often been asked if I had to choose one thing to do in a home program, what would I choose; and the answer is: stretching. If you are going to choose stretching, choose to do it regularly and consistently. You should stretch in the morning, stretch during the day, and stretch at night.

There are some general rules with stretching. Always move slowly and gently without jerking motions, and make sure there is no restrictive clothing or jewelry. Wear comfortable clothing. When you stretch, hold to a slow count of 3 to 10. When you first start, hold for only 3 seconds, and when you become more experienced, gradually increase your ability to hold for the full 10 seconds.

How does one begin a stretching program? I like to begin by teaching my patients passive stretching techniques. These do not require any specific equipment and can be done anywhere.

There are some general rules with stretching. Always move slowly and gently without jerking motions, and make sure there is no restrictive clothing or jewelry. Wear comfortable clothing. When you stretch, hold to a slow count of 3 to 10. When you first start, hold for only 3 seconds, and when you become more experienced, gradually increase your ability to hold for the full 10 seconds. Find a feeling of stretch within your comfort zone. Remember to practice deep breathing exercises as part of your stretching.

Repetitions should be started at a low number and increased. If you have been sedentary for a long period of time, you should begin with a schedule of doing all the stretching exercises, but each one only once, holding each stretch for 3 seconds. Over the first week, progress from stretching once a day to stretching twice a day, each stretch up to 3 seconds of holding. During the second week, progress to stretching twice a day, holding for 5 seconds, and repeating each exercise 3 times.

In each successive week, increase the time held in each stretch by 2 seconds, and the number of repetitions by 2, until you reach a maximum of 10 seconds and 10 repetitions twice a day.

These above guidelines are for a person who has been sedentary for a long while and is just beginning to exercise. Note that I have emphasized slow, gradual stretching over an entire month before even adding any type of conditioning-type exercise. A controlled, gradually increasing stretching program as described should minimize the pain and still allow progressive improvement. Ice after stretching, muscle creams, and over-the-counter antiinflammatory medicines can be used to help smooth over the transition period.

Certainly one can speed up the progression and perform stretching numerous times during the day. I recommend stretching at least twice a day in the training process, and increase as tolerated. I encourage people to always think about stretching as part of their daily routine.

Passive stretching exercises can be done on different body parts: head, neck, trunk, shoulder, upper body, low back, hip, and legs. Dozens of stretching exercises are possible, and all of them can be beneficial if done properly. The following are descriptions and diagrams of these types of passive stretching exercises.

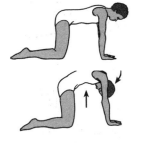

Head and neck forward stretch:

Lie on your back with your knees bent and feet flat.

Place hands behind head with fingers on head and thumbs at the bottom of the skull.

Gently lift head with hands forward and chin toward chest and go to the comfort zone; hold to a count of from 3 to 10 as tolerated.

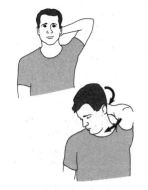

Head and neck lateral stretch:

Place one hand on the opposite side of head below ear, gently pull and turn head so nose points to underarm.

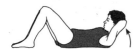

Thoracic or trunk stretches:

Cat back on all fours. Start with hands and knees on floor, head positioned between shoulders. Let back sag, keep head parallel to floor. Lower head with chin to chest, tighten stomach and arch back as high as possible.

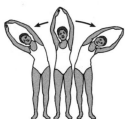

Lateral side bends:

Lateral side bends. These are performed against the wall and are called teapot exercises. Stand so your back and shoulders touch the wall. Cross your arms over your head making sure that your elbows and your head touch the wall, slowly bend your upper body to your right and then to your left, keeping your feet on the floor.

Shoulder girdle and upper body:

Hold a towel overhead with hands at either end of it, and gently pull from side to side.

Another exercise is to clasp your hands behind your back and lift your arms upward until you feel a comfortable stretch.

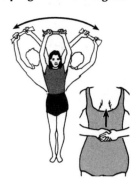

Pectoral stretch:

Stand facing a wall and place both hands on the wall at shoulder height. Turn body away to one side, keeping the shoulders in the same position and keep turning until a stretch is felt in the pectoralis muscle. Lean the body towards the wall to increase the stretch. Repeat the steps for the opposite side.

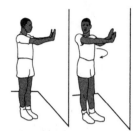

Latissimus dorsi stretch:

Kneel on the floor with elbows and hands placed together on a chair. Slowly move your chest towards the floor and sit back towards your heels until the stretch is felt.

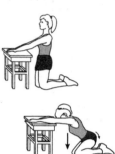

Low back:

Single knee to chest, and then both knees to chest.

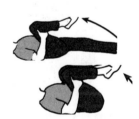

Low back and hip:

Lie on back with knees bent and feet flat on the floor. Rotate knees from one side to the other.

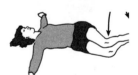

Piriformis stretch:

Start on your hands and knees. Place the left foot across your body and directly in front of the right knee. Turn your left knee out slightly to the side. Keep your shoulders and hips square and slide your right leg backwards, gradually sinking down until you feel a stretch in the left buttock/piriformis muscle. Resting on your elbows as you sink down is more comfortable. You should not feel pain in the low back or during this stretch. Reverse technique to stretch the opposite side.

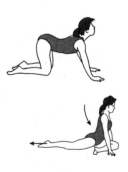

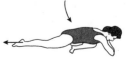

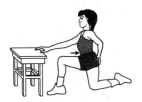

Kneeling hip flexor stretch:

Kneel with the right knee on the floor and the opposite hip and knee flexed to 90 degrees. Maintain an upright trunk and hold onto a chair with the left hand. Position the right leg so the right hip is rotated inward. Place the right hand on the right buttock and flatten the stomach. Contract the right buttock muscle and feel the stretch in the right front thigh. Reverse the process for the other side.

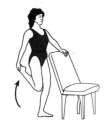

Quadriceps:

While standing, stabilize yourself with a chair or table.

Pull your foot up towards your buttock and keep your hip as straight as possible.

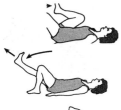

Hamstring stretch:

Take one knee to the chest and slowly straighten out the knee while allowing the leg to return to floor.

Hold the leg as high as possible with the knee straight to a count of 3 to 10 as tolerated.

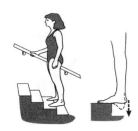

Calf-Step stretching:

Any step will work, but it is best to use stairs that have a railing for better support.

Place the ball of the foot (the padding just before your toes start) on the step, letting your heel sag over the edge of the step and press down until you feel a comfortable stretch.

Bed stretches:

Passive stretching should start in bed before getting up in the morning. Following are suggested bed stretches. These should be done while lying in bed prior to getting up. Stretch and hold each position for 3 seconds.

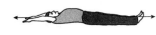

Arm and leg reach:

Reach your arms up as far as you can with your legs straight out and feet and toes pointed ballet style.

Chin tuck:

Place your arms behind your head and push your head forward so your chin touches your chest.

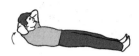

Neck push back:

Look up and back as far as you can, pressing your head into the pillow. Turn your head to the side, pressing your cheek into the pillow. Repeat with the other side.

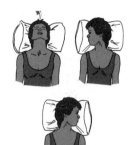

Neck extension with chin press:

Start to tilt your head backward, and at same time try to press your chin into your chest.

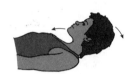

Alternate knee to chest:

While lying on your back, bend your knee to your chest, holding with the arm on the same side. Repeat on the other side.

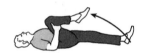

After your stretches are completed, log roll out of bed using proper body mechanics.

Good morning!

Stretching in the shower can be especially effective since you can use the warm water. In addition, it helps you start off your morning with stretching at a time when your muscles are usually the tightest.

These pages have given examples of stretches in different situations. One can stretch any part of the body, and I have not demonstrated every possible stretch. An excellent reference book is *Stretching* by Bob Anderson.

Therabands

Exercise using elastic bands (Therabands) can provide dynamic stretching to increase strength and flexibility of our muscles. These are not aerobic exercises, but can be very effective. The rubberized elastic bands come in different colors which represent different strengths or tensions. These bands look flimsy, and one may wonder how they can be effective in an exercise program, but they can provide excellent resistance for the muscles. The harder you pull and stretch them, the more the tension on the muscles. Thicker bands provide more tension.

I have found theraband exercises to be effective for many patients. These exercises require instruction and practice to work best. Sometimes you don't realize how hard you are working with the bands, so you need to be careful not to overdo the first few times you use the bands. Once the exercises are learned, the individual can perform them as part of a self-program.

Here are some examples of basic theraband exercises that can be helpful in stretching and strengthening the upper body and arms especially.

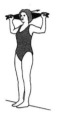

1. Place the theraband behind your head. Your knees should be slightly bent and your back flat. Push your head into the band so that your chin stays parallel with the floor. Push straight back. Don't forget to breathe!

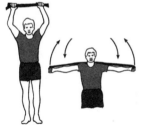

2. Take the theraband in both hands; start with your arms straight out in front and pull them backwards until they touch the wall.

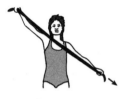

3. Take the theraband in both hands. Start with your arms straight out in front of you diagonally. Pull your arms backwards until they touch the wall.

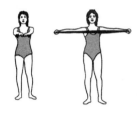

4. Start with your arms overhead holding a theraband. Pull downward until your arms are level with your shoulders. Hold your shoulder blades down as you relax your arms and move them upwards.

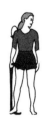

5. Place a theraband under one foot. Turn your head so that your chin is over the opposite shoulder and look down. Grasp the theraband and roll your shoulder up, back and down without bending your wrist.

Practice deep breathing techniques while doing these theraband exercises. Once you are comfortably instructed, begin a regular theraband program ranging from 3 times a week to every day. Like stretching exercises, the theraband should be slowly moved to position and then held to the count of 3 and slowly returned to the starting position. There is resistance from the bands during both the stretch and return. An exercise session can include an increasing number of repetitions up to 10 of each exercise if the individual can tolerance it. I advise my patients to perform therapy and exercises regularly whether or not they are having pain.

One woman with upper back pain found theraband exercises very effective in keeping her pain under control. However, she stopped doing the exercises in January because of various other projects and experienced a flare-up of upper back pain in February. Her flare-up persisted in spite of continuing the other components of her program. Once we realized that she had stopped her theraband exercises, she resumed them and reported that her upper back pain decreased and stabilized again. This is an example of how a particular exercise can be helpful, but it needs to be continued on a regular basis. If the exercises work, do them!

Massage

Massages are a wonderful way to decrease pain, relax muscles, improve blood circulation, passively stretch muscles, and overall, let you feel good.

Massotherapy could be done daily if a person had access to this treatment. However, our health care system does not usually pay for such daily intensive treatment. If massotherapy works for you, try to have it done once or twice a month at least. (If you've won the lottery, have it done weekly!) Family members or significant others can be trained to perform therapeutic massages for you.

It has been my experience that massotherapy does not aggravate the muscles, even though the first 1 or 2 treatments may cause increased muscle soreness, so ice, heat, creams or medicines afterwards may be helpful. Once the muscles become used to the technique, the usual response is one of considerable relaxation and decreased pain. Usually people leave the massotherapy room with a natural euphoric feeling.

Self-massage is a fairly simple procedure that can be learned and performed effectively. Self-massage can be performed any time, but is often best done in the shower where the hand can glide easily by using soap. Stretching is easily combined with self-massage. One massotherapist who has worked with hundreds of fibromyalgia patients likes to instruct patients to give themselves a hug when taking a morning shower. This provides stretching, self-massage — and starting the day off with a hug! Remember to hug thyself frequently!

Light Conditioning

People with fibromyalgia may not tolerate a lot of exercise, as a general rule, but a little bit of exercise is helpful. A light conditioning program means enough exercise to stimulate the cardiovascular system and strengthen the muscles without overworking or exhausting them and causing increased pain. When we resume exercising, our muscles have to go through a "learning curve" again. So expect to be sore at first. Some people with fibromyalgia are exercise intolerant, and any exercise, or even stretching, will aggravate the pain. Most people will be able to find some exercise/stretching program that helps (not hurts!) them. Any increased activity is better than no activity.

Set realistic goals for the body that are well beyond high school! We have to realize what we can reasonably accomplish, for example, a good workout for 30 minutes, 3 times a week. Don't put pressure on yourself to exercise longer and harder in order to feel better. I always tell patients that the amount of time spent exercising is not as important as the actual effort to exercise.

The keys to a successful exercise program are as follows:

1. Emphasize stretching and flexibility exercises of all major muscle groups and focus on a warm-up period that consists of stretching only.

2. Add a low impact, aerobic type program (light conditioning). Such a program can include walking, water aerobics, using an exercise bicycle, or performing a low impact aerobic program.

3. Gradually progress in an exercise program as tolerated. The goal is to achieve improvement and a stable baseline.

4. Continue a regular exercise program at least three times a week, even on days when there is increased pain.

5. Follow proper posture and body mechanics to minimize strain of the muscles and joints.

Light conditioning involves periods of stretching, strengthening, relaxation, and actual conditioning. Any conditioning program involves proper warm-up, breathing techniques, good posture, awareness of the body's response, and a cool-down period. Forms of exercise that fall into the category of light conditioning include weights, walking, cycling, stair machines, arm pulleys, aquatics, aerobics, and dancing.

A light conditioning program should not be started until you are comfortable with a regular daily stretching program. For individuals who are more active, a light conditioning program can be started soon after completing a regular instruction program. Perform light conditioning exercises for 20 to 30 minutes at least 3 times a week. As a rule, one should skip every other day to allow the body a chance to rest and recuperate, but this differs according to the individual's abilities and needs. When beginning, it is best to exercise about 10 minutes per session for the first week, and then gradually increase 5 to 10 minutes each week until you reach at least 30 minutes 3 times a week.

Light conditioning does not necessarily entail intensive aerobic activity for 30 minutes. It can involve periods of stretching, strengthening, relaxation, and actual conditioning. This alternating strategy usually works best for fibromyalgia muscles that do not like too much of one thing at any given time. Any conditioning program involves proper warm-up, breathing techniques, good posture, awareness of the body's response, and a cool-down period. Forms of exercise that fall into the category of light conditioning include weights, walking, cycling, stair machines, arm pulleys, aquatics, aerobics, and dancing.

Weight-lifting

Weight-lifting is a category of exercise that emphasizes strengthening, but there are stretching and conditioning components as well, especially if the exercise is repeated a number of times. People with more severe forms of fibromyalgia usually do not tolerate any type of weight-lifting, either free weights or machines. It appears that the continuous resistance on the muscles overstimulates them and increases the pain.

For individuals who have tried weight-lifting and continue to experience increased pain, I usually recommend avoiding weights altogether. These people should use alternative exercises which allow variable resistance on the muscles and are usually tolerated better.

Many people with milder forms of fibromyalgia can develop a very successful weight-lifting program without muscle flare-ups. In these people, the practice should be to use less weight and more repetitions to minimize microscopic tears or strains to the muscles and increase endurance and energy. Free weights and variable resistance weight machines seem to work best. If your fibromyalgia has reached a point where you have difficulty doing any type of exercise, I would not advise a weight-lifting program.

Walking

Walking is a very effective form of light conditioning exercise. Wear soft cushioned comfortable shoes. Rubberized tracks are the best surfaces to walk on as they minimize the impact to your feet and ultimately your back. Walking with a buddy is a great way to motivate and commit yourself to this type of exercise.

When beginning a walking program, you can alternate 5 minutes of brisk walking with 5 minutes of leisurely walking, and repeat this cycle. The goal is to gradually increase your brisk walking to at least 20 to 30 minutes 3 times a week.

Some people do not tolerate walking because of particular pain in the low back, hip, or leg areas. However, others who have predominantly upper body pain may find walking the best way to loosen up these sore muscles. The upper body and arms can get involved with walking, particularly brisk walking with a lot of arm swinging. Increased heart rate and stimulated respiratory drive makes this exercise a beneficial cardiovascular and aerobic activity as well.

I am frequently asked if any certain exercise equipment is helpful in fibromyalgia. I always advise people that anything can be tried, but before making a large purchase, one should try several sessions of exercise on that particular piece of equipment, either at a health spa or at a friend's house. If you like the exercise, tolerate it well, and feel it is helpful, then you can consider purchasing it. Too many of my patients have unused exercise equipment sitting in their basements. Try before you buy!

Here are some considerations for different types of exercise equipment:

Treadmill

Many people prefer to use a treadmill for controlled walking exercise. I thought I would enjoy this type of activity, but after I purchased a treadmill, I found this type of walking to be too artificial. There is something about walking but not seeing things move past me that bothers me. I have a hard time maintaining an exact rhythm as I prefer to be able to vary my pace and I tend to lose my balance every so often. I found that a slight loss of balance on the treadmill could throw me off it entirely! Even though I prefer natural walking, I still encourage people to consider treadmill walking if they are interested, but try it before you purchase the machine. If you like your trial, I know where you can get a cheap treadmill that has hardly been used!

Exercise cycle

The biggest potential problem with an exercise cycle is malpositioning on the unit. If the seat is too narrow or the handlebars are too far out in front, you could be in a position where you are leaning forward and reaching out with your arms, creating a lot of neck and back strain. Wide, comfortable seat and handlebars that reach out so you can hold them and still be in a comfortably aligned position are necessary. Persons with painful knees may not tolerate stationary bikes at all, although the seat height can be raised to decrease strain and painful movements of the knees. Exercise cycles that allow a reclined position can be very effective for fibromyalgia patients since they minimize the strain on the low back and arms.

Stair machine (StairMaster)

This equipment emphasizes strengthening the gluteal and leg muscles. Many people with fibromyalgia can only handle this type of machine for a short period of time before cramping increases, especially in the calves. Those with knee pain may find this exercise too aggravating. If you can tolerate and progress with this machine, it is an excellent workout.

Arm pulley systems

These systems may be part of a treadmill, stationary bicycle, or other leg exercise apparatus. The main problem with this type of system, for people with fibromyalgia, is that it puts a lot of strain on the arms, particularly with all the reaching, pulling, and squeezing involved. The arms usually tire very quickly. People who have difficulty reaching out with their arms will usually not tolerate any arm pulley system as part of an exercise program, but some systems, which don't require as much reaching, are tolerated well.

Aquatics

Another popular form of exercise is aquatics. Water exercises provide an opportunity to stretch, strengthen, and condition the body. The water supports the spine and extremities and acts as a brace and massager. Those who have difficulty holding their arms out in front may do so more comfortably as the water buoys the arms. Standing chest high in water will remove much of the gravity in the lower back area, which may dramatically reduce pain.

Numerous aquatic exercise classes are available for people with arthritis and fibromyalgia. Warm water is necessary. Ideally water temperature should be 88 degrees or higher, although many pools keep the temperature for these types of classes around 85 degrees. Various aquatic equipment is available to help work out in the water.

Like other forms of exercise, one needs to first try the water program to determine if it is helpful. Some individuals do not tolerate the cold feeling in the water or the air drafts that cool the skin. Wearing a wet suit or long sleeve shirt in the pool and having lots of dry towels ready as soon as you get out can help avoid the cold.

Others describe the process of changing into a bathing suit, getting into the pool, getting out of the pool, showering, drying the hair, and getting dressed again to be too much of a hassle even though there may be some benefits. However, many people, particularly those who have tried land exercises without success, and who may have particular problems with the low back, pelvic, hips, and leg areas, respond very nicely to an aquatics exercise program. I recommend that these exercises be done first with an aquatics instructor, usually in a class. Choose a pool with warm water and warm, still air around it! Individual programs can be developed if group aquatic exercises are helpful.

Aerobics

Traditional aerobics are not tolerated very well by people with fibromyalgia, since it involves a lot of exercises with the arms out or overhead, prolonged standing, and high bodily impact. Low impact aerobics may be better tolerated. Arm exercises and standing still are difficult for many people. Step aerobics are popular, and some individuals with milder fibromyalgia may do well with these.

Modified aerobics, if tailored to the individual, can provide effective light conditioning. Chair aerobics is an example. The individual sits as much as possible to unload the spine. Activities are done primarily from the chest level and below, avoiding any overhead arm activities. Higher impact movements are modified. For example, walking movements may be simulated by "marching" while seated. Stretching is emphasized and problem areas are moved slowly. Exercises are designed to stretch the tight muscles, usually the chest and quadriceps, while strengthening the weaker muscles, usually back and hamstrings, and also to achieve a better posture. Therabands are commonly used in chair aerobics.

Dancing

Many of my patients have found dancing to be a great workout that they tolerate well. Jazzercise, line dancing, polka dancing, and good old rock and roll are examples of light conditioning and aerobic exercises that have worked for various people. Some dance to video tapes and others go to public dance floors. Remember to stretch and warm up before turning yourself loose!

Summary

As always, the key to the numerous types of exercise is to actually do something! Professional guidance and supervision are available to help you find the right program for you, but it is your responsibility to do something, and to do it regularly and consistently. You should stretch before and after exercising, and you should stretch just about any other time in between! You may prefer to exercise at home because you can be more independent and flexible in a convenient location. You also don't have to worry about being embarrassed by others watching you, if that is a concern.

On the other hand, working out in a gym or spa allows you to get away on a predictable schedule and be in a social setting. Paying for a membership often motivates a person to follow through regularly, and positive results will increase your confidence and self esteem.

Activating muscles can be painful at first, but it is not harmful. You are not hurting yourself and you will be able to work through this initial pain. Temporary flare-ups can occur when one is starting an exercise program, but support and supervision from your medical professionals will enable you to overcome any initial difficulties and "get over the hump," so to speak.

Once a successful exercise program is underway, I believe that subsequent flare-ups are very rarely due to the actual exercise program. (See Chapter 35, Handling Flare-ups). You may need to modify your exercise program during the flare-up, but it is important that you continue exercising in spite of the flare-up. If you stop using or exercising the other muscles, they will get tighter and will quickly become unconditioned, that is, they will get weaker and have less stamina. It then becomes even harder to reactivate the muscles. Muscles that are flared-up need to be exercised to keep them as flexible and conditioned as possible, even though they hurt more.

Adding extra modalities can also help you return to a stable baseline. Don't stop everything, though. You will be surprised to find you can still follow through with an exercise program even when you have more pain.

Chapter 22 — Survival Strategies

Home Program

1) Realize your muscles are painful, tight, and easily fatigued, and that is before exercising!

2) Accept that we cannot do what we did in high school.

3) Understand that people with fibromyalgia have a limited tolerance for exercise.

4) Our home program is our responsibility.

5) Redefine what exercise means.

6) Expect a 30 minute activity to have periods of stretching, relaxation, and conditioning. 30 minutes start to finish, not 30 minutes of intensive aerobic activity. Continue to exercise in spite of flare-ups.

7) Consider stretching as a form of exercise.

8) Expect some discomfort when beginning exercise.

9) Work through that period.

10) Explore the use of massage in your home program.

11) Remember that the amount of time spent exercising is not as important as the actual effort to exercise.

12) "Try before you buy" any exercise equipment.

13) Consider walking, aquatics, dancing.

23 ▸ Managing Fatigue

Chronic fatigue syndrome (CFS) is a condition that is very similar to fibromyalgia. In fact, many medical professionals believe that the two are actually the same condition. CFS may be a subset of a broader fibromyalgia syndrome.

In the fibromyalgia spectrum I've described (Chapter 10), I would put chronic fatigue syndrome in subset 6: fibromyalgia with a particular associated condition. The particular associated condition is chronic fatigue syndrome.

In CFS support groups and fibromyalgia support groups I have attended, both pain and fatigue are frequent topics of discussion. A person with CFS who sees me usually has other associated conditions including sleep disorder, headache, muscle pain, joint pain, difficulty concentrating, and neurologic symptoms. Not surprisingly, the exam usually reveals typical painful tender points. Overall, I treat patients with CFS pretty much the same way I treat patients with fibromyalgia, especially if those with chronic fatigue syndrome are having a lot of pain.

I think one person describing her fatigue said it best. She said her eyelids felt like cement weights. Fatigue can be an overwhelming problem in fibromyalgia, and unfortunately many people get the double curse, both severe pain and severe fatigue. Why do patients with fibromyalgia (and CFS) have such a problem with fatigue? There are probably multiple reasons and a combination of contributing factors. These reasons include:

1) **Non-restorative sleep disorder.** Restoration that should be occurring during the deep stage of sleep is not happening. Manufacture of proteins, replenishment of energy stores, and repair of tissues are incomplete. (Chapter 26 will review in more detail.)

2) **Deconditioned muscles.** Deconditioned muscles in fibromyalgia have lost their ability to make the body's energy molecules called ATP (adenosine triphosphate). This energy molecule is stored in our tissues, particularly muscles, and is used as fuel to enable the body to perform all of its functions, including muscle contractions. The less ATP around, the less energy available, and once the stored supplies are used up, fatigue occurs. If this process occurs quickly, one may feel a sudden, unpredictable energy crash.

3) **Constant pain.** The body's process of monitoring pain, recording pain, and expressing pain is energy consuming and involves nerves, neurotransmitters, and other enzymes and hormones. The patient in constant pain will use up more energy and have less stored energy than normal.

4) **Decreased oxygen use by the muscles.** Studies have shown that muscles with fibromyalgia do not use oxygen as well as normal muscles. This may reflect a

problem with the muscle mitochondria, the small organelles that use oxygen and manufacture ATP. A biochemical problem may prevent the available oxygen from being used efficiently and adequately to create ATP.

5) **Associated clinical depression.** Depression is seen in nearly half of patients with fibromyalgia and can cause extreme mental fatigue.

6) **Associated chronic conditions** such as arthritis, hypothyroidism, or other disease. People with fibromyalgia may have other conditions that consume a lot of energy and contribute to excessive fatigue.

7) **Cognitive factors.** An inherent neurasthenia factor with fibromyalgia causes difficulty with concentration and attention, increased anxiety, increased sensitivity to depression, and absentmindedness. This is our fibro-fog.

8) **Dysfunctional autonomic nervous system.** We are more prone to anxiety and panic attacks, Raynaud's phenomenon, fast heart rate (especially in response to stress), rashes on the skin (especially in response to touch), throat tightness, and other symptoms that are all consequences of an over-sensitized autonomic nervous system.

   The autonomic nerves, as you may recall, are the small nerves in the body that interconnect the major nerves with the various tissues such as blood vessels, bones, muscles, and organs. These nerves are responsible for keeping the internal body in harmony with the outside environment. Body functions that are managed by the autonomic nerves include sweating, digestion, pain regulation, and blushing. The dysfunctional autonomic nervous system demands and depletes more energy, thus less is available for muscle activity and movement.

9) **Visual overload.** I use this term to describe the overwhelming information our eyes receive and have difficulty interpreting, as I reviewed in Chapter 4. We try to spot a particular object but are confronted with a variety of shapes, sizes, colors, and lines in different directions that literally overwhelm our visual senses and at times cause a feeling of dizziness, light-headedness and increased anxiety. I believe this contributes to fatigue by demanding so much energy to sort out this information.

10) **Decreased respiratory endurance.** Many patients with fibromyalgia complain about their shortness of breath with short bursts of activity such as climbing steps, running or walking swiftly. They may actually have difficulty catching their breath. This respiratory complaint may be from sudden exercise-induced fatigue of the respiratory muscles that disrupts the breathing rhythm. The complaint seems to be independent of whether or not the person is out of condition or living a sedentary life-style. Since an efficient breathing process is necessary to deliver oxygen to the bloodstream, any problem in this area will certainly create potential for fatigue.

11) **Constant muscle movements.** People with fibromyalgia are frequently shifting their bodies to find more comfortable positions. Habitual movements such as tapping fingers on the table, tapping or bouncing the feet on the ground, frequent crossing of the legs, and kicking out a leg are probably subconscious movements to relieve muscle stress, keep the blood flowing, and readjusting the muscles and posture to try to decrease the pain. How-

ever, the side effect of these movement patterns is increased energy consumption.

12) **Hormonal problems.** Decreased supply of hormones or inefficient use of available hormones may factor into fatigue. Low growth hormone and low thyroid levels are common in fibromyalgia and can decrease energy metabolism and hence increase fatigue. Altered stress mechanisms in our bodies will increase energy consumption and interfere with efficient use of energy, hence fatigue is worsened. Other hormones that can cause fatigue when in short supply are estrogen and serotonin (a brain hormone).

Whatever the cause of fatigue, it creates problems in our daily activities. The major negative effect of fatigue is increased pain which in turn consumes more energy and causes further fatigue — a self-perpetuating cycle of pain and fatigue.

Fatigue interferes with our ability and motivation to socialize, carry out daily routine chores, and perform our jobs properly. When one is fatigued, it is difficult to converse or communicate, thus interfering with our relationships. Muscles become more deconditioned and we experience decreased overall cardiovascular fitness. We may develop feelings of depression and overall decreased well-being. Even if we have no energy, we still tend to feel stressed and, like the pain, the additional stress consumes more energy and further increases our fatigue.

There are some strategies for treating fatigue. Fatigue will probably never be completely eliminated, but many things can be done to control its consequences and minimize its impact on everyday life. Your doctor may first want to investigate for underlying diseases such as hypothyroidism, sleep disorders, anemia, and connective tissue disease, which involve different treatment approaches. If there are no significant underlying diseases present, the fatigue may be attributed to the fibromyalgia syndrome (or chronic fatigue syndrome).

What steps can be taken to minimize the potential debilitating effects of fatigue? Below is a list of strategies that I have found helpful.

1) **Develop good sleep habits.** Quality sleep is necessary for the body to manufacture energy. Develop a good sleep routine.

2) **Avoid long daytime naps.** Although fatigue may be compelling at times, it is best to try to avoid taking naps since this alters the body's sleep rhythm. Naps are often non-refreshing and time-consuming. Upon awakening, many people feel even less energetic and have more difficulty getting going again. They may even have a period of increased confusion and mental fogginess.

In some people, however, a strategic nap (less than one hour) accomplishes its goal by refreshing and restoring the individual for more successful completion of the rest of the day. As long as the primary nighttime sleep is not disturbed any more than usual, these naps are not to be discouraged. However, it is my experience (and sleep studies show) that most people who try to overcome fatigue with a nap actually do not accomplish the refreshing and restoring mood that they are seeking, and the evening sleep pattern is disrupted.

3) **Proper nutrition.** I reviewed a dietary strategy in Chapter 14. A high protein and low carbohydrate diet has helped many people improve their energy.

Diets too rich in fat can put the body into a lazy mode, but if you reduce your fats at the expense of getting too little protein, you may have more fatigue, so find your balance.

4) **Medications (natural and prescription).** The dozens of natural supplements advertised to increase energy are successful for some people. However, many energy products contain the stimulants caffeine or ephedrine, which can have long-term adverse effects on the body and can be dangerous if taken together. Before trying any natural energy product, I recommend first consulting with your doctor.

Certain prescription medicines (*i.e.* Cylert, Ritalin) can be prescribed by your doctor in cases of extreme fatigue causing debilitating functional problems. These medicines are the same ones used for children with attention deficit disorders. If underlying depression is a problem, your physician may opt to prescribe an antidepressant medication because improving the depression will usually improve the fatigue as well.

My advice is to routinely plan some activity, especially for after supper, that includes running errands, getting outside, visiting people, or just staying up on your feet. You will be surprised to learn how frequently a second wind will come. Many people have a natural rhythm that causes low energy in the late afternoon and early evening, but then the mood and energy level swings back up again.

5) **Follow proper fibronomics.** Maintaining proper body posture at home and at work will not only conserve energy, but decrease pain.

6) **Plan scheduled activities,** especially in the evening. The late afternoon and early evening are often the most difficult times for persons with fatigue. After supper can be an especially difficult time, especially if the person sits down to relax or lies down to read the paper. "Crashing" and inability to do any useful activity for the rest of the evening may occur.

My advice is to routinely plan some activity, especially for after supper, that includes running errands, getting outside, visiting people, or just staying up on your feet. You will be surprised to learn how frequently a second wind will come. Many people have a natural rhythm that causes low energy in the late afternoon and early evening, but then the mood and energy level swings back up again. If you are a night owl, you tend to feel better and more energetic around 9 p.m. and may have a few good hours where you feel alert and can accomplish a lot. Recognize your own biorhythm and take advantage of it to plan your best work around your high points and to try to stimulate yourself through the low points by involving yourself in an activity.

7) **Divide your task into smaller projects** instead of one big one. Do a little at a time and do more at your best time. For example, yard work can be divided into specific chores for different nights of the week. You may mow the front lawn one night, the back another, and trim on a third night, instead of doing all three in one day. If we are moving and decide to do our own packing, it is much easier to pack a box per day for the six weeks prior to the actual moving date, than to try to do all the packing in one or two days before the actual move. This type of self-discipline is also needed when vacationing and decorating for the holidays. (Actually, self discipline could help a lot of things!)

8) **Perform regular exercise and relaxation.** Exercise increases endurance, cardio-vascular conditioning, and a sense of well being. Relaxation decreases stress and reduces pain. A 30-minute brisk walk after supper provides exercise and mental relaxation and counteracts the low biorhythm point at the same time. One does not have to sit perfectly still to physically and mentally relax; in fact, this often increases fatigue and the tendency to sleep. Remember to relax, not nap.

9) **Make a daily schedule** and check off things as you accomplish. Allow plenty of time to complete the task. By keeping a structured list, you have a better chance of motivating yourself to reach daily goals.

10) **Delegate chores to others.** One of the best energy-saving techniques known is to have someone else use his or her energy to do your task. While delegating responsibilities is difficult for many people, there are others who will gladly perform certain chores for you. It is best to be as independent as possible, but it is better to allow someone else to help if it means you will have energy for a longer portion of your day.

Hopefully, some of these weapons can help you combat fatigue. Remember that fatigue, like pain, is a "relative" problem (no, I don't mean cousin Vito!). The problem is always there, but you try to achieve a lower, more functional state that, relative to the previous level, is considered a successful, manageable level.

Chapter 23 — Survival Strategies

1) Avoid the cycle of pain and fatigue by identifying the major-energy draining activities in your day.

2) Delegate those identified activities to others when possible.

3) Minimizing fatigue's impact on every day life is your goal.

4) Work with your doctor and investigate whether any underlying diseases or conditions are contributing to your fatigue.

5) Review fatigue factors such as sleep habits, nutrition, medications, fibronomics. Work to change or eliminate negative factors.

6) Practice "self-discipline" in dividing tasks into smaller projects. Resist that "urge" to do "just one more thing." You only have so much energy per day. Think and plan how you will spend it.

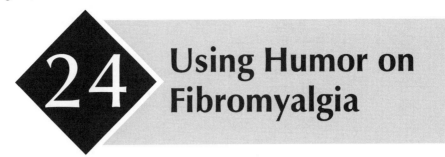

24 Using Humor on Fibromyalgia

Fibromyalgia is not a funny condition. It causes severe pain and disabilities, and it affects every aspect of our lives. Sometimes, however, we need to take a break from our pain and try to laugh.

Laughing is therapeutic, especially when we can laugh at ourselves. Norman Cousins wrote a classic article in the *New England Journal of Medicine* that became the first chapter of his book, *Anatomy of an Illness.* In it he describes how laughter helped him overcome a painful connective tissue disease. Physiologically, laughing helps us by:

- Increasing release of endorphins, our natural painkillers.

- Improving blood flow and relaxing muscles.

- Stimulating the brain centers that tell us to feel good.

- Temporarily blocking pain signals.

- Improving body's homeostasis, including our immune

  function.

If we can learn to laugh at ourselves, we may find it easier to cope with fibromyalgia. I've always tried to keep my sense of humor in spite of my pain, and I've appreciated over the years that people with fibromyalgia, as a group, have a great sense of humor. You know all of the bad things about the condition and how it affects your everyday life. Whenever we think we are feeling a little bit better, something will happen to remind us we still have pain. There is so much we can't control: the weather, what others think or do, and what life's next surprise will be.

Maybe, though, we can learn to approach our fibromyalgia with a lighter attitude. I say that if we are stuck with this miserable daily pain, we should try to laugh at it. It is like dark humor. In some aspects it is sad, but we can make humor of the situation to better cope with it. Plus, we are more fun to be around if we are funny or at least trying to be positive.

There are various ways we can poke fun at our fibromyalgia, you know, take a light look and lighten up.

1) Think of advantages of having fibromyalgia.

Perhaps not all of fibromyalgia has to be bad. Think of some good things that happen from having fibromyalgia. It provides convenient excuses for our mistakes: "I forgot the meeting? Oh, sorry, must be my fibromyalgia, it affects my memory."

"Darn, I broke the glass. That fibromyalgia makes me drop things."

It saves you money. No need to purchase alarm clocks, self-installed appliances, or vacuum cleaners.

Since you can't do anything else, it enables you to spend more time watching TV and adding to your knowledge. You can learn all about what movie stars like to eat and what cars they drive, natural habitats for iguanas and other lizards, and other interesting information.

It allows you to eliminate unenjoyable activities such as mowing the lawn, visiting certain relatives, and cleaning out the garage.

The best reason of all for making jokes about our fibromyalgia is that only people with fibromyalgia will understand. We have our own club. We're special indeed!

2) Look at things from a different light.

Think about situations you get into with fibromyalgia and add your own unique flavor to emphasize a point and make it humorous. One way to do this is to come up with some funny definitions of common situations that happen with fibromyalgia.

Here are some examples.

Fibronyms: Words that take on a unique meaning when pertaining to our fibromyalgia.

Mack truck: A popular vehicle that frequently runs over fibromyalgia patients while they are asleep.

Groan-up: Adult fibromyalgia patient.

Pain pal: A fibromyalgia colleague who understands what we are going through.

Pain in the neck: A fibromyalgia person who has a whiplash injury.

Painstaking: The diligent care and effort taken when palpating and mapping out the painful tender points.

Ambidextrous: The ability to be equally clumsy with both hands.

Etiquette: Knowing the proper way to tell people you have completely forgotten their name.

Expert: Someone who doesn't know any more than you do about fibromyalgia, but uses slides.

Fibro-fog: Mental state where 60% of the time, one is confused and absent minded, and the other 60% of the time, has difficulty concentrating and remembering things.

3) Make up a funny list.

Write down a list of things that you would like to see or how you would like something to be. These are things you can't change, but describing something that bothers you in a different way. A funny list can help. Here are some examples of Top Ten lists:

Top Ten Fibromyalgia Self Help Books That Never Became Best Sellers

1. How to Cure Fibromyalgia.

2. Learn to Speak Assertively to Your Muscles.

3. How to Blame Others For Your Fibromyalgia.

4. Be Positive in Spite of Miserable Depressing Pain in Every Despicable Muscle of Your Body.

5. Yes, Every Problem You've Ever Had is From Fibromyalgia!

6. Teach Your spouse, Family, and Friends to Completely Understand Fibromyalgia.

7. Smother Your Pain With Love.

8. Planning a Vacation? Don't Forget to Bring Along Your Fibromyalgia.

9. Use Your Pain to Win the Lottery!

10. How to Function on Only Two House of Stage IV Sleep.

Top Ten Rejected Theories on the Cause of Fibromyalgia

1. Oxygen allergy.

2. Watching TV too close as a child.

3. Firefly radiation.

4. Eating too much microwave cooking.

5. Microscopic defects in teeth enamel.

6. Wet earthworm smells.

7. Over exposure to sneezes from inconsiderate people who didn't cover their mouths.

8. Too many refrigerator magnets.

9. Mother overslept during pregnancy.

10. Drinking too much water.

Top Ten Complaints About Sleeping in the Same Bed with Fibromyalgia Patient

1. Every night: Same old, same old.

2. Continuous tossing and turning causes motion sickness.

3. Restless legs activate security system motion detectors.

4. Racing thoughts create annoying draft.

5. Acts too dopey from all of the night medicines.

6. Too many pillows impair breathing.

7. Nocturnal myoclonic injuries.

8. Prays too loudly for stage IV sleep.

9. Noisy, hissing electric blanket.

10. Cold feet cause frostbite.

Top Ten Pain Behaviors to Let the Doctor Know You Hurt

1. Keep saying, "this pain is killing me."

2. Limp out of the office.

3. Slouch and walk slowly into the exam room.

4. Cry out loudly as soon as the doctor touches your skin.

5. Sigh frequently during the interview.

6. Squirm and fidget in the chair.

7. Begin hyperventilating halfway through the physical exam.

8. Grab the doctor's hand when ever he tries to press on your muscles.

9. Grimace whenever touched (watch so you don't strain your face muscles).

10. When asked to bend forward, move a few inches and say "that's it."

Top Ten Ways to Know Your Brain Is Affected by Fibromyalgia

1. You confuse your right arm with your left leg.

2. You discover fourteen different routes home from work, when in actuality there are only two.

3. You avoid salad bars because too many decisions are involved.

4. Pre-schoolers challenge you to chess games.

5. The national weather forecast issues a fog warning in your brain.

6. You get distracted by clouds while driving.

7. People seem more interested in talking to your pets than to you.

8. You write yourself daily reminders that read "don't forget to breathe, eat, and sleep today."

9. You consistently lose memory games played with your two-year-old son.

10. You've made mistakes on your last fifty checks written.

Top Ten Signs That Your Autonomic Nerves Have Gone Astray

1. You have anxiety attacks while napping.

2. Clam fishermen gather around and stare at your hands.

3. Your sweat freezes.

4. When you get embarrassed, neighbors plan impromptu cookout and barbecue hot dogs on your face.

5. The pounding in your head drowns out the loud music.

6. When taking a leisurely stroll, you uncontrollably scream out "I can't stand it anymore!"

7. Puncture wounds from the hair standing up on your arms.

8. Skin rashes begin to form messages like "I hurt all over."

9. Entomologists request permission to study "whatever is crawling under your skin."

10. Your teeth begin to sweat.

Top Ten Fibromyalgia Treatments That Did Not Work

1. Hot motor oil bath.

2. Surgical excision of tender points.

3. Gentle pressure massage by ex-Olympic wrestlers.

4. Microwaveable ice pack.

5. Daily vegetable soup soaks.

6. Drinking daily 8 ounce mixture of wine, fish oil, broccoli juice, dissolved aspirin and holy water.

7. Prolonged underwater exercises.

8. Acupuncture by ancient Antartican technique.

9. Combined electric current and aquatics therapy.

10. Hanging upside down by your ankle tendons.

Top Ten Things Overheard from Muscles at Their Annual Board Meetings

1. Remember our motto: No Mercy.

2. Hold on, everyone will get a chance to speak.

3. Let's discuss ways to recruit new members to our club.

4. We've agreed to continue the rotating leadership format.

5. The muscle maintenance contract has been cancelled.

6. We've gotten numerous complaints about the excessive pain you have been causing: Keep up the good work!

7. Congratulations to the Paraspinals on the birth of their new tenderpoints.

8. Don't forget to mark your calendars for the upcoming Family Flare-up Night.

9. Mr. Trapezius has agreed to cover for Max Gluteus when he goes on vacation.

10. All in favor of mandatory monthly flare-ups, say "Aye."

Top Ten Vacation Activities to Avoid

1. Annual North Pole Expedition, Fort Yukon, Alaska.

2. Cross-country Unicycling Tour: starting point, Plymouth, Indiana.

3. Human Mannequin Contest, Los Angeles, California.

4. Moose Hunting from Trees, Northern Canada.

5. Family Triathlaon Olympics, Steubenville, Ohio.

6. Amateur Lumberjack Festival, Spokane, Washington.

7. Drywallers' Fantasy Camp, Iowa City, Iowa.

8. Backpacking with the Pack Backers, Green Bay, Wisconsin.

9. Marathon Rock Climbing, Bryce Canyon National Park, Utah.

10. Camping Stargazer's Reunion, Eureka, Nevada.

Signs That Your Child May Have Fibromyalgia

1. Has growing pains without actual growth

2. Says your perfume makes him "puke his guts out."

3. Says when she grows up, will consider numerous jobs as long as they are classified as sedentary.

4. Only kid in the school history to flunk gym.

5. Volunteers in school to be in a sleep study.

6. For Christmas, all he wants is a hot tub.

7. Selective memory loss (can't remember homework assignment).

8. Complains of constant hairballs in her throat.

9. Gets upset if you don't park exactly between the lines, get completely embarrassed and refuses to get out of car if you straddle a line.

10. Spends more time in the bathroom than the classroom.

Fibromyalgia Hazards Found in Church

1. Petrified pine pews and kneelers with scant, if any, padding.

2. Speakers too loud for uninterrupted snoozing.

3. Burning, perfumed incense entering dry nasal and eye membranes.

4. Long, single-file communion lines.

5. Single antique ceiling fan that serves as entire church's climate control system.

6. 30 inch leg room space for 34 inch legs.

7. Noxious mix of smelly cosmetics used liberally by attendees.

8. One toilet for 300 parishioners.

9. 517 page song books that have fallen under the pew.

10. Weekly ritual struggling to remember names of all those familiar faces.

4) Use humorous reinforcement.

We know ways to increase our pain and cause flare-ups, and we need to continuously remind ourselves of things to do and not to do. To lighten your view, think of funny ways to cause increased pain and flare-up.

To demonstrate this I've come up with FLAWS, which stands for Fibromyalgia Famous LAst WordS. FLAWS are what we say or hear just before a flare-up.

"This shouldn't take too long."

"No thanks, I can lift this myself."

"Mom, throw us the frisbee!"

"That car is coming awfully fast, I don't think it is going to stop in time."

"Forty bucks to install! Forget it, I'll do it myself."

"I haven't tried a somersault since high school."

"Game of one-on-one, old man?"

"Hey, old buddy, good to see you again. Let me give you a big slap and hug."

"I'm going to put up all of the Christmas decorations now."

"No, that's not where it goes. No, you're not doing it right. Here, I'll just do it myself."

Humor has its proper place. It is not to be used inappropriately or to offend anyone. Humor is a choice. You can choose whether or not to read something, and you decide whether or not you find it funny. It is your choice and your responsibility. Humor is not something that should ever be thrust in your face, because it can offend or shock you. Fibromyalgia humor is truly only understood by people with fibromyalgia, everyone else will just look at you with a confused expression.

"Good night, Dad. Thanks for camping out in the backyard with us."

"The weather forecast this morning — cold and damp."

5) Mentally send funny messages.

People are always trying to think of clever and humorous greeting cards and answering machine messages. Imagine funny messages that you would send someone with fibromyalgia about some aspect of fibromyalgia.

Personalized fibromyalgia greeting cards:

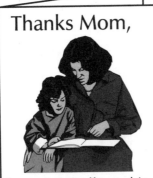

Thanks Mom, for passing your fibromyalgia genes onto me.

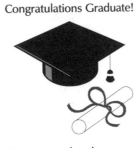

Congratulations Graduate! You've completed your physical therapy and counseling programs!

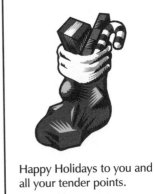

Happy Holidays to you and all your tender points.

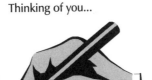

Thinking of you... I'd write more often but my arm is continuously numb.

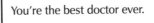
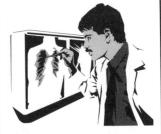

You're the best doctor ever. Hey, can I get an early refill on my Darvocet?

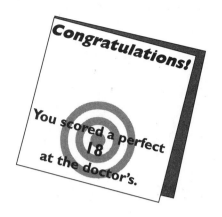

I know you have an
important event happening

I forgot which one though.

Please check which one
applies...
❏ Happy Birthday!
❏ *Happy Anniversary*
❏ Congratulations!
❏ Other

Personalized answering machine messages related to fibromyalgia:

a) Hello, you've reached the Smith residence. I'm unavailable because of my fibromyalgia. I'm either at the doctor's, getting massotherapy, taking a hot shower, or spending time in the bathroom. Leave a message, and if I remember to check the machine, I'll call you back.

b) I can't come to the phone right now. In fact, I can't move from the couch because I hurt all over. If I reach for the phone, it would hurt my arm, so I'm just lying here instead. My ears are fine, though, so feel free to talk away when you hear the beep.

c) Hello, it's Arlene. I'm here but I can't find my cordless phone. I always misplace the dang thing. Just leave a message. When I find the phone, I'll call you back.

d) (Digital computer voice) The person you have reached at 555-1234 has been changed. The new person has fibromyalgia and feels disconnected as if she is no longer in service.

6) Pain Power.

Imagine how your pain can cause you to create situations and have power. Because of your pain, you are able to create unique and humorous situations. Pretend that you have a lot of control over your fibromyalgia rather than no control.

I came up with "how bad is my pain..." to give us some power! Patients will always say to me, "my pain is so bad that..." Common examples include, "My pain is so bad that it feels like a hot poker is sticking me." Or, "My pain is so bad I feel like a Mack truck ran over me."

So here is how I imagine what you may really want to tell me to give your pain more power:

"How bad is my pain?"

"My pain is so bad that...A hot poker tickles me."

"My pain is so bad that...Semi trucks swerve to avoid running over me."

"My pain is so bad that...Others take narcotics when they see me."

"My pain is so bad that...The sound of a dental drill is actually soothing to me."

"My pain is so bad that...In the Complete Encyclopedia of Pain, I am Volumes 7–12."

"My pain is so bad that...Hungry mosquitoes avoid me."

Humor has its proper place. It is not to be used inappropriately or to offend anyone. Humor is a choice. You can choose whether or not to read something, and you decide whether or not you find it funny. It is your choice and your responsibility. Humor is not something that should ever be thrust in your face, because it can offend or shock you. Fibromyalgia humor is truly only understood by people with fibromyalgia, everyone else will just look at you with a confused expression.

I have been in situations where fibromyalgia humor was thrust upon unwitting people who did not have it. This has occurred on several occasions in a court room setting. I would be providing medical testimony about a particular fibromyalgia patient that I am treating, and the opposing attorney would begin to question me using humor that I had written. Imagine the jury members' surprise, shock, and disbelief when an attorney introduces a fibromyalgia humor book in a setting as serious as a court room. I never imagined that my attempts to help patients use humor would ever be used in such a shocking and negative way in a court room.

I realize now that attorneys will use whatever they can to influence the jury. So, remember that humor, especially humor about a serious medical condition, needs to be used appropriately and responsibly so as not to offend anyone.

Fibromyalgia makes us more understanding, compassionate, appreciative and perceptive. When we are laughing, there is a period of time when we aren't noticing any pain. And every time we laugh, we send a message to our muscles and nerves that we are not going to let them win. Don't be afraid to use humor to help you manage your fibromyalgia.

Chapter 24 — Survival Strategies

1) Try to laugh, it's therapeutic.

2) Discover new ways of coping with fibromyalgia through humor.

3) Approach your fibromyalgia with a little lighter attitude.

4) Use humor in its proper place.

5) Avoid offending other fibromyalgia sufferers who are not ready to laugh.

6) Don't be afraid to use humor to help manage your fibromyalgia.

7) Have fun!

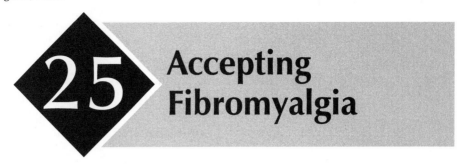

Accepting Fibromyalgia

Now that you have read about strategies to mentally and physically cope with fibromyalgia, it is time to start accepting this condition.

Acceptance is the ultimate mental coping mechanism where we validate who we are. Unless we can accept ourselves, we cannot expect the rest of the world to do so. I think the people who have the most difficult time dealing with fibromyalgia are those who can never truly accept it. They may read everything about it and know a lot, but they refuse to accept themselves with the condition. Fibromyalgia is not something we would ever choose to have, but if we have it, we must reach a point where we accept the condition as part of ourselves. I try to help people realize they need to reach this stage in order to become a true fibromyalgia survivor.

Acceptance is actually the end result of going through various mental stages in coping with a bad situation. Five classic stages of grief have been described as denial, anger, bargaining, depression, and acceptance. For example, when a person learns that he is dying of cancer and has only a certain amount of time to live, he will demonstrate typical coping behaviors. These stages are as follows:

1) **Denial:** The person does not believe this is happening to him and denies that the cancer even exists. The diagnosis is simply a mistake, as the doctors will soon realize.

2) **Anger:** This is the "Why me?" stage. A person asks, "How could I get this?" and "What have I done to deserve this?" He is very angry with the world.

3) **Bargaining:** The person is beginning to feel more hopeless and desperate. He promises to be a better person if only this cancer would be cured.

4) **Depression:** The person realizes that the cancer is incurable and goes through a period of clinical depression.

5) **Acceptance:** The person finally accepts his incurable disease and prepares for the end. He tries to appreciate the quality of the life that he has left.

These five stages are also experienced with other losses, such as the death of a loved one, or with debilitating diseases (for example, spinal cord injuries, stroke, rheumatoid arthritis).

Stages in Fibromyalgia

Persons with fibromyalgia can also experience these different stages because of the chronic pain and loss of function.

Denial

We frequently try to detach ourselves from our fibromyalgia and ignore it or pretend we don't have it. Denial may be reinforced by others who tell us we look normal, or doctors who tell us that there is nothing wrong. The mysteries, confusions, and controversies surrounding fibromyalgia make it difficult to acknowledge and easy to deny. When we are feeling better or have little pain, we might think we have gotten rid of it.

To get past this stage, we need to REcognize and REdefine (see Chapter 21). There may not be a cure yet for fibromyalgia, but there is a lot that can be done to treat it and help heal it. Facing any problem head on instead of denying it is harder. But we need to eventually face the facts so we can move on with our coping strategies.

Anger

Patients will usually confront fibromyalgia with questions such as, "Why me?" or "How did I get a condition for which there is no cure?" When a flare-up occurs, people often get very upset and angry. Fibromyalgia makes one more irritable, frustrated, and temperamental.

People can get caught up in this cycle and start feeling desperate and panicky. Doctor/therapist shopping, compulsive shopping, eating binges and other types of "desperate" behaviors are common when people get caught up in these confusing cycles. We need to realize this and be warned that this is the time when we are vulnerable and may try any therapy at any price. Allow your health professionals to help you resolve these cycles and point you towards acceptance.at any price. Allow your health professionals to help you resolve these cycles and point you towards acceptance.

All five REpairs are needed to address the anger. REcognize the anger and REdefine how you will handle it. Find a place to put your anger and REdirect it from your body and your loved ones to something more constructive. Take a walk or write a scathing letter to yourself. If you are angry at a person, imagine you are talking to this person and actually talk out loud (make sure you are alone!). This is one argument you will always win! You can REtrain yourself to let the anger go or to plan to address the source of your anger (after you've rehearsed strategies). Let your significant others help you. The RElaxation REsponse is an ideal way to deal with the anger response. REspect how fibromyalgia can cause anger and be REsponsible for controlling it.

Bargaining

The fibromyalgia patient often feels hopeless and desperate and will be vulnerable to making "deals." An example might be promising to start a new diet and exercise daily in attempt to cure the condition. Or the person might try a product they heard of on the Internet to cure pain. Many hopes and wishes are not realistic, which a person usually realizes, but she/he still allows the emotions to take control.

REcognizing and REdefining, and REalistic REtraining are helpful in this stage. REdefine what REalistic goals and expectations are appropriate with your fibromyalgia. Control what you can and appreciate what your abilities are rather than focusing on your inabilities. Remember fondly the way you used to be before fibromyalgia, but realize you have to do things differently now.

Depression

Half of the people with fibromyalgia will experience clinical depression. Even more will have depressed moods, decreased self-esteem, feelings of worthlessness, and a sense of failure.

REliable RElationships are helpful for managing depression. REspect and REsponsibility are also important. Depression can require its own separate medications and professional counseling, and you need to respect these needs and be responsible enough to ask for and receive the necessary treatments.

With fibromyalgia, these classic adjustment stages exist, but individuals have a harder time progressing through them in an orderly fashion to reach acceptance. They often move back and forth among the various stages, and may never reach the acceptance stage. I believe this happens because fibromyalgia is not as predictable as other incurable conditions or irreversible outcomes (such as death or paralysis). With these conditions, there is usually a defined pattern or course that the disease will take, and an anticipated end point. With fibromyalgia, there is no way to predict what will happen, when a flare-up will occur, or how a person will be twenty years from now. Consequently, it is difficult to progress through various stages systematically.

What often occurs is that a patient with fibromyalgia displays denial, anger, bargaining, and depression at different times. If the condition is relatively stable, there may be a return to denial because the person finds it to be the best mental coping mechanism. "I'm feeling better, therefore I must not have a problem anymore." Once a flare-up occurs, however, the person may return to anger, bargaining, and depression. This "bouncing around" in various stages makes it difficult to reach the final stage: acceptance.

People can get caught up in this cycle and start feeling desperate and panicky. Doctor/therapist shopping, compulsive shopping, eating binges and other types of "desperate" behaviors are common when people get caught up in these confusing cycles. We need to realize this and be warned that this is the time when we are vulnerable and may try any therapy at any price. Allow your health professionals to help you resolve these cycles and point you towards acceptance.

Acceptance

Because acceptance is such an elusive prize to many people who are trying to manage their fibromyalgia, I think that once this level is truly reached, it is most appreciated and people will maintain it. Once acceptance is realized, you can appreciate all of the things you've accomplished.

- You have gained an inner strength that will enrich other aspects of your life.

- You have made a decision to become an active participant in your healthcare decisions.

- You have stopped looking for someone to help you and have taken on the job of helping yourself.

- You have stopped trying to overcome fibromyalgia and instead work toward peacefully coexisting with it.

- You have made changes in your life-style and changes in your attitude, good changes!

- You have redirected your anger and hate, and have more energy available to appreciate simple things, educate yourself, and laugh.

- You have set up a support system that you can rely on for physical and mental support.

- You have learned to let go of anger and grudges and to forgive those who don't understand your illness.

- You have gotten out of the victim mode.

I have accepted my fibromyalgia. Mentally, I educated myself, reviewed and rehearsed strategies, and continue to "challenge" myself (and the fibromyalgia) to think of how to keep it under control. Physically, I've followed through with my mentally rehearsed strategies. I try to maintain proper posture (Fibronomics), stretch daily, exercise regularly. I accept the ongoing mental-physical/mind-body connection with fibromyalgia. I accept the periodic flare-ups and stable baselines that come with it.

When you've accepted your fibromyalgia, you are allowed to give yourself credit and to pat yourself on the back. You have been through a lot and have overcome many obstacles. But it was worth it, because you're worth it! By achieving acceptance, you have provided yourself with a powerful tool necessary to mentally and physically manage fibromyalgia and reintegrate into the world. Allow yourself to be proud of yourself, allow yourself to love yourself. You can make a positive contribution to your community, be an important and valuable part of your circle of family and friends, and have a positive quality of life.

Fibromyalgia Acceptance Affirmation:

To be able to accept fibro as a part of you, you must be able to understand and accept important fact. Once you begin to work on accepting these facts, you will be on the path to accepting your fibromyalgia.

These affirmations can help with that process:

1) Having fibro is not my choice. It is something I would never choose, but I need to reach a point where I can accept this condition as a part of myself.

2) I did not receive fibro as a punishment. I am a good person. I do not understand the reason I was destined to have this condition. Instead of wondering "why," I will focus on "where I can go from here."

3) Denial is unproductive. I am here, I have this condition, there are many things I can do to "heal" myself.

4) I cannot make fibro go away. I cannot "bargain" it away. I will control what I can. I will appreciate my abilities instead of focusing on my inabilities.

5) I will take depression seriously. If I begin to suffer from depression, I will quickly seek medical and/or counseling treatment. I will accept the responsibility to ask for and receive treatment deemed necessary.

6) There are things about my illness I cannot control. There is no way to predict what will happen, when a flare-up will occur, or how my health will be 20 years from now. I will not use valuable energy for unproductive thoughts.

7) I take responsibility for the things about my illness I CAN control. I will do my best to "heal" myself through: education, stress reduction, following a home program, and setting realistic goals and expectations.

8) I have decided to become an active participant in my healthcare decisions. I will educate myself so that I can be a good medical consumer and make clear, informed decisions about my treatment.

9) I will stop looking for someone to help me, and take on that job myself. I will attend support group meetings. I will help others who also have fibromyalgia.

10) I have stopped trying to be "cured" of fibromyalgia. Instead, I am working towards peacefully coexisting with it.

11) I will learn to forgive others. I will let go of anger and grudges and redirect that energy. I will appreciate the simple things, learn to love myself, and enjoy laughing.

Chapter 25 — Survival Strategies

1) Work towards acknowledging you have fibromyalgia instead of denying it.

2) Recognize and acknowledge its existence and how it affects your life.

3) Understand that there is no cure for fibromyalgia today, but you can do a lot to treat it and help heal it.

4) Redirect anger to something more constructive.

5) Focus on abilities rather than inabilities.

6) Responsibly treat depression.

7) Avoid doctor shopping, compulsive shopping, overeating.

8) Accept and love yourself; you cannot expect others to accept your illness until you do.

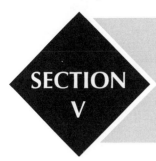

SECTION V

Handling Specific Situations

You've already read about prescribed and self directed strategies for managing fibromyalgia. In this section, I want to focus on some specific situations you encounter with fibroymalgia, and see if you can pick up some tips on how to handle them. This section has new information combined with informtion you've alread read; I've done this to reinforce what you've learned and to apply the information to specific, unique situations. (I'm not trying to confuse you or bore you, honest!) Some of the chapters in this section may not apply to you, so you can browse past them if you wish. You should not be offended when you get to Chapter 31, OK? Don't be making fun of the stick diagrams in Chapter 31. (I said "stick" not "sick") Chapter 35 addresses flare-ups and specific locations of flare-ups designed to be a reference guide.

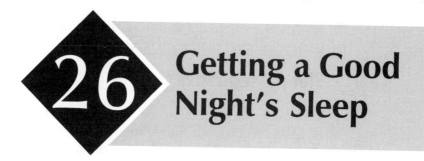

26 Getting a Good Night's Sleep

Most of us with fibromyalgia complain about our sleep, whether it would be difficulty falling asleep, frequently waking at night, or both. It is during sleep, and particularly deep sleep, that our body repairs itself, makes vital proteins, and replenishes our energy supply. Thus, we need to devise some strategies to ensure the best and most restful sleep.

In 1975, Dr. Moldofsky proposed the term "non-restorative sleep syndrome" as a name for fibromyalgia. When he studied ten patients with the diagnosis of fibromyalgia, he found that seven had an abnormality in the Stage 4 delta sleep (the deep sleep stage). There was an intrusion of alpha rhythms into Stage 4 delta sleep, and this alpha-delta sleep pattern at first was thought to be diagnostic and possibly the cause of fibromyalgia. However, this finding is not unique to fibromyalgia. It can be found in other conditions that cause chronic pain.

Five stages of sleep have been defined. When a person is relaxed but still awake, alpha waves are present on an EEG. As the person begins to fall asleep, the alpha waves disappear (Stage 1). In Stage 2 sleep, bursts of sleep spindle waves occur. Stage 3 is the beginning of deep sleep, and Stage 4 is deep sleep where delta waves predominate on the EEG. The last stage (Stage 5) is called REM sleep, or rapid eye movement stage where most dreaming occurs. Fibromyalgia people dream most about trying to get into Stage 4 sleep and staying there!

Pre-Sleep Routine

The first step in sleeping better is preparing to sleep better. Fibromyalgia doesn't like change, so a consistent sleep schedule, going to bed and getting up at the same times, is helpful. If you want extra sleep, it is better to go to bed earlier than to sleep late. What you do prior to going to bed is important to your sleep routine.

You have to unwind and cleanse the mind before lying down to sleep. Taking all of your problems to bed with you only heightens anxiety and makes it difficult to relax your mind. Allow yourself to get as much accomplished as you can in the evening, but reach a "limit" where you allow yourself to say, "I've done as much as I can on this for now, and I'll address it further tomorrow." By reaching this limit, you can close the book for the night and plan to open the book the next day. Do something relaxing before going to bed: listen to music, read a book, watch a TV program, or take a hot bath. Writing a list of things to do the next day and then "clearing the mind" is helpful to me and enables me to close the day. Practice some of the relaxation techniques that you have learned. Avoid caffeine in the evening.

People who work during the night and sleep during the day have even more difficulty getting restful sleep. Our bodies prefer to sleep at night. The pre-sleep routine needs to be followed if you work the evening shift, and it is especially important to allow your mind to unwind when you get home from work.

Sleep Medicines

Many medications are used to treat sleep disorders. Some of these medicines can be habit forming, but if they are used as prescribed and used judiciously, very rarely do I find any problems with side effects. The logic is that fibromyalgia is a chronic condition associated with a chronic sleep disorder; therefore, one is expected to sleep poorly most of the time. Given this, I believe an individual is justified in taking a nightly medicine to improve sleep as long as the beneficial effects far outweigh the potential risks.

I advise my patients to try to use sleeping medicines on an as-needed basis, perhaps during a flare-up or a persistent period of poor sleep. I also "rotate" different medicines (prescribed or natural) for sleep. One medicine may be used during the week, and a different one used on weekends. This enables the beneficial effects of improved sleep, but also allows the body a periodic wash-out effect, and decreases the chance of developing a tolerance to, or side effects from, the medicines. Weekends are not the time to try to "catch up" on your sleep; you need to stay in a consistent pattern all week.

An ideal prescribed sleep modifier would be one taken at bedtime that starts working when you have "naturally" reached deep sleep, and acts to continue deep sleep for several more hours. Instead of waking up at 4:00 a.m., you wake up at 7:00 a.m. and feel refreshed. The medicine shouldn't cause any morning sedation, confusion, or hangover effects. I prescribe a number of sleep modifiers; Sonata is probably my current "favorite" because it most consistently meets this "ideal" criteria.

Many recommended natural sleep modifiers are available over the counter. They include melatonin, valerian root, 5-HTP, St. John's Wort, Passiflora, and Kava Kava. Some people do well with over-the-counter medicines that contain diphenhydramine (Benadryl). Others can get headaches, morning hangovers, or increased fatigue when taking Benadryl at night. I always advise that you work with a knowledgeable medical professional when considering natural sleep modifiers. Natural medicines can interact with prescribed medicines or have side effects that can cause problems. You want to sleep well, not for all eternity!

The Bed

The first step in sleeping better is preparing to sleep better.

I'm frequently asked what type of bed is best. Should a water bed be considered or a mattress? I personally have found the most comfortable bed to be one that has a good firm mattress with a soft mattress pad or eggcrate pad. This type of mattress provides good support for the spine, but also provides some cushion effect on sore skin. Many people report that water beds are hard to get in and out of and do not support the spine as well, so they are not as comfortable. If your mattress is soft and you sink into it, or if you find that you are more comfortable with sleeping on the floor instead of on your bed, you need to consider investing in a firm new mattress.

Some patients like to use magnetic mattress pads and say their pain is decreased and energy level improved. Consider a one week trial for this type of mattress before you purchase one.

The Pillow(s)

You probably have seen hundreds of pillows offered to improve your sleep. I prefer the old-fashioned, lightly packed feather pillow that I can mold and fluff to fit. Your goals for proper head position during the night include:

1) The pillow should be soft and comfortable.

2) Your head and neck should be supported in a natural position. The pillow shouldn't be too thick or fluffy as to push your neck upward, or so flimsy that your head sinks down too much, but just right so that you head is in the neutral position, centered between your shoulders when you are lying on your side.

3) Your pillow should adjust to your changing positions during the night. A pitfall of customized, fabricated pillows is they work great for one position only. In reality we shift into many positions during the night.

Your pillow should be shaped so that it allows your head to be in the neutral position and properly centered, yet it should have a fullness to support the neck gap between your head and shoulders when you are laying down (on your side or your back). This "neck gap" support is important to enable the neck muscles to relax during the night by having some support. If you change positions, you naturally adjust your pillow. A customized pillow can be moved as needed. I've had many patients tell me that the water/gel pillows are not comfortable for them. A specialized head pillow containing biologic magnets have been helpful to a number of people.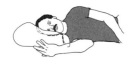

Body pillows can be added. Some people do well with the very long body pillow that intertwines the head, neck, arms, and hip areas. Others prefer to have a separate head pillow and arm and leg pillows. Other people have gotten lost under a pile of pillows in their bed!

When lying on the side, a pillow should be placed between the knees to properly align the hips and pelvis. This reduces the stress on the hips and sacroiliac areas and increases comfort.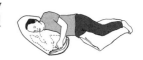

Many patients have discovered that an extra long pillow, not a body pillow, will help with the head and neck positioning and arm cushioning and support. I prefer the extra long pillow to position my head and neck, and also to cushion my arms. You may need to experiment with different pillows and be creative. If you are not comfortable with a particular pillow, no matter how highly recommended it comes, get rid of it and find another one. Likewise, if you find a perfect pillow, take it with you wherever you go, and guard it with your life!

Other Sleep Necessities

Other sleep necessities in terms of equipment include a bed sheet and a blanket. If you are bothered by hot flashes when you first lay down at night, use the sheet only, but have the blanket ready to cover yourself in the middle of the night when you start to feel the other extremes of your autonomic nerves kicking in, the cold limbs. An electric mattress pad or an electric blanket, when used properly can help keep you warm. Many people have done well with a magnetic mattress pad, but others, including me, find that it makes them too hot and causes uncomfortable night sweats, particularly in the neck and upper back areas. An eggcrate mattress can be helpful. These are available in medical supply stores. A clock is optional since we all have excellent internal alarm clocks, and we simply will ourselves to get up at a certain time. However, to keep us company while we are clock-watching during the night, it is not a bad idea to have a clock with nice big numbers so we can easily see what time it is that we are not sleeping! To minimize the cold chills, keep our limbs

> What is the best sleeping position with fibromyalgia? I believe it is lying on the side in a modified fetal position.
>
> If you haven't been sleeping in this position, it can take about a week to become accustomed to this new position. Once you make the change, your body will adapt to this new position and automatically make the adjustments while you are asleep. You can train your subconscious to minimize pain while you are asleep.

covered with long sleeves and long-legged clothing, and wear cotton socks to bed. The tubular athletic socks work well when it comes to keeping your feet warm. The higher the socks, the warmer the legs!

Keep the room temperature comfortable, about 72° F. During winter, be sure to keep warm; you may have to turn the thermostat up during the night. You can always turn it back down in the morning after you are up and about. NEVER sleep with an open window or be in the path of direct drafts from vents. Central air conditioning is okay, and is preferred by those who do worse with temperature fluctuations, but avoid the direct cool air drafts. Air drafts are synonymous with muscle spasms!

Body Position

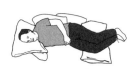

What is the best sleeping position with fibromyalgia? I believe it is lying on the side in a modified fetal position. To assume this position, you lie on your side with your knees bent up, tilt your head forward, and place your arms to your side, bent at the elbows (see diagram). The hands and wrists need to be in the neutral positions though, because the fetal positions of these joints (fingers curled and wrists bent down) are usually painful. So sleep like a baby but keep your wrists and hands neutral.

If you haven't been sleeping in this position, it can take about a week to become accustomed to this new position. Once you make the change, your body will adapt to this new position and automatically make the adjustments while you are asleep.

Sleeping on the stomach usually hurts. In this position, your stomach sinks into the bed and arches the back, which puts strain on the back during the night. Likewise, sleeping on the back causes your shoulders and buttocks to arch your back and form a "bridge" which can increase pain. Bending the knees can help relieve some of the low back pressure when laying on your back. In the stomach or low back positions, the muscles in the neck and back are working hard instead of relaxing even though you may be sleeping.

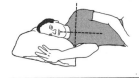

The head and neck should maintain neutral position. Once you are in the final sleeping position, the head and neck should be aligned properly with the shoulder. In this position, individual neck muscles are not strained. Make sure the pillow does not allow the head to sink too far into the bed or be pushed too far away from the bed once your comfortable position is assumed so as not to cause unnatural positioning of the head and neck (see diagram).

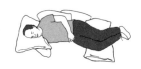

Another position that can be comfortable is lying mostly on the back but tilting to the side with a pillow under both knees (see diagram). This pillow under the knee prevents the legs from straightening out and thus arching the back. Remember your fibronomics.

The arms and legs also need to be positioned as part of the overall proper sleep posture. Your arms are not pillows, so avoid laying on them or resting your head on your hands. This puts pressures on the muscles and nerves and will often cause you to wake at night with a numb arm. Avoid stretching your arms over your head also. If you are lying on your side, the arm closest to the bed can be tucked under the pillow. Be careful to keep your elbow out in front of you so you are not laying directly on the elbow. The other arm can be draped over the pillow, if you have a longer pillow, which prevents the arm from resting on your body (see diagram).

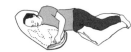

The legs seem to do best in a bent position, with the knees separated by a pillow as mentioned above. If the knees are on top of each other, the hardness of both knees can often cause pain, and the pillow between the knees helps this problem. The ankles can be overlapped so they are not directly on each other, of if you are using a pillow between your knees that reaches down to the ankles, cushion the ankles with this pillow. If you are laying on your back, keep the knees bent. Remember, it takes some time to train yourself to become comfortable in these new body positions; then your subconscious will take over and put you into these positions during the night.

Getting Back to Sleep

Invariably, for one reason or another, we awaken during the night. Our goals are to decrease the number of times we wake at night, and increase the speed at which we can fall back to sleep. If you are on prescription sleep medicines, it is usually easier to fall back to sleep quickly. If you wake up, don't make a big deal about it; just tell yourself you will quickly fall back asleep. If you need to use the bathroom, have a night light in the bathroom. Some studies have shown that a red light minimizes eye glare and "irritation" at night, so try a red night light. The key is to not turn on a bright 150 watt light, twelve inches from your eyes! Make sure there is enough lighting so you can see and don't fall over something.

If you get back in bed but find yourself unable to fall asleep again, repeat your relaxation strategies, or try a mental rehearsing strategy. That is, think about something that might involve numbers and calculations and trying to do mental math. You know, boring stuff that hopefully will signal your body to get so bored that it just falls back asleep. Some prescribed sleeping medicines can be repeated in the middle of the night from time to time. Your doctor may allow you to take an extra dose of sleep modifier if everything else fails.

Hopefully, you can develop good sleep habits and go through the various sleep stages. Ultimately, you can experience good Stage 4 sleep!

Chapter 26 — Survival Strategies

Night's Sleep

1) Prepare a pre-sleep routine that can be repeated nightly.

2) Discuss with your physician available medications to improve sleep.

3) Investigate over-the-counter sleep modifiers including natural medicines and herbs.

4) Evaluate your sleep area:

    a) Check bed for comfort, firmness.
    b) Choose pillows to support neck and body.
    c) Consider an electric blanket or mattress pad.
    d) Adjust room temperature.

5) Increase your awareness of good sleep habits.

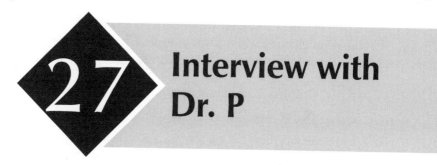

27 Interview with Dr. P

<u>Location</u>: Dr. Pellegrino's office in Canton, Ohio. Dr. Pellegrino is sitting at his desk being interviewed by Mary King as part of the Mary King Live show. Dr. Pellegrino has agreed to this interview to discuss fibromyalgia and particularly how he deals with it. Let's now go to the interview...

Mary: Good afternoon, Dr. Pellegrino. Thank you for agreeing to be interviewed. My name is Mary King and this is Mary King Live. You certainly have a beautiful office here. Thank you for agreeing to let us use your location for our show.

Dr. P: You're very welcome, Mary.

Mary: You are a fibromyalgia doctor, aren't you?

Dr. P: Yes, I am.

Mary: Why did you become a doctor?

Dr. P: I've wanted to be a doctor since I was fourteen years old. I broke my shoulder, and the orthopedist who fixed me was fascinating, and I thought I wanted to become an orthopedist. After I went to medical school, I became fascinated with the Physical Medicine and Rehabilitation specialty, and I decided I wanted to become a physiatrist.

Mary: Well, I want to ask you about your fibromyalgia and how you deal with it. You have fibromyalgia, don't you?

Dr. P: Yes, I do.

Mary: How did you discover you had this?

Dr. P: I was diagnosed by one of my residency doctors, Dr. George Waylonis, during my third year of residency. I was experiencing a lot of shoulder and back pain that just wouldn't let up. I thought the pain was due to my coat which was a standard white doctor's jacket, only I had books, equipment, and anything you can imagine stuffed in the pockets; you know how insecure residents can be! I weighed my coat once and it weighed 14 pounds, fully loaded. Dr. Waylonis examined me and found the typical painful tender points and determined I had fibromyalgia.

Mary: The coat that caused fibromyalgia, huh? You mentioned shoulder and back pain, do you have any other pains with the fibromyalgia?

Dr. P: Growing pains.

Mary: Groin pains?

Dr. P: NO, growing pains. GROWING pains! I had a lot of leg cramps and pains at nighttime when I was young. When I was told they were growing pains, I thought, oh great, I get to have this pain for another ten years. But those stopped.

Mary: Any other problems you remember as a kid that may have suggested you were going to get fibromyalgia?

Dr. P: There have been several things that I can recall. I could never hold my arms out in front of me for very long. It wasn't painful, but I just felt like all of the strength left my arms. I particularly noticed this if I would change a light bulb or something like that. I knew then that I wasn't going to be painter or a dry-waller.

I remember when I got a brand-new ten speed bike with rams horn handle bars and a narrow seat. I was forced into a hunched over position when riding, and my neck and shoulders would hurt. I learned how to ride my bike sitting more upright and extending my hands and fingertips to the top of the rams horn handle to avoid this hunched over position. I got pretty good at steering and turning with just my fingertips, until I hit a bump and fell off. In fact, I don't think I've ridden a bike since I was a kid.

I can remember having episodes where I would get really tired. I didn't start getting the persistent pains until my late twenties, so that would have been about two or three years ago. But I can look back now and say that I probably had some childhood symptoms that made me at risk for ultimately getting fibromyalgia.

Mary: So what do you think caused your fibromyalgia?

Dr. P: Mine, genetics. I was destined to have this! Various members of my family have fibromyalgia, in fact, it spans four generations. I'm thinking about proposing a TV miniseries!

Mary: Wow. You know, you are really a funny guy with your funny stories. So what have you done since you have been diagnosed with fibromyalgia?

Dr. P: I try to learn everything I can about it. Half of the battle is won once you learn about fibromyalgia and try to understand it.

Mary: Do you know a lot about fibromyalgia now?

Dr. P: Sometimes.

Mary: What do you mean?

Dr. P: Heck, I can't remember everything. Fibro-fog is a problem, so I'm forgetful and absentminded at times. Did I mention that yet, Diane?

Mary: It's Mary, and no you didn't mention that. So does this Fibro-fog cause other problems for you?

Dr. P: Yes, I make wrong turns or drive past stores, or get lost in my car.

Mary: So, it is hard driving through the Fibro-fog! (Mary laughs).

Dr. P: Oh, aren't you funny.

Mary: Sorry, couldn't resist that one. So I'd better not ask you for directions on how to get back home today. (Mary laughing out loud)

Dr. P: Excuse me, can we continue please?

Mary: I'm really sorry. Oh boy, okay, here we go. (Mary looking at notes) Are there any other brain problems?

Dr. P: Yes, I get right and left confused at times. This is actually embarrassing, so make sure this is between you and I, okay? I don't want anyone to think that Dr. Pellegrino gets his right and left sides confused.

Mary: This will be our secret.

Dr. P: Good, I don't want to seem paranoid. But I say you've got to be a little paranoid with fibromyalgia and wear a mental seat belt.

Mary: What do you mean?

Dr. P: Pretend everything you do is a flare-up waiting to happen. You have to watch your posture and follow fibronomics. It is bad enough that you have to hurt everyday, but you need to do what you can to prevent flare-ups and to keep the pain more manageable.

Let me tell you one of my favorite tricks for fibronomics. Oh, I can see you look confused, Mary. Fibronomics is the art of properly manipulating our fibromyalgia bodies in the environment to complete an activity without aggravating our fibromyalgia.

I realized a long time ago that when I was putting my ties on in the morning, I would aggravate my neck and shoulder pain. You see, I'm a bit of a perfectionist, and my tie has to be tied just right, and as you men know out there, it is sometimes hard to get the tie tied just right on the first try. You look at what needs to be adjusted, and then you make the adjustment and tie the tie again. Hopefully, you will get it right on the second time. If you don't get it right by the third time, you have no business wearing ties.

Well, as part of my right-left confusion, I cannot look in a mirror and tie a tie. I have to look down to tie my tie, so here I am putting my head in an awkward position trying to look down and tie my tie, sometimes up to three times before I get it just right. So no wonder I have increased pain.

I discovered a trick. Once I got the tie tied right and went through my day, instead of unraveling the tie at the end of the day, I would just loosen the noose enough to slip it over my neck, then I would place the tie on my tie rack, still tied. That tie will await its next turn, and a few weeks later, I simply take the tie off of the tie rack, slip it over my neck, tighten it up, and I am ready to go. See this tie I am wearing?

Mary: Yes.

Dr. P: Looks pretty good, huh?

Mary: Yes, it does. It looks like you tied it this morning.

Dr. P: It does, doesn't it? But I tied this six months ago!

Mary: Amazing. What else do you do for your fibromyalgia?

Dr. P: Regular stretches. I try to do a regular exercise program of walking and playing basketball.

Mary: I've heard about you and your basketball skills. You're pretty good, aren't you?

Dr. P: Well, ...hey, how tall are you?

Mary: 5 feet 8 inches.

Dr. P: Ever play basketball?

Mary: No.

Dr. P: Then I could beat you one-on-one.

Mary: You're so funny, Dr. Pellegrino. So you watch your posture, stretch, and exercise. What do you do to relax?

Dr. P: I like to write, and I spend time with my family.

Mary: How do you find time to write?

Dr. P: I give my family money to go outside and leave me alone. No, just kidding. (Mary laughs).

Most of the writing is actually imagining what you want to say. It is like creative daydreaming, I think of what I want to say and imagine what it would look like. Then I write down notes and ideas and try to keep them organized in places where I can find them.

Mary: Did you recently write a note about describing different types of pain sensations?

Dr. P: Yes! How did you know that?

Mary: I can read the Post-It note that's stuck on your jacket sleeve.

Dr. P: Oh this, heh-heh, I was looking for this. I misplaced it, I guess. Thanks.

Mary: How do you remember what to do each day?

Dr. P: I use a Day Planner.

Mary: Is that what that black book is you're holding?

Dr. P: No, this is a phone book. I forgot to order my Day Planner this year.

Mary: So tell me about your family.

Dr. P: I have a great family. I have three kids, a girl and two boys, and they keep me busy. My wife and kids are supportive.

Mary: Your eyes are getting teary, is that because you're talking about your family?

Dr. P: No, I think your perfume is causing my eyes to water. I'm really sensitive to odors.

Mary: But I'm not wearing any perfume.

Dr. P: Well, I'll figure this out. (Dr. Pellegrino, looking around the room and sniffing) Fibromyalgia makes me more sensitive to smells, and I can usually spot anything with my nose, whether it be smoke, chemicals, spoiled food. Is that your briefcase, Mary?

Mary: Yes.

Dr. P: Well, it looks like you have a news magazine in there, would you care to take that out please?

Mary: Sure, what does this magazine have to do with your eyes watering?

Dr. P: Open it up and see that advertisement there for cologne, they actually put a sample of the cologne in the magazine. I hate when they do that.

Mary: Yes, you're right, I never even noticed that.

Dr. P: Excuse me a second. (Dr. Pellegrino removes the cologne advertisement page with sample on it and leaves room and returns a few seconds later empty-handed.)

Dr. P: Fibromyalgia people are very sensitive to smells. As I'm getting a little bit older, I noticed that I am having more problems with odors.

Mary: I'm glad I didn't have any garlic for lunch. (Mary laughing out loud)

Dr. P: You're funny.

Mary: Do you eat any special foods?

Dr. P: All foods are special to me. I think people with fibromyalgia do better if they eat a diet that is higher in protein and lower in carbohydrates and particularly try to avoid sugars such as doughnuts and cookies. Those happen to be some of my favorite foods though, by the way.

Mary: Do you take any specific medicines or nutritional supplements?

Dr. P: Yes. I use magnesium and malic acid combinations, colostrum, and will occasionally take a sleep modifier. I found this great nutritional supplement for memory. I think this is the one, it is fantastic.

Mary: So that is why you are so smart. Tell me, what is this memory supplement called?

Dr. P: It is called ...darnit, I can't remember. I'm drawing a blank here. Sorry. (Dr. Pellegrino scratching head)

Mary: Well, let me know if you think of it. Now we have time for some questions from callers. Thank you, Dr. Pellegrino, for allowing us to set up this phone system in your office here. I know you tripped over one of the cables earlier; is your knee feeling any better?

Dr. P: Yes, thank you.

Mary: Okay, let's here from the first caller. Hello?

Caller #1: (Very stuffy voice) Hello, I'm sick with the flu. I'm calling from bed in Boise, Idaho. I want to know if I should be getting the flu vaccine if I have fibromyalgia. Can it cause flare-ups?

Dr. P: Hey, I'd better not get too close to the phone so I don't catch anything, ha-ha. People with fibromyalgia can have bad flare-ups if they get the flu, and in the past many people could get flare-ups with the flu vaccine. The newer flu vaccines, however, are more refined, and I'm not seeing them cause as many flare-ups as they did a few years ago. So if you are one who gets the flu every year, you might want to consider getting the flu vaccine. Check with your doctor.

Mary: Let's hear from our next caller. Ma'am, can you identify yourself?

Caller #2: Yes, I'm Gina from Moosecreek, Alaska. I have fibromyalgia, and mine is particularly aggravated by cold weather. How I can learn more about fibromyalgia?

Dr. P: Hi, Gina. There are a lot of great newsletters that can give you updated information including the latest research. If you have access to a computer, there is a lot of free information available on fibromyalgia. I'll bet you're not the only one in Moosecreek who has fibromyalgia, too. Check around, and you may find out in your area that there are a few others who know exactly how you feel. Try to find a doctor who is willing to work with you on your fibromyalgia. Hopefully, there are more people living in Moosecreek than you! Good luck, Gina.

Mary: We have time for one more call. Who is this?

Caller #3: This is Michael. I hear you want to play me one-on-one. You'd better stick to fibromyalgia, dude, before you really get to hurting.

Mary (hurriedly interrupting): Okay, that's all the time we have for questions and comments from our callers.

Well, Dr. Pellegrino, just a few final questions. Thank you for taking this time. You are a funny guy, and smart too. Is your fibromyalgia getting worse?

Dr. P: It is stable. I stick with my routine and have been lucky to have a program that currently works. I work together with my patients to find out what works, and I try to help them, and in turn they help me as well. I hope I can continue to do well and help people and learn.

Mary: You always joke about your age. How old are you really?

Dr. P: I'm in my fifth decade now.

Mary: You look much younger than fifty-something.

Dr. P: I am younger than fifty-something. Fifth decade means 40-49 years old.

Mary: Sorry about that, what I meant was that you look younger than your age.

Dr. P: Okay, Mary Ann, I think that was a little too much on how young I look. I appreciate you doing this interview, but don't feel obligated to say all of this just because you are my wife.

Mary (Ann): I'm only trying to help. And I'm reading exactly what you told me to ask. I feel silly enough, Mary King Live! I mean, you think that's funny? Why don't you get one of the kids to finish up?

Dr. P: No, no, you did good. I'm done now. Let's go for a walk and stretch out.

Mary (Ann): All right, but leave the basketball home this time.

(End of Interview).

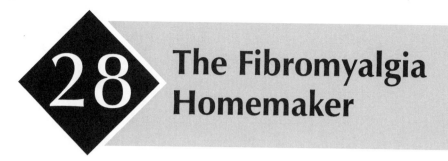

The Fibromyalgia Homemaker

One of the most frequent complaints made by women with fibromyalgia is their inability to perform standard homemaking chores. The bending, reaching, lifting and pulling required of these tasks causes increased pain and often leads to painful flare-ups. The fibromyalgia homemaker is faced with the dilemma of wanting to have a clean home, but not having the physical abilities to complete these routine tasks without pain. What does the homemaker do?

Options to consider:

1) **Stop doing housework altogether.** Yes, just go on strike! See if the work gets done by others. Watch as nothing gets done and your house becomes a health hazard! You can't stop everything, but daily or weekly tasks can be analyzed to determined if they can be done less frequently. Consider a rotating system where different parts of the house are cleaned on different days and not all at once. Instead of doing one heavy task in one day, spread it out into several mini-tasks over the course of a week. Your whole house may not be perfectly clean all the time, but parts of your house are perfect every day!

2) **Have someone else do it, with you supervising.** This is a good way to teach responsibility to your children (or your spouse, the biggest kid of all). The shared housework concept divides the responsibilities among the entire family, and you do the share of tasks that you can comfortably handle. The heavier tasks (vacuuming, carrying laundry loads) should be delegated to other family members. You supervise — and be sure to look busy at all times!

3) **Pay someone else to do it, if you can afford it.** Try to have the paid person come weekly or every other week to do the major cleaning, scrubbing and vacuuming. You can do the minor "touch-up" work in between visits. Bribe your kids to work cheap!

4) **Modify the way you are doing particular tasks.** This allows you to continue doing the homemaking, but do it in a way that is kinder to your muscles. Since homemaking chores are done with your body in unusual and awkward positions that aggravate your fibromyalgia, proper attention must be paid to fibronomics.

Probably a combination of these options works best for each homemaker. New strategies can be learned and used successfully.

Below is list of usual homemaking tasks that individuals with fibromyalgia have difficulty performing.

- Running the vacuum cleaner

- Doing dishes

- Ironing

- Dusting

- Scrubbing

- Laundry

- Washing windows

- Getting objects in and out of high or low cupboards

- Lifting or moving heavy objects or furniture

- Prolonged writing

- Yard work of any type

- Buying, carrying and unloading groceries

Sometimes unusual projects cause flare-ups. For example, one patient described how she spent several hours decorating cakes for her boy's basketball team and had severe pain in her shoulders and arms. Another woman had a flare-up in her back when she was lifting heavy bird seed bags into the trunk of her car. Both ordinary and unusual homemaking tasks and projects can cause flare-ups, so you must be constantly on guard to try to prevent them. Wear your mental seat belt and follow fibronomics.

The following pages are devoted to showing you some strategies and homemaking fibronomics to apply to usual tasks.

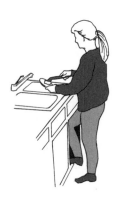

1) **Problem:** Vacuuming is Housework Enemy Number 1. It can aggravate pain in the back, shoulders and arms because your arms are reaching out to push and pull the heavy vacuum and you are bending forward while pushing which puts stress on the back.

Solutions:

a) Obtain a lightweight vacuum cleaner to minimize the load on the arms and back.

b) Hold the vacuum cleaner by holding arms down against the side and lightly holding the vacuum handle but not squeezing hard. The handle of the vacuum cleaner rests against the upper thigh and hip area. Walk forward with back maintaining a normal curvature to push the vacuum cleaner forward, and then backing up, squeeze the handle harder and pull the vacuum backwards with steady force. Repeat these steps to cover different areas of the carpet. Be sure that the arm does not reach out away from the body, but that the whole body moves forward along with the arms (see diagram) .

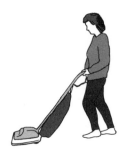

2) **Problem:** Standing at the sink washing dishes hurts your lower back because you have to lean forward.

Solutions:

a) Alternate leg on a stool or inside sink cupboard to unload the back and decrease the pain.

b) Use disposable paper plates, paper cups, paper cereal bowls. (Don't hurt your back throwing them away!)

c) Do a few dishes at a time, do something else, then do more dishes. The alternating method helps reduce prolonged back strain.

d) If the sink is too short for your height, place a large plastic dishpan on the counter top and wash dishes in this.

e) Use one of those sponges that have dish detergent in the handle. You can rinse and wash dishes easier.

f) Cook and eat from same dish. Use a microwave bowl to cook and then eat out of it. If you're eating alone, just eat out of the pan.

g) If cooking for your family, serve from the stove so you don't have extra serving dishes and spoons to wash.

h) If using a dishwasher, have family members load their own dishes, and assign the job of unloading clean dishes to children or spouse.

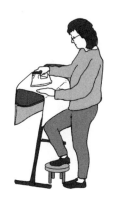

3) **Problem:** Ironing. Bending forward increases back strain and repetitive arm reaching hurts.

Solutions:

a) Alternate leg on a foot stool to unload the back.

b) Avoid overextending the arm; keep the elbow bent and the iron as close to the body as possible.

c) Use a drive-through dry cleaning service.

d) Buy fabrics that don't need ironing.

e) Wash clothes at home; hang dry so you don't have to use dryer. Take them to the cleaners for pressing.

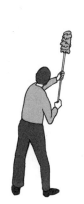

4) **Problem:** Dusting. The major problems with dusting are reaching for the tops of shelves and bending to reach difficult low areas of furniture.

Solutions:

a) Use a longer handled dust mop to allow the equipment, not your arm, to reach the spots.

b) Use a hair dryer to blow dust off.

c) Store all knick-knacks in glass-enclosed shelving.

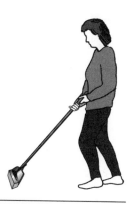

5) **Problem:** Scrubbing. Scrubbing the floor, furniture or countertops is an invitation to a flare-up. You bend and reach and you hurt!

Solutions:

a) Use a long-handled mop when scrubbing the floor. Take advantage of any cleaning solvent that will perform the chemical scrubbing for you, so all you have to do is wipe up.

b) Use an electrical device that does the scrubbing for you.

c) Hire someone to clean your floors yearly.

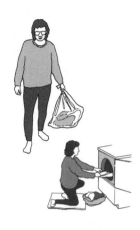

6) **Problem:** Doing laundry. There are various components to laundry that cause problems, including gathering up dirty clothes, carrying them up and down stairs, and loading and unloading the washer and dryer.

Solutions:

a) Use dry cleaning services whenever possible, especially the drive-through or pick-up and delivery service.

b) Instead of using the laundry basket to carry clothes up and down steps, place the clothes in a mesh laundry bag and throw them down the steps. Drag them up the steps behind you.

c) Dryers that have front openings are preferred. You can get closer to the opening to pull out the clothes, making it easier on your low back and arms.

d) Do one or two loads at a time; wash enough clothes for 2 or 3 days, instead of a week.

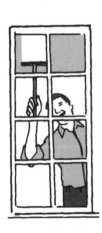

e) Use an assistance device (a reacher/grabber device) to reach into the washer or dryer and avoid bending over.

7) **Problem:** Washing windows. Another enemy of housekeepers and almost everybody else! Reaching, straining the back, wiping; it hurts me to write this, and I don't do windows!

Solutions:

a) Use a long-handled window cleaner with a squeegee to clean the outside windows so you can observe proper fibronomics.

b) Don't try to do all your windows in one day; wash only one window every other day.

c) Hire window cleaners once a year.

8) **Problem:** Getting objects in and out of high cupboards. The reaching and lifting can hurt your shoulders and back.

Solutions:

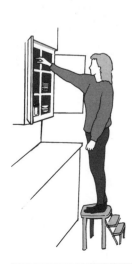

a) Use footstools or kitchen step ladders so you can practice fibronomics when getting objects out of cupboards.

b) Store your everyday pots and pans in the most accessible cupboards; the rarely used and heavy cooking items can go in the higher cupboards or less accessible locations.

c) Store all cooking utensils in a basket on your kitchen counter so they are always accessible.

d) Use a reaching device.

9) **Problem:** Lifting or moving heavy objects or furniture. Every once in a while, we decide it's easier to move something ourselves and we usually will pay the price.

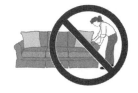

Solutions:

a) Do not buy heavy objects unless they can be placed in a permanent resting spot, and I do mean permanent, forever, always, OK?

b) Do NOT lift heavy objects; leave them where they are as long as they are not bothering anything.

10) **Problem:** Prolonged writing. This might include bill paying or writing letters. Also, frequent typing on computer keyboards can increase neck and shoulder pains.

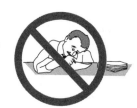

Solutions:

a) Instead of paying bills all at one time, designate two nights a week for the task.

b) Use marker pens or pens with a medium point to minimize the amount of pressing required.

c) Reduce the total number of checks to be written by consolidating loans or using automatic deductions. Some banks offer online bill paying services that might save you time and effort.

d) Write or type a "master" letter and photocopies for your different friends, adding personal tidbits to the individual's copy.

11) **Problem:** Yard work. This can be especially challenging since many patients with fibromyalgia love being outdoors and working on the flowers, garden, or lawn. Rather than giving this up completely, I encourage patients to find ways to enjoy some aspects of yard work without doing work that is too strenuous or painful.

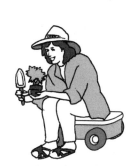

Solutions:

a) Buy a garden seat and cart to allow sitting and other proper fibronomic techniques.

b) Don't be a yard warrior. Break up large tasks into a series of smaller tasks and spread them over a longer period of time. Cut the front grass one night, the back the next, and do the trimming on a third night instead of doing it all in one day.

c) Hire a lawn service for heavy duty tasks, like spring clean-up, edging, or mulching. You do what you enjoy.

Grocery Shopping with Fibromyalgia

Grocery shopping can be a dreaded activity with fibromyalgia. The fibromyalgia homemaker should prepare some shopping strategies. One of the first steps is to choose a time to arrive at the store when no one else wants to shop. It is that simple! During early morning or late evening, most stores are not crowded. Determine the peak shopping hours at your favorite stores and avoid those times. Those times are usually during the lunch hour, after school and work, and Saturday. It is easier to pick a small store that does not have miles of parking lots to cross just to get to the front door. Thus, the super store is usually out. Even if they have a better selection and price, what good is that if you are exhausted even before you get into the store!

Remember where you park your car. Park in the same section all the time if you can.

A shopping list is a must. To make your shopping fast and easy, prepare a master list of all of the products that you will use and purchase. Then, in your mind, go through the store and write down the items in the order that the aisles are arranged in the store. You've made your grocery map from your master list. Check this "master map" before you leave home, and when you arrive at the store you will be organized and can shop fairly quickly with a minimal amount of walking. Conserving your energy is important so you can get those newly purchased groceries into your car!

So you park close, get to the store quickly, avoid any long lines, and keep a list. What other strategies can be helpful to get your groceries into your home? Consider these tips:

1) When you enter the grocery store, look for those small plastic baskets you can carry, and put one in the bottom of the shopping cart basket. Thus you only have to bend and lift one time at the checkout to place the items on the counter, and your grocery cart is easier to unload.

2) Buy smaller amounts of groceries. Beware of quantity. It is better to make two or three trips a week than to buy jumbo sizes of laundry detergents, cereal boxes, and milk containers that are too heavy to handle on a daily basis.

3) Ask for help to get your groceries into the car. The bagger can pack them lightly and in paper bags so they are easier to handle.

4) Keep small laundry baskets in the trunk of your car. These baskets can keep grocery bags upright and prevent them from sliding to the back of the trunk where it is hard to reach. Keep a reacher/grabber (an assisting device) in the trunk to get items you can't reach.

5) Once you arrive home, take the bags containing items that need refrigeration inside; you can unpack the rest at a later time. Or bring the bags into the house and put them away later. Or have a family member or friend carry the bags into the house. You might even pay someone to go out and get your groceries in the first place!

Conquering Cooking

Getting groceries is a challenge, but cooking is a true adventure. The fibromyalgia homemaker may have chosen to not work outside the home, but still have difficulty finding time, energy, or physical stamina to prepare meals. You can cook and not feel guilty in spite of your fibromyalgia.

Prepare meals that can be done quickly and do not require extensive physical labor. Choose recipes that you can rely on when you are tired and operating on very low energy reserves, and prepare meals with ingredients that you have on hand. Avoid meals that require standing for long periods of time to cut vegetables or stand with arms extended over a kitchen counter.

You can keep it simple. Adding items to the meal directly increases the time needed for preparation, serving, and cleaning up. Try to use foods that are already prepared such as salads in a bag, cole slaw, macaroni, and bean salad. Use paper plates, napkins, salad bowls or whatever you can throw away.

Choose meals that can be prepared the night before. Salads, desserts, and vegetables can be prepared early and refrigerated overnight. Make sure you have all of the ingredients as nothing is more frustrating than making a mad dash to the store when you are trying to prepare a meal.

Any job can be made easier if it can be broken down into smaller tasks. Divide and conquer is a good plan. If you've picked a meal that is "fibro-friendly," gathered the necessary ingredients, prepared some items the night before, all you need to do is divide and delegate the work. If you are preparing the meal for yourself, you can take it one step at a time and rest in between. Prepare your salad, sit, eat, then take a short rest, and then progress to the next item. Clean-up can always be done the next day. If you are preparing for others, divide the task so that each person has a job. Remember, clean-up tasks are to be delegated as well.

Make sure your body is in the best possible position while you are in the kitchen to help avoid increased pain. Remember the rules of fibronomics, (see diagram).

Four Rules of Fibronomics:

1) Arms stay home.

2) Unload the back.

3) Support always welcome.

4) Be naturally shifty.

Examples of Fibronomic Applications in the Kitchen:

1) Use disposables to save time. Paper towels, paper plates, paper napkins, paper cups, etc.

2) Use reacher/grabbers and long-handled items.

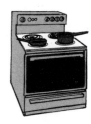

3) Avoid hanging things over the stove or places where you have to lean or reach.

4) Use the front burners on the stove, less reaching is involved.

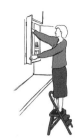

5) Store items in mid-range, avoid using the top or bottom shelves. If you must use high shelving, use a step-ladder. Use a plastic basket on each shelf so you can pull it out and search through it.

6) Store items in the same place everyday (remember, we have fibro-fog).

7) Wash dishes a few at a time. Use a sponge with soap in the handle. Place a container on top of the sink and wash.

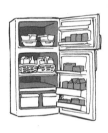

Sit down to clean up spills on the floor. Or use the Ann Evans Bath Towel Method (A.B.T.) to clean up spills. Stand on a towel and use the foot to wipe up the spill!

Buy a refrigerator with the freezer on the bottom. The fridge will be at a more comfortable height, and the lesser-used freezer will be out of the way. Don't forget to put a magnetic notepad (your Fibrominder!) on the refrigerator.

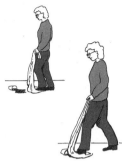

Before doing any type of housework, both physical and mental preparations are necessary. Pretend that you are about to perform an event in the Homemaker Olympics and you are representing your fibromyalgia. In order to make the best representation, you should make certain that adequate time is allowed for warm-up exercises that include stretching and flexibility. Emphasis is placed on the muscles that are going to be used most, and stretching should be done just prior to the event. Mentally visualize how you will perform from start to finish, seeing yourself cross the finish line free from flare-up. Psyche yourself up and tell yourself that you will do the best you can and that you anticipate no surprises.

Hopefully, you will be successful in all your homemaking events and win a lot of gold medals. Who knows, you may even be inducted into the Fibromyalgia Homemaker's Hall of Fame where each recipient is honored with a bronze dust pan!

Grocery Shopping and Cooking Survival Strategies

1) Prepare shopping and cooking strategies to accommodate your fibromyalgia.

2) Develop realistic expectations considering your limited time and energy.

3) Simplify tasks as much as possible to save time and energy.

4) Delegate as much as possible.

5) Remember to use fibronomics.

6) Erect a sign on the front door that says, "Martha Stewart doesn't live here!"

Chapter 28 — Survival Strategies

1) Apply fibronomics to household tasks.

2) Accept that your house cannot always be perfect
— people will still love you anyway!

3) Remember that you have chosen to put other people
or tasks as a higher priority than housekeeping.

4) Divide and delegate as many tasks as possible.

5) Instead of having friends visit at your home - meet them
at a restaurant.

6) Remember that women are no longer measured by the
house they keep or the meals they prepare. If your
home is not perfect, it doesn't mean you are not a
good mother, spouse, person; it means you are a
person who chooses to spend energy on more
important things.

The Fibromyalgia Homemaker   Inside Fibromyalgia with Mark J. Pellegrino, M.D.

244

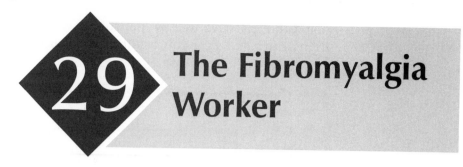

29 The Fibromyalgia Worker

Fibromyalgia plays an important role on the job. Whether the fibromyalgia was actually caused by work injuries, or whether the work is aggravating the pre-existing fibromyalgia, the worker has to make changes in the way he or she approaches work to minimize pain and functional impairment.

Post-traumatic fibromyalgia due to work injuries is being seen more frequently. There may be a single trauma such as a back strain from lifting, or it may be a cumulative trauma that appears over time from continuous performance of specific job activities. The number of cumulative trauma cases has increased. Improved technology has caused jobs to become more repetitive while work speed has increased, work places have become more specialized, and workers and physicians are more aware of symptoms.

Various risk factors are involved in developing post-traumatic fibromyalgia or aggravating pre-existing fibromyalgia. These risk factors include:

1) **Repetitions:** Jobs that require a lot of repetition put continuous strain on soft tissues. Many manufacturing, assembly line, and secretarial jobs involve frequent use of the hands and arms and are examples of jobs that are risky.

2) **Excessive force:** Jobs that require excessive force also increase the risk. Activities such as power gripping or movements against gravity (lifting objects off the ground or pushing up on tools) are examples of activities requiring excessive force on the muscles.

3) **Unnatural positions:** If joints are not in the neutral or natural position, more strain is exerted on them and on soft tissues. The arms outstretched or overhead, elbows away from the body, wrists bent up or down, palms facing up, or leaning forward and bending are various unnatural positions that increase the risk of injury and subsequent post-traumatic fibromyalgia.

4) **Cold, damp environments:** Jobs that require a lot of outdoor exposure, particularly in the winter time, or changing temperatures within the workplace itself (going from a freezer to a refrigerator to a heated area at various times during the course of the day) will increase fibromyalgia symptoms.

5) **Stress:** Increased stress on the job can occur for a variety of reasons. Working long hours or overtime, working strictly night shift, worries about job security or financial issues, and extra responsibilities in management positions are a few examples of stresses on the job that can increase fibromyalgia symptoms.

Various work categories exist and are determined by the amount of lifting and carrying required. They range from sedentary work to very heavy work. Often, light duty is not tolerated well by individuals with fibromyalgia. Even though no heavy lifting is involved, light duty requires a lot of arm repetitions, which can increase pain in people with fibromyalgia.

Job Considerations

Individuals with fibromyalgia must consider various factors when looking for a job. First, one must develop a realistic outlook for the type of job that he or she would qualify for from a physical standpoint. Since individuals with fibromyalgia have a difficult time performing activities that require reaching, overhead use of the arms, bending and heavy lifting, certain high risk jobs would not be considered realistic.

Examples of high risk jobs involving a lot of reaching and overhead use of the arms include assembly line jobs, dry-walling, hair styling, secretarial, computer programming, transcription, carpentry, and bricklaying. These types of jobs are more demanding on the neck, shoulders and upper back. I have seen a number of women hair stylists and school bus drivers who gradually developed fibromyalgia over the years. Some of them had to give up their jobs because of the pain. Examples of jobs that require a lot of bending and heavy lifting include construction workers, welders, truck drivers, and movers. These jobs are more demanding on the low back. You need to know the risk factors and risky jobs and try to avoid them as much as possible when looking for a job.

Job hunting is difficult enough, even without fibromyalgia. *Know your strengths and weaknesses, and know that, in spite of fibromyalgia, you can be a reliable, dependable, efficient and intelligent worker who would be an asset to any company.*

Job hunting is difficult enough, even without fibromyalgia. *Know your strengths and weaknesses, and know that, in spite of fibromyalgia, you can be a reliable, dependable, efficient and intelligent worker who would be an asset to any company.* Research the companies and fields that particularly interest you and take advantage of any professional guidance that might be available through various schools, career centers, and reference books. Let your natural ability to be organized, concise and "perfect" help you in developing a professional resume and plan.

The web site of the President's Committee on Employment of People with Disabilities gives job links of employers who have indicated interest in recruiting and hiring qualified individuals with disabilities. This web site is: http://www50.pcepd.gov/pcepd/joblinks.htm.

Explore the type of hours available at any prospective job. Part-time, flexible hours might suit you best compared to a full-time job. Swing shifts and strictly night jobs are more difficult due to the disruption it causes on the already impaired sleep pattern. Even persons who work permanent night shifts never develop the quality of sleep of persons that work the day shift, so keep this in mind and seek stable daytime hours if you can.

Health insurance is certainly an important issue. Persons with fibromyalgia require periodic medical attention ranging from seeing the doctor, taking medication, participating in therapies, to taking time off work altogether. A job that provides adequate health insurance and acceptable sick time is certainly a plus.

Checklist to Think about when Considering a New Job:

Hours:

- What type of shift?
- How many hours over 40?
- Flexible schedule?
- Commute time?
- Part time vs. fulltime?
- Can you make up missed time on weekend?

Building:

- Can you park close?
- Stairs, elevator?
- Climate, cold, damp, basement?
- Furniture, ergonomic?

Physical:

- Standing too much?
- Sitting too much?
- Can you pace your work?

Work Load:

- Can you rotate tasks?
- Are deadlines critical?
- Are others depending on your work before they can finish theirs?
- How much pressure?
- How much politics
- Work quotas?

Work Environment:

- Lighting?
- Heating?
- Cooling?
- Drafts?
- Quiet?
- Disruptions?
- Phones?

Insurance:

- Is it adequate?

- Long term paid medical leave?

- Pharmacy plan?

Should You Reveal FM?

A frequently asked question is whether an individual should reveal his/her fibromyalgia to a potential employer. I always advise my patients not to volunteer any information regarding their health, specifically as it relates to fibromyalgia, because chances are a potential employer will not know what the condition is and will consider it something negative. The Americans with Disabilities Act, otherwise known as ADA, protects people who have disabilities from job discrimination. A potential employer is not supposed to ask about any medical condition, either on the application or during the interview, according to the ADA. However, the employer can perform medical testing on a newly hired employee to make sure the employee is medically able to perform the job for which he/she was hired.

I understand that both the potential employer and potential employee have specific interests and concerns. The employer does not want to hire someone who may have a pre-existing medical condition which will worsen once the individual begins a new job, thus costing the employer. From this standpoint, any medical information about the employee might be harmful to him/her, particularly if the employer were to assume that fibromyalgia, because it causes pain, would mean that the employee would not be able to perform a particular job. Of course, the potential employee wants to be honest and not hide anything, but why should you volunteer information that could cost you a job? I feel the potential employee should receive the benefit of the doubt.

> I always advise my patients not to volunteer any information regarding their health, specifically as it relates to fibromyalgia, because chances are a potential employer will not know what the condition is and will consider it something negative.
>
> A potential employer is not supposed to ask about any medical condition, either on the application or during the interview, according to the ADA. However, the employer can perform medical testing on a newly hired employee to make sure the employee is medically able to perform the job for which he/she was hired.

By law, this question should never come up before a job is offered, but if it does, you need to answer in the manner in which you are most comfortable. If you choose to reveal your fibromyalgia, it should be done in a manner that focuses on your abilities, not your inabilities. I would try to convince the employer that you have a good understanding of your condition and know your limitations. Point out that you are capable of handling the job, and that you consider yourself a responsible, reliable and efficient individual who would be an asset to the company. An honest and confident approach is probably your best long-term strategy even though this approach could still scare away some potential employers. But don't offer anything about your fibromyalgia unless you have to. If you are hired, you may be asked to undergo a medical evaluation to assure you are medically fit for a particular job.

Once an individual finds a job, what can be done to prevent fibromyalgia from developing or flaring up? Preventive measures focus on stopping the problem from ever developing in the first place, or in the case of the fibromyalgia worker, preventing flare-ups from occurring. Maintain a regular stretching and exercise program to reduce the chance of injury. A worker should approach his or her job in the same way a trained athlete approaches a sporting event. Prior to attempting any sport, the athlete will perform warm-up exercises, especially those that include stretching. The fibromyalgia worker must also perform warm-up stretching exercises prior to performing the daily event. The stretching exercises will improve flexibility and circulation, decrease the tendon tightness, and decrease the chance of stretch and tear injuries.

Pay attention to increased pain and early symptoms of a flare-up. The company doctor or nurse should be notified. Contact your personal physician, if available. Over-the-counter pain medications, modalities

The Americans with Disabilities Act requires employers to provide equal employment opportunities for people who are able to do the job, but who are limited by physical disabilities. The employee has a right to reasonable accommodations provided by the employer to help overcome any physical limitations.

(heat, ice or muscle creams) and work restrictions can be part of the initial treatment. If the flare-up worsens or a new problem develops in spite of what you do, further medical evaluation by your own physician will be necessary. The earlier a flare-up or injury is treated, the better the chance of resolving the problem.

Ongoing training and education involves periodically analyzing your work site and recognizing and correcting any ergonomic or fibronomic hazards. Work positions, power tools, ergonomic chair, telephone headset, or other adaptive equipment may be helpful. Working with your company's safety committee to review any injury trends or identify any patterns that can be further analyzed and remedied, if possible, is part of the ongoing follow-up needs.

Reasonable Accommodations

The employee, the employer and the doctor can work together to create a safe, pain-free workplace. The Americans with Disabilities Act requires employers to provide equal employment opportunities for people who are able to do the job, but who are limited by physical disabilities. The employee has a right to reasonable accommodations provided by the employer to help overcome any physical limitations.

Examples of reasonable accommodations for fibromyalgia workers (and all workers) in an assembly line setting might include:

1) Rotating jobs to minimize the chance of flare-ups rather than performing a single job all the time.

2) Rearranging work stations and providing ergonomic tools to optimize proper body mechanics and use of the rules of fibronomics.

3) Providing rubber mats where prolonged standing is required.

4) Allowing frequent breaks during the work day.

5) Allowing scheduled time for stretching exercises.

6) Forming an education and prevention committee.

Examples of reasonable accommodations for a clerical worker might include an ergonomic chair, a phone headset, a couch in the break room to lie down, and allowing frequent stretch breaks at the workstation.

In general, patients of mine who work in small business or professional offices report that their employers are very understanding and cooperative. From patients who work in larger corporations, I frequently hear that an employer is not as receptive and responsive to some of the individual issues. Know what your legal rights are under ADA and work with your union representative or legal advisor if necessary.

The fibromyalgia worker's personal physician has an important role in helping the worker preserve gainful employment. Flare-ups of fibromyalgia occurring at work need to be evaluated by the physician and treated aggressively. Most of the time, a flare-up is related to a temporary situation that can be successfully treated. The person can resume a normal baseline and return to regular job duties. Specific treatment depends on the specific area or areas of flare-up as addressed in Chapter 35.

Part of the treatment approach of a fibromyalgia worker who is experiencing a flare-up is the need to consider work restrictions. These can range anywhere from complete time off work to limiting certain activities.

The Family Medical Leave Act (FMLA) was passed to allow workers to take time off work when they (or family members) are incapacitated and require medical treatment for a serious health condition. An employee who takes an FMLA leave is assured that his/her job will remain available once the medical condition has disappeared or stabilized. A health care provider must certify a FMLA leave. I complete FMLA forms for my patients when necessary.

On the FMLA form fibromyalgia is defined as a serious health condition under Category 4: Chronic Conditions Requiring Treatment. This chronic condition requires periodic visits for treatment, continues over an extended period of time and may cause episodic incapacity (flare-ups that make the person unable to work). I describe the medical facts supporting the diagnosis of fibromyalgia and the need for FMLA certification and would indicate if the condition is incapacitating or can cause intermittent inability to work a full schedule. I usually state that fibromyalgia is a condition that may unpredictably flare up from time to time resulting in impairment of work ability and may require a time off work on a temporary basis. I describe the health services needed, such as medications, therapies, or injections, and explain the justifications for a leave from work. A leave from work may be brief — one or two days — or may require a few months. The patients and I work together to keep time off work to a minimum and prioritize returning to work and staying there as much as possible.

If the patient is able to continue working, work restrictions may be necessary. Examples of work restrictions specific to a patient with fibromyalgia include:

1) Not working more than eight hours a day, five days a week; specifically, no overtime or weekends

2) Working part-time hours, working day hours only, or working flexible hours

3) Avoiding temperature changes (no exposure to cold or damp weather)

4) No direct air-conditioning drafts

5) No repetitive reaching or overhead use of the arms

6) No repetitive bending or leaning forward

7) No sitting, standing, or walking for a certain period of time before alternating positions

In addition to work restrictions, a prescription for specific adaptive devices may be necessary. This could include:

1) Phones with headsets to minimize the reaching and bending required to manually hold the phone

2) An ergonomic chair

3) A modified typing station that includes a drop keyboard, wrist bars, and arm rests

4) A back brace to be worn at work only

Many times I will place absolute restrictions on patients in terms of weight lifting (no lifting more than 20 pounds frequently and 50 pounds occasionally). If a person is experiencing a flare-up, I may temporarily place more restrictions depending on the individual situation. If the flare-up resolves and the person returns to baseline state, the restrictions can be removed. I prescribe rest often as part of a treatment program. If repeated flare-ups are occurring within a certain job description, it may be necessary to place permanent restrictions on the worker.

Quite often a person can be off work, obtain therapy and treatment, and feel pretty good. But if no attempt is made to alter the job situation, it is not surprising that when he/she returns to work, another flare-up occurs. The flare-up may occur within days or may take months. Long-term strategies are vital in helping a fibromyalgia worker sustain gainful employment.

Most patients will indicate that their pain level is less when they are not working. When a person returns to work, the pain baseline creeps up. Hopefully, it stabilizes at a level that enables one to continue working at a comfortable baseline.

I frequently write letters to patients' employers on their behalf to explain what fibromyalgia is and how it causes muscle pain and interferes with certain activities. I will indicate restrictions, but at the same time focus on what the person is able to do. Employers who are receptive to open communication between patient, doctor, and employer usually make every effort to facilitate effective strategies at the work site.

The fibromyalgia worker is responsible for continuing his or her regular home program even though he or she may be working full time. If this home program is not maintained, the work pain baseline will probably creep up even higher and be very easily triggered into a flare-up or recurrent flare-up.

If various treatments such as modifying the physical stresses at work, rearranging the workstation, placing work restrictions, prescribing rest, or completing a physical therapy or occupational therapy program does not help the fibromyalgia worker maintain a regular job, a different job altogether needs to be considered. Vocational counselors can help persons find different jobs that allow for medical restrictions, retrain for new skills, or pursue educational programs for entirely new careers. There are vocational bureaus at the state level that offer qualified vocational counselors.

It is my experience that the majority of fibromyalgia workers are motivated and determined to maintain their jobs, but issues of disability may need to be pursued. I think that total disability should be rare in fibromyalgia, and despite all the problems, there should be something that the individual should be able to do. However, the economy is not always receptive to a worker with various restrictions due to a medical condition, and all factors have to be considered when determining whether total, partial or no disability applies to a person with fibromyalgia.

> The fibromyalgia worker is responsible for continuing his or her regular home program even though he or she may be working full time. If this home program is not maintained, the work pain baseline will probably creep up even higher and be very easily triggered into a flare-up or recurrent flare-up.

The patient and doctor need to work together to reach these difficult decisions.

I believe in maximizing one's abilities despite his or her medical condition. In an ideal situation, there will always be some type of job an individual with fibromyalgia could perform despite the pain. Individuals with pain who are gainfully employed will think less about pain. I recognize a big difference between the ideal situation and the real world, and I certainly work with each individual's situation to try for the best possible quality of life.

I'm often asked how I can continue a hectic full time schedule with my fibromyalgia. I remind them that everyone's fibromyalgia is different. My job is a sedentary one. I'm supposed to be using my brain mainly. I am able to shift my body positions to avoid strains. I can control my hours to allow rest times. Sure, I get flare-ups like everyone else, and I deal with them when they happen. I hope I can continue to work for a long time. I always think ahead, but I take one day at a time.

Chapter 29 — Survival Strategies

1) Develop a realistic outlook for the type of job you would qualify for from a physical standpoint.

2) Know your strengths and weaknesses both physically and mentally.

3) Realize that even with fibromyalgia you can be a reliable, dependable, efficient and intelligent worker.

4) Take advantage of any career guidance provided through schools, career centers, and books.

5) Develop a professional resume and plan.

6) Research companies and fields that interest you.

7) Continue your home program with the same intensity.

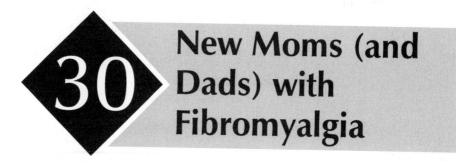

30 New Moms (and Dads) with Fibromyalgia

Fibromyalgia affects mostly women, and many of them are first bothered by symptoms in their early reproductive years, so it is common for issues regarding pregnancy to surface. This entire chapter is devoted to mothers-to-be or new mothers who have fibromyalgia. New dads with fibromyalgia will also benefit from reading this chapter.

A frequent question is whether or not a woman should consider getting pregnant if she has fibromyalgia. From a medical perspective, there is no contraindication or unusual medical risk involved with fibromyalgia and pregnancy. Fibromyalgia has not been shown to cause infertility or increased miscarriages. Endometriosis frequently occurs with fibromyalgia and may cause problems with getting pregnant. Fibromyalgia has a hereditary component and could be passed on from parent to child, but this is not considered a dangerous medical risk or a reason to avoid pregnancy.

Another concern is whether or not the pregnancy will cause a significant flare-up for the pregnant woman, or perhaps aggravate the condition to a more severe level that persists after the pregnancy. I have treated many women for whom pregnancy has played a major role in the onset of fibromyalgia. A number of women in my practice have indicated that they were never bothered by any symptoms before pregnancy, but since then, they have had persistent muscle pains and have been diagnosed with fibromyalgia. Surprisingly though, I find that more women who develop fibromyalgia from pregnancy do so after their second pregnancy, not their first.

Another group of women have indicated that they had some pre-existing mild muscle pain, but pregnancy worsened their overall condition and led to fibromyalgia. A few individuals traced the onset of their initial low back problems and generalized fibromyalgia to their epidural procedure during delivery. Overall, a large number of women with pre-existing fibromyalgia state that their condition flared up during the pregnancy. In some, the condition became worse overall, but most have said their conditions returned to their previous stable baseline after the baby was born.

Because many people seem to have problems with increased pain, does that mean the hopeful mother-to-be should be advised not to consider pregnancy because of her fibromyalgia? Absolutely not! Despite the numerous reports, these same women will also tell you that the reward, a beautiful baby, was well worth any pain and suffering they had to endure. The benefit far outweighed the risk. Their advice to mothers or potential mothers with fibromyalgia is this: "Go ahead with it, you will be glad you did. I have no regrets and I would do the same thing all over again." (And many do!) I think that the more sophisticated one's knowledge, the better she will anticipate and deal with any increased pain during the whole process of making a new family member.

The woman with fibromyalgia must consider many issues when deciding whether or not to have a child. There may already be a strained marital relationship, which could be further strained by adding a child. The potential mother needs to know how much help the spouse and relatives are willing to give, especially if extra help is going to be needed because of fibromyalgia. Finances can be a big concern. Will the mother still be able to work and care for the baby? These issues and many more need to be carefully considered when making the decision.

Once the decision is made, the first thing that should be done, even before becoming pregnant, is to review all the medications related to fibromyalgia. Very few medications have been found to be completely safe during pregnancy; so as a rule of thumb, all prescription medicines should

> From a medical perspective, there is no contraindication or unusual medical risk involved with fibromyalgia and pregnancy. Fibromyalgia has not been shown to cause infertility or increased miscarriages.

be reviewed with the primary care doctor for advice on whether or not they can be discontinued altogether. Some medicines can be completely stopped. Others have to be weaned gradually. Remember that medicine should be completely out of her system before the woman attempts to become pregnant (about a week after stopping medicines). If one waits until the pregnancy is confirmed, the fetus will already have been exposed to the medicine for a month. Vitamins and nutritional supplements also need to be reviewed with the doctor prior to actual pregnancy. Don't just stop medicines as some may need to be gradually weaned off: check with your doctor first.

Fibromyalgia dads should review their medications as well prior to actual attempts to impregnate their partners. Sperm cells are well protected from medication side effects, and the chance of causing a defective sperm that will affect the fetus at the time of conception is very remote.

If medications were a crucial part of the overall pain management, there may some increased pain once the body realizes the medicines are no longer in the system. However, there is also a readjustment phenomenon. The pain settles down again after it rebounded upward, and levels off to a more stable baseline, even though the baseline may be a little higher than the one achieved with medication. This is the time to take advantage of more natural measures to control pain, such as using moist heating pads, hot baths, ice packs, massage, or trying to get pregnant! Certain over-the-counter pain medications may be allowed during pregnancy. Check with your primary care physician.

A hopeful mother-to-be can take several measures to decrease the risk of fibromyalgia flare-up, whether or not medications were being used. Here are a few tips.

1) **Exercise.** Stay with a regular exercise program that includes stretching and conditioning exercises, with emphasis on the back. This is always easier said than done, but hopefully the mother-to-be will already be performing a regular exercise program.

   This program does not have to be time-consuming. Our studies have shown that 20 minutes of exercise three times a week will significantly improve overall conditioning and strength. Stretching exercises should be done daily, however, and the trick is to integrate an overall program into your lifestyle and then continue even after the baby is born.

2) **No smoking or exposure to secondhand smoke.** Nicotine decreases the blood flow to the muscles by constricting the arteries, which decreases the oxygen and increases the pain in the muscles. Cigarette smoke can also be harmful to the fetus. Frequent coughing can strain the back and cause exacerbation of the fibromyalgia.

3) **Follow fibronomics.** The mother-to-be needs to perfect the techniques of proper posture and body mechanics (and fibronomics). She will really need to call upon these skills once she has the baby.

4) **Get proper rest.** Proper rest resets the body's physiologic mechanism to help ward off injury, illness, and stress, and reduces the chance of a flare-up.

5) **Schedule time for yourself.** The mother-to-be should try to set aside at least an hour a day for her own private time. This is the time to relax, listen to music, read a book, work on a hobby, or enjoy recreational activities. This will help deal with physical and emotional stress.

Pregnancy Changes

What happens to the body during pregnancy as it relates to fibromyalgia?

At the beginning of pregnancy, the body's hormones are undergoing rapid changes. The changes in the blood level concentration of various hormones such as estrogen and progesterone are necessary to enable the fetus to grow in a proper well-balanced environment and to prepare the mother for the birth. Surging hormonal changes in the first trimester can have opposite effects on the muscles of women with fibromyalgia. About half of my patients state that their muscles become more painful and they experience an overall aggravation of their fibromyalgia. In addition, many types of smells and various foods are not tolerated well, especially in the morning. These symptoms lead women to describe a feeling that they have the flu.

About half of the women, however, actually feel better from a fibromyalgia standpoint during the first trimester of pregnancy. This is somewhat surprising since, normally, any type of change in the body causes increased muscle pain. However, not all changes must be bad, since a good percentage of women actually feel better. The reason for this improvement is probably due to hormonal changes that cause positive psychological mood changes and decreased sensitivity of the muscle pain receptors. Your body physiologically tries to make you feel "happy" during pregnancy.

The woman with fibromyalgia must consider many issues when deciding whether or not to have a child. There may already be a strained marital relationship, which could be further strained by adding a child. The potential mother needs to know how much help the spouse and relatives are willing to give, especially if extra help is going to be needed because of fibromyalgia. Finances can be a big concern. Will the mother still be able to work and care for the baby?

During the second trimester of pregnancy, the stress to the body slowly increases. As the fetus grows, the resulting protrusion shifts the body's center of gravity forward. In order to compensate for this shifting weight, the lumbar spine must curve backwards, and in doing so increases the swayback posture, also known as lumbar lordosis.

This position creates unusual strain on the back muscles as they work harder to maintain a balanced erect posture, and the risk of back pain increases.

For every pound of extra weight in the front of the body, there are more than two pounds of extra force exerted on the low back to compensate; so there isn't an even trade-off. The back works harder. These muscles become stressed and are more likely to cause pain and fatigue. Also, the back is more vulnerable to injury and strain. This is true for overweight people as well.

Hormonal changes during pregnancy cause the back and pelvic ligaments to soften to enable easier stretching during delivery. However this softening alters the structural balance of the back, increases the mechanical stress, and results in more back strain.

As the pregnancy progresses, the fibromyalgia mother-to-be becomes more at risk for increased generalized pain, especially in the low back area, and increased fatigue. It is important to continue the regular stretching and conditioning exercises during pregnancy, especially for the low back.

About half of the women, however, actually feel better from a fibromyalgia standpoint during the first trimester of pregnancy.

Towards the end of pregnancy all the muscles, especially the spinal muscles, are more strained. The physiologic weight gain during pregnancy has increased the energy demands and requirements on the muscles. The extra breast weight further destabilizes the upper spine and mid-back area and contributes to an unnatural strained positioning. The muscles are becoming overwhelmed and aren't "happy" anymore.

The majority of fibromyalgia women report increased muscle pain particularly in the low back towards the end of pregnancy. By then, all of the various factors have compounded to cause increased pain. It is difficult for the new mother-to-be to find comfortable positions or control her pain. I have had many of my patients participate in a supervised physical therapy program that includes heat and massage to the low back during the later stages of pregnancy. Also, trigger point injections have been helpful. This technique is not contraindicated during pregnancy, but the obstetrician and the fibromyalgia doctors need to carefully review this possible treatment method and indications for each individual patient.

Although late pregnancy may be a difficult time, it is almost the end. The mother can call upon all of her tricks and techniques to control the pain, with a little extra help from therapy or other medical treatments if needed, and hopefully keep the condition manageable.

After childbirth, additional factors can cause acute exacerbation of back pain or fibromyalgia symptoms. During labor and childbirth, sudden strenuous contractions pull on the back structures. If the labor is prolonged, the already vulnerable low back can sustain acute injury.

There is no evidence that natural childbirth versus epidural versus C-section makes any difference in terms of whether or not the woman will experience a flare-up of fibromyalgia back pain during childbirth. There are several patients in my practice who feel that the epidural itself was the cause of the fibromyalgia, first starting off as back pain, then generalizing. It is theoretically possible that there could be a "trauma" associated with the epidural, particularly difficult epidurals as my patients described, to result in a post-trau-matic fibromyalgia. How-ever, epidurals are gener-ally safe and only rarely result in complications, and may be necessary and recommended for child-birth. I think the poten-tial benefits of epidurals, such as decreased pain, far outweigh any potential risk concerning fibromyalgia.

Towards the end of pregnancy all of the various factors have compounded to cause increased pain. I have had many of my patients participate in a supervised physical therapy program that includes heat and massage to the low back dur-ing the later stages of pregnancy. Also, trigger point injec-tions have been helpful.

Fibromyalgia mothers become fatigued easily during labor. However, there is no evidence of defective uterine contraction pattern unique to fibromyalgia mothers, nor has there been any evidence showing that fibromyalgia mothers should have more C-sections compared to vaginal deliveries.

Post-pregnancy Factors

Back pain may develop within hours after delivery, whether it was a vaginal deliv-ery or a C-section. The abdominal and pelvic muscles stretched and weakened during the pregnancy and delivery are not able to balance the spine well, and painful muscle spasms can occur. After delivery, there is decreased mobility and activity as the new mother adjusts to the post pregnancy changes and restores the body's energy supply. This is a risky time for flare-ups.

Back stretching and strengthening exercises should be started within a few days after delivery, with an attempt to resume the fibromyalgia home program as quickly as possible. Sometimes extra support is needed, such as a back brace or abdominal binder for a few weeks until the muscles can regain their strength and provide support. Larger breasted women who are nursing should wear a supportive bra so the extra breast weight does not further de-stabilize the spinal balance and increase neck, shoulder, or back pain.

By far the biggest challenge on the new mother's fibromyalgia is the newest mem-ber of the family, the infant! This lovable, irresistible little person who weighs less than 10 pounds manages to locate him or herself into strategic positions that are most challenging to the new mother's ability to maintain proper low back and body pos-ture. Whether the baby is in a crib, on the floor, or nestled in a car seat, the new mother must bend, and bend frequently, to a level below her waist. Twisting and reaching go hand-in-hand with bending, and all three of these positions are hazardous to the vulnerable back and the fibromyalgia mother. Carrying the infant is also diffi-cult and the burden on the back increases as the child grows.

Both physical and emotional stress can cause a flare-up of pain. As we know, people under stress often tense their muscles, which causes spasms and pain. New mothers are certainly under a lot of stress due to the physical and emotional responsibilities of a newborn. Even though this type of stress may be considered good, the fibromyalgia muscles do not make a distinction.

An additional imposed stress on the new mother is sleep deprivation. Lack of sleep is synonymous with being a new mother! Increased pain and fatigue result.

Mothers who breastfeed their babies are at particular risk for sleep deprivation and this is a factor to consider when deciding whether or not you want to nurse your baby. Mothers who nurse will probably not get back on medications as quickly as mothers who choose to bottle feed. Most of my patients choose to bottle feed, particularly after the first pregnancy, because it causes fewer sleep problems and enables the partner to be more involved in the nighttime feedings.

There is no evidence that natural childbirth versus epidural versus C-section makes any difference in terms of whether or not the woman will experience a flareup of fibromyalgia back pain during childbirth.

Postpartum depression is also common, and can lead to additional poor sleep, increased fatigue, and increased pain. Fibromyalgia women don't seem to be more prone to postpartum depression than their non-fibromyalgia counterparts but I wouldn't be surprised if future research shows otherwise since people with fibromyalgia are more prone to clinical depression. Given all of these stresses, it is no wonder that a new mother is more vulnerable to pain. If all of these stresses overwhelm the muscles, acute flare-ups can occur.

How does the new mother decrease her risk for an acute injury or flare-up as she cares for her new baby? Here are a few tips.

1) **Resume your regular exercise program of stretching and conditioning exercises as soon as possible.** Start with five minutes of stretching twice a day for a week and then increase ten minutes twice a day the second week. During the third week and thereafter continue with fifteen minutes a day.

   The second week after delivery, begin a regular exercise program which might first include casual walking for ten minutes three to four times a week, gradually progressing to at least twenty minutes three times a week. The trick is to integrate a regular exercise program into your new mother's lifestyle.

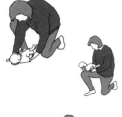

2) **Follow fibronomics** (Moms and Dads). Although it is impossible to avoid dangerous positions (bending, twisting, reaching, lifting), a new mother can learn to practice proper posture and body mechanics, specifically fibronomics, when lifting and carrying the child or engaging in other activities.

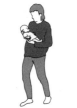

   To properly place the infant on the floor, or to pick the infant up from the floor, avoid bending at the waist; instead, bend at the legs and allow the legs to do the lifting while maintaining a natural back position. The one-knee lift technique allows you to bring your baby close to the body before completing the lift. Keep your elbows close to your sides.

   To properly carry the infant, always hold the child close to your own center of gravity, which is from the chest to the naval area. Keep your elbows at your side and avoid reaching out and lifting.

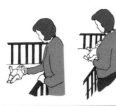

   To place in or pick up from the crib, first drop the crib side to the lowest position possible to minimize the bending required. Spread your legs apart and bend your knees slightly to lower your chest and the infant as much as possible. Keep back in neutral position. Slowly bend forward with the infant still held close to your chest and then slowly open the arms, keeping your elbows against your abdomen. Set your infant down on the crib and gently ease into the proper lying position.

To adjust your baby's position once in the crib, try using a technique called the Golfer's Lift, (see diagram in Chapter 20, page 163). To place the infant into the car seat, put your foot onto the car floor, and lean as close as possible to the car seat. Try to keep your elbows as close to the side as possible during the transfer into the car seat. Since baby's car seat has to go in back because of front seat air bags, it is hard to turn around and see the baby. Many new mothers say turning the neck causes pain to flare up. A trick is to secure another mirror below the rear-view mirror to allow you to see into the middle of the back seat, (see diagram). You can glance in this mirror and monitor your baby without twisting your neck.

As your child gets older (and heavier), take advantage of his/her developing motor skills to protect your back. Let your child crawl onto your lap instead of picking him up. Whenever possible, sit instead of stand to hold. Encourage your child to walk from point A to B instead of carrying her.

3) **Get proper rest**; proper sleep resets the body's physiologic mechanisms. Avoid caffeine at night. You may take naps during the day as needed.

4) **Schedule your own time.** Try to set aside at least an hour a day that you consider your own private time. This is when you should achieve relaxation, and do other leisurely activities such as reading a book, listening to music, or working on a hobby.

5) **Pain relief can be obtained by various measures.** Check with your doctor to see what over-the-counter medications may be allowed. All of these medicines, except Tylenol, can help decrease both pain and any acute inflammation. (Tylenol decreases pain but does not help inflammation in a strained muscle.) Application of light heat or an ice pack can help decrease pain and spasms and increase blood flow.

Sleeping medications should usually be avoided. A sleeping medicine may prevent the mother from hearing the infant cry or have side effects such as drowsiness,

Although it is impossible to avoid dangerous positions (bending, twisting, reaching, lifting), a new mother can learn to practice proper posture and body mechanics, specifically fibronomics, when lifting and carrying the child or engaging in other activities.

confusion, or impaired balance. If the new mother is not nursing, she should try to work out a call schedule with her husband to handle night time feedings so she can get a good night's sleep. Although a new mother with fibromyalgia may be at a higher risk for developing flare-ups or acute low back strain, she can learn how to prevent or minimize these consequences so they do not interfere with the wonderful task of having and raising a new baby.

6) **Consider taking longer than the usual 6 week medical leave to recover.** Sometimes fibromyalgia delays recovery and you may need a few more weeks before you are ready to return to work.

Fibromyalgia Fathers

Fibromyalgia fathers certainly experience a lot of stress and anxiety during the wife's/partner's pregnancy. It is natural to have concerns about the well-being of the developing fetus and the mother's health, and these natural stresses can cause fibromyalgia flare-ups.

The fibromyalgia father needs to pay special attention to proper fibronomics just as the mother does. If the mother chooses to bottle feed, as my wife did, the fibromyalgia father should be involved in the bottle feeding. I took on feeding responsibilities particularly on weekends. I am not sure which was worse, my weekend night call duties feeding the baby, or my medical on-call duties! Truthfully, I didn't mind the night feeding call duties at all because I was happily fulfilling my duty as a new parent. I was able to psyche myself up for these upcoming weekend duties, and my wife and I worked out an arrangement so I could catch up on my sleep when I was "off duty." This helped me to minimize potential fibromyalgia flare-ups.

Chapter 30 — Survival Strategies

1) Consider that as a mother with fibromyalgia, there is no medical risk involved with fibromyalgia and pregnancy.

2) Realize fibromyalgia has a hereditary component and can be passed from parent to child, but this is not considered a dangerous medical risk or reason to avoid pregnancy.

  a) Discuss with your spouse how fibromyalgia will affect your pregnancy. Ask the following questions: Is the marital relationship already strained because of fibromyalgia? Will that strain increase with the baby?

  b) How much help can you depend on from spouse and relatives?

  c) What will happen financially if you are unable to work during part of the pregnancy?

  d) Will you physically be able to work and take care of a baby?

3) Expect some increase in pain during the pregnancy. Your goal will be to keep your condition "manageable."

4) Once you decide to become pregnant, review all medications with your doctor and discontinue most or all medications before conceiving.

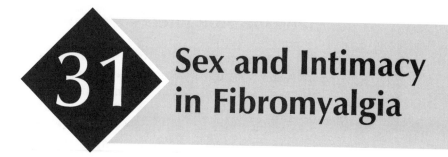

Sex and Intimacy in Fibromyalgia

Chronic pain and illness can affect sex and intimacy in a relationship. Fibromyalgia and its chronic pain often intervene and introduce new fears, concerns, and anxieties into a relationship. Fibromyalgia affects everything else, so why shouldn't it cause some unique problems with sex and intimacy as well? The main problem is pain, and pain is the physiological equivalent of a cold shower!

Pain

Muscle pain can result in painful intercourse. People with fibromyalgia hurt all over and are more sensitive to pain. Muscles are particularly sensitive to pressure and squeezing, and these muscles usually "talk louder" during attempts at intimacy. Sometimes, no matter how careful or gentle you may be proceeding, each and every muscle that gets involved or is touched will scream out. This is a distraction, to say the least.

The muscles can hurt with any pressure or weight on them, and that makes it difficult to be on the bottom. Many women with fibromyalgia have pelvic pain due to the involvement of the pelvic and sacroiliac muscles as well as the low back muscles. This can cause pain during intercourse attempts. Men with fibromyalgia may have severe low back pain, particularly when the man is on top. Sometimes intimacy is moving along fairly smoothly, then suddenly a muscle develops a painful cramp right in the middle of intercourse.

Fatigue

Fatigue is also a problem. Energy is required to be sexually active, but there is very little energy at times with fibromyalgia. This physical fatigue makes it difficult to feel like moving your body at all, much less being sexually active. The mental fatigue is just as bad as it can result in decreased motivation and loss of libido.

The person with fibromyalgia may be going to bed several hours before the partner and is asleep by the time the partner gets ready for bed. It is difficult to have a successful sexual intimacy when one person is asleep! For persons in a deep sleep stage, this particular sleep stage is highly coveted for it is short-lived. I guarantee this deep sleep will be more desired than sex at 11:30 p.m.!

Associated Conditions

Irritable bowel syndrome can cause nausea, abdominal pains, and more bowel alertness than sexual alertness. Depression can cause additional loss of motivation, loss of interest, and loss of libido. Frequently, weight gain is a problem with fibromyalgia, and this can lead to further loss of interest due to low self-esteem or embarrassment.

Medicine Side Effects

The medications used to treat fibromyalgia can cause side effects that interfere with sexual abilities. Specific medicines, particularly those that increase the serotonin level, can decrease the sexual response. In women, this means decreased sexual desire, responsiveness, or inability to achieve orgasm. In men, there may be decreased libido or difficulty achieving erections. Other medicines can cause extreme sedation, which prevents sexual alertness. Some medicines cause nausea or gastrointestinal side effects, which shift the focus of attention to the bathroom rather than the bedroom.

Fibromyalgia does not physiologically interfere with the sexual function, however, even though there may be some problem because of the pain, fatigue, or treatments.

Benefits of Sex

If you focus on the benefits of sex rather than the problems, you can reassure yourself that becoming intimate is good for you and your relationship. Think of sex as being therapeutic. It is a physical activity that increases the body's endorphins (natural pain killers). It improves blood flow, removes toxins from the cells, and boosts the immune system. The physical activity provides stretching, conditioning, and relaxation of the muscles. Plus, one tends to forget about pain during intimacy.

Strategies to Improve Sex and Intimacy

You need to be reassured that you are not hurting yourself by being intimate; rather you are helping both your fibromyalgia and the relationship. Your partner is also dealing with fears and anxieties about hurting you, so you both need to be reassured about the positive aspects of being intimate.

Open Communication

Open communication is the most important factor in dealing with sex and intimacy problems. Talk to each other and discuss what hurts and what helps, and attempt to overcome any fears and anxieties that are present. Frequently, couples tell me that they are not comfortable having conversations about sex and may find it embarrassing to speak freely at first. If a couple's relationship is already built on solid communication, talking about intimacy will be more comfortable. Begin discussion and communication gradually, then become more open in your sharing.

Re-discover the Romance

Intimacy does not mean sex alone or having sex at all. Men seem to be confused at times regarding this concept! I frequently hear women complaining that their husbands ignore them during the day, or don't bother to say two words to them, but then when they get into bed, they expect a switch to turn on and proceed with sexual activity. Intimacy does not happen in the bedroom only; it is something that occurs throughout the day.

Men need to learn that what they do during the day is the most important factor in whether or not they will be intimate (by man's definition) that night. Women must realize that they too need to be responsive to their mate throughout the day. Make sure you notice your significant other, compliment him or her, smile to send intimacy signals, and be a loving mate.

Touching, hand-holding, kissing, couples massage, and couples hot tub can be excellent forms of intimacy. Stroke gently and massage to rediscover touch, and make sure your significant other learns the definition of the word gentle. Educate your partner to not poke, squeeze, or slap playfully.

Take more time to get ready. Yes, I'm talking about foreplay, remember this? Sex or intimacy is natural and needs to be felt as such. The physical environment should have a comfortable room temperature without drafts. If you need more time and attention to get aroused, let your partner know. Remember that sexual activity will not damage fibromyalgia muscles, so have fun.

Find Comfortable Positions

Certain positions may be painful for the person with fibromyalgia. Examples of common positions that are painful include:

1) The missionary position. For the woman with fibromyalgia who has pain with any pressure on the muscles, being on the bottom can be very painful. Men with fibromyalgia who have particular low back problems may find this position too painful because it requires arching of the back.

   And how did the missionary position get its name? Supposedly, when missionaries came to America, they saw the native Americans copulating in all types of unusual positions. These missionaries apparently observed these native American practices, and trained the native Americans in a new "traditional European" sex position with the woman on the bottom. Apparently this training was done by actual demonstration. Being a missionary at that time must have really been a tough career!

2) Positions that involve arching the back, straightening the legs, twisting the spine.

3) Positions that involve an unsupported dangling leg, or require supporting or holding up the weight with arms, or positions that require body weight on an arm or a leg.

Experiment with different positions and find out what will work for you. You need to redefine what is "traditional" for you. Lying on the side, positions with the knees bent, sitting positions, or positions where there is support of the back or neck usually work better for those who have fibromyalgia.

You need to follow your fibronomics during sexual activities as well. Remember to be naturally shifty, that is, don't be in one position too long as it can cause muscle cramps, so rotate different positions just like you would rotate between sitting, standing, and walking. Remember that support is always welcome, whether it be a chair, a pillow, or your partner's arm, leg, or body. Train your partner to support your back or hips during sexual activity to minimize pain.

Specific Examples

I was debating on whether or not to include diagrams in this chapter. I don't want this chapter to be censored! On the other hand, diagrams can be helpful in demonstrating specific types of information, in this case specific sexual positions that may be less painful and more pleasurable for you. I played it safe, however, and used stick people.

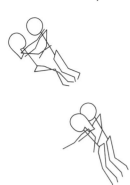

A) Lying on the side.

1. Partners facing each other. Man and woman on their sides facing each other. The bottom arm of each partner is placed under the neck or under the armpit to minimize direct pressure on the arms. This position allows for pleasurable body contact without forcing the body to bear weight.

2. Partners in the same direction (overhead view).

This position likewise avoids weight on the body and allows for rear entry vaginal intercourse with the knees and hips in a bent position that may be more comfortable.

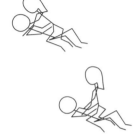

B) Fibromyalgia partner on top.

1. Man is on the bottom with knees straight or bent. His hands are holding and supporting her lower back. Woman is on top with knees bent, leaning forward with back in a natural position, arms forward providing some support.

2. Man on the bottom, woman sitting straight up with back naturally supporting itself. This position takes pressure off the lower back, and both the man and the woman can move with minimal strain on the back and pelvis.

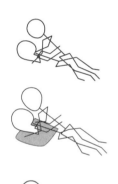

C) Fibromyalgia person on the bottom.

1. Woman on the bottom with knees bent. Man on top with arms supporting him. This position unloads the woman's back and pelvis and avoids weight pressure on the woman because the man is holding up his weight with his outstretched arms.

2. Woman on the bottom with knees bent and a large pillow supporting her upper back and neck, man on top. This position provides support to the woman's upper back and enables the couple to have more physical contact with upper body as the full weight of the male partner is disposed in this angle twist position. Closer intimacy is allowed.

3. Woman on the bottom with a pillow supporting the low back and hips, man on top. This position relieves the pressure on the woman's back and hip areas and allows more tolerance of her partner's weight. This position allows for maximum body contact between partners.

4. Woman on her back at edge of bed, knees bent, and legs supported by partners upper body.

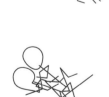

D) Sitting positions.

1. Partners facing each other. Man sitting, woman on the top, chair for support. Partners arms embrace each other for additional support. The floor can support the legs.

2. Partners facing the same direction.

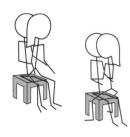

Professional Counseling

Sometimes it may be necessary to work with a health professional who is experienced in treating problems related to sex and intimacy. As I've mentioned, it may be difficult to talk about intimate, personal problems to each other, or even to a doctor. Many physicians and health professionals are skilled and comfortable discussing sexual matters. They have expertise and training to provide valuable insight and recommendations. Counseling is a definite option. Don't be reluctant to see someone who might be able to help you.

Showing love is a mental and an emotional process, not just physical. If fibromyalgia has interfered with your total process of showing love, then you and your partner need to acknowledge this and make a commitment that the interference will only be temporary as you learn to redefine intimacy on your own new terms.

Your new terms can include oral sex, masturbation of each other, or other sexual activities if intercourse is too difficult or painful. It's okay to do other things and not have intercourse. An intimate relationship does not have to focus all on sex, so don't base a successful relationship on whether or not you have intercourse. But most importantly, don't let fibromyalgia rob you of the pleasure of enjoying each other.

Chapter 31 — Survival Strategies

1) Educate yourself as well as your partner about how fibromyalgia causes problems with sex and intimacy.

2) Make a firm commitment with your partner to identify and communicate needs and desires.

3) Work together to achieve comfortable solutions for both parties. Experiment with new techniques and positions.

4) Increase intimacy in the relationship.

5) Re-discover the romance.

6) Agree to seek help from a professional if your attempts to make changes are unsuccessful.

7) Place sex into the proper perspective. It's a small part of a big picture.

8) Determine with your partner realistic expectations about how sex fits into your relationship.

Sex and Intimacy in Fibromyalgia   Inside Fibromyalgia with Mark J. Pellegrino, M.D.

266

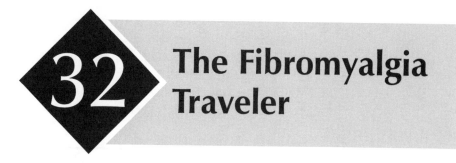

The Fibromyalgia Traveler

Vacation time should be relaxing and free from pain. Many of my patients complain that they have more pain or flare-ups from their vacations than other situations. One particular woman was surprised at the severity of her fibromyalgia flare-up, but when I asked exactly how she spent her vacation, she explained that she jetted to Europe, walked in five different countries in seven days, returned to the U.S. and flew across the country to California for a reunion with family members, many of whom she had not seen in years. She then returned home to help her daughter move to a college dormitory for the fall semester. My back started to hurt just listening!

Vacation time can be extremely stressful. Remember, fibromyalgia does not distinguish good stress from bad. They both hurt. There are many reasons why vacations cause paradoxical flare-ups of our fibromyalgia: Happy stress, a hectic schedule, increased physical activities (walking, hauling luggage, etc.), and changes from our proper posture. In our eagerness to take our vacation, we often forget our necessary daily routine for controlling fibromyalgia. We must remember that we are bringing our fibromyalgia with us, and we have to make sure our fibromyalgia has a good time too!

Planning

Vacations, like everything else, have to be planned in detail. We need to think of as much as possible ahead of time to anticipate potential problems and avoid surprises. Always try to plan a few days at home after the vacation, strictly to rest and recover before returning to work or whatever you do in the "real world." Getting home from vacation on Sunday night and returning to work Monday morning will only invite a prolonged fibromyalgia flare-up.

Decide What You Want to Do

So how does one prepare for vacation to include fibromyalgia? We can't fly to Europe and then see how it goes. Trying to decide what to do after you are already there is inviting stress, confusion, disagreements and, of course, pain.

First, decide on a **suitable vacation spot** for both you and your fibromyalgia. Locations with hot, dry climates are best. I haven't met anyone who has taken a vacation to Siberia. However, I have met a city employee with fibromyalgia who has traveled all over the world, including Antarctica, Indonesia, Uganda, Brazil, and Portugal! Another patient plans a local getaway where she checks into a local hotel for one week a year from Monday to Friday. No one stays there during the week so it is quiet and she has the pool to herself. There is no long drive, minimal packing and expense, and lots of rest and relaxation!

If you like to stay busy, pick locations that offer a variety of attractions or events involving sitting as well as standing. Theme parks can be difficult places because of all the required walking and standing in lines. Avoid locations that require sleeping on the ground (camping out in a tent!) or sleeping on an impossible bed (recliner cot in an RV, Aunt Mae's sofa, etc.). My idea of camping is fishing, hiking, and boating during the day, and at night staying in an air conditioned hotel with a king-sized bed (firm mattress) and my pillows from home. You're allowed to get away to some relaxing resort and do absolutely nothing.

Some people have a difficult time planning for a major vacation and this stress can increase pain even before the vacation starts. I've had several patients tell me they were so overwhelmed by everything that had to be done beforehand, that they chose not to take a vacation at all. Or they didn't want work to pile up while they were gone, so they never left!

> Avoid locations that require sleeping on the ground (camping out in a tent!) or sleeping on an impossible bed (recliner cot in an RV, Aunt Mae's sofa, etc.).

One way to avoid being overwhelmed by the big picture is to plan and organize (and write down) every detail of your trip as exactly as possible, and try to follow this agenda. Take care of all your home activities such as paying the bills, doing the laundry and shopping. Prepare a list of various vacation packing duties and spread out these duties each day for two weeks before you actually leave on vacation. Arrange for coverage at work so you can minimize the dreaded work pile-up.

By planning each day and activity, you can keep your mind occupied and off the pain as much as possible. This also breaks down the very big stressful vacation into a series of small mini-events that are not as intimidating and seem possible to accomplish and enjoy. Organizing your vacation into a series of smaller events allows you to focus your attention and energy on smaller tasks that can be accomplished, whereas if you look at the whole vacation and what you are trying to accomplish you may be overwhelmed and not feel that you have the energy or motivation to do it.

Taking Care of Yourself

Since the majority of vacationers often spend several hours more on their feet during each vacation day than they would under non-vacation circumstances, we need to recognize the potential for aggravation of back, hip and leg symptoms. Carefully organize the vacation event so that you allow frequent breaks between walking, sitting and standing. It is a good idea to plan a rest day every third day for sitting and browsing only. Plan on watching a show, taking a seated sightseeing tour, or lounging at pool side. Planned rest breaks in a hectic schedule are very much appreciated by our muscles.

If you are **traveling by car**, make sure you allow plenty of extra time so you can give proper attention to your fibromyalgia. A good rule of thumb is to add 10 extra minutes per every hour of travel. Ideally, we should stop the car for every hour of driving and take a two-minute stretching break and a five-minute walking break before resuming the trip. Every four hours we should take a five-minute stretching break, a five-minute walking break and at least a 30-minute seated break (eating a meal in a restaurant).

Watch your position and body mechanics while you are seated in the car. Don't turn your head in an awkward position to talk to someone for long periods of time. Likewise, if you are taking a nap, try not to lean on a pillow with your head tilted for a long period of time.

Many fibromyalgia patients are bothered by **motion sickness**, especially those who try to read while riding in the car. Some patients don't even attempt to take cruises because they have overwhelming motion sickness. An airplane ride is usually tolerated better except during prolonged turbulence. The apparent increased motion sickness probably relates to a hypersensitive vestibular system that overreacts to extra signals.

There are several strategies for minimizing motion sickness. If you are prone to developing motion sickness, your doctor may prescribe a pill or patch to use as needed. Avoid reading while riding in the car; be especially careful when looking at maps while riding. When it's necessary to look at a map, look at it for no more than 15 seconds at a time before shifting your focus to outside the car at moving scenery for 15 to 30 seconds; then look at the map again, no more than 15 seconds at a time. Breathing fresh air, getting out of the car and walking, and switching roles with the driver are all helpful in combating motion sickness.

> Carefully organize the vacation event so that you allow frequent breaks between walking, sitting and standing. It is a good idea to plan a rest day every third day for sitting and browsing only. Plan on watching a show, taking a seated sightseeing tour, or lounging at pool side. Planned rest breaks in a hectic schedule are very much appreciated by our muscles.

Watch out for drafts; vacation time seems to be a drafty time! Avoid direct air conditioning drafts in the car or in the restaurant and have a light coat to keep your arms and neck covered if it is chilly or drafty in an area. Don't roll windows down, especially when driving on the freeway.

If you are bothered by a lot of neck pain and fatigue during prolonged driving, you would be a good candidate for wearing a soft cervical collar during your trip. A soft collar can help rest the neck muscles while supporting the head; it can be particularly effective while driving over bumpy areas where there are more demands and strains on neck muscles. I recommend that the collars not be worn more than 50% of the time while driving or riding, and no more than one hour at a time to prevent the neck muscles from getting stiff.

Help your fibromyalgia in any way you can while driving or riding in a car. Taking over-the-counter pain medications 30 minutes to an hour before an anticipated strenuous activity may help dampen the pain. Rubbing muscles with creams that generate either heat or cold can help. Bring along a tape player with earphones and play your favorite music or relaxation tape.

If you are **traveling by airplane** you need to maintain proper body mechanics and frequently reposition your body. An aisle seat is best so you can stretch out your legs and alternate positions, especially on long flights. Take your Walkman with you. If you hate flying like I do, practice your deep breathing exercises especially just before take-off. Bring your own comfortable pillow to increase the chance of getting some restful sleep during those transcontinental or transoceanic flights at night. Your doctor may be willing to prescribe a sleep modifier to use especially on the plane to help achieve good quality sleep. In planes with larger aisles, walk around frequently. If your budget permits, buy first class or business seats simply for the extra space. Watch out for those air blowers above you so they don't shoot cold air right onto your neck.

Luggage can cause special problems. If you are loading your own luggage into the trunk or carrying it around for long distances, you are particularly prone to developing increased pains in your neck, shoulder, back and arm muscles. Take less! Use luggage racks, carts, and wheels whenever you can. Don't sling straps over your shoulders as this will aggravate your trapezius and back muscles. The best way to transport luggage if you have fibromyalgia is to let someone else carry it for you. The next best way is to push a luggage rack on wheels in front of you. Pulling it behind you is harder. If you have to carry your own luggage, make sure that you switch arms frequently, take rest stops every hundred yards and actually set down your luggage, stretch your arms and massage your shoulders.

If you are bothered by a lot of neck pain and fatigue during prolonged driving, you would be a good candidate for wearing a soft cervical collar during your trip. A soft collar can help rest the neck muscles while supporting the head; it can be particularly effective while driving over bumpy areas where there are more demands and strains on neck muscles. I recommend that the collars not be worn more than 50% of the time while driving or riding, and no more than one hour at a time to prevent the neck muscles from getting stiff.

In addition to taking your own **pillows**, remember that many hotel air conditioners blow air directly on the bed, so be certain that you either block or redirect the air to avoid direct drafts. Have a VCR set up in your room so that you can play your favorite exercise video that you have remembered to bring. Always make sure that the hotel you will be staying in has a hot Jacuzzi so you have a relaxing, deep heat modality. Pack your bathing suit. If you like ice packs, bring some instant cold packs or a Ziploc plastic bag to make your own.

Don't forget to take your medicines along, especially sleeping pills or medicines that you use only for flare-ups in case you need them. I have had patients call me from different states wondering if I could prescribe something because they forgot to bring their medicines. Never leave drugs in visible areas where they could be stolen.

There is no need to let fibromyalgia ruin a perfectly good time. Nor should you let it prevent you from taking a well-deserved vacation. Bon voyage!

Chapter 32 — Survival Strategies

1) Remember that vacations can be stressful. Fibromyalgia does not distinguish good stress from bad stress.

2) Plan and anticipate potential problems.

3) Organize and write down every detail of your trip.

4) Organize your vacation into a series of smaller events so that you can focus on smaller tasks.

5) Plan a rest day every third day.

6) Add an extra 10 minutes per hour when traveling by car: 1 fibro hour = 70 minutes.

7) Remember to take medicines for sleeping and flare-ups in case you need them.

8) Give yourself permission to relax, enjoy, and do absolutely nothing.

The Fibromyalgia Traveler   Inside Fibromyalgia with Mark J. Pellegrino, M.D.

272

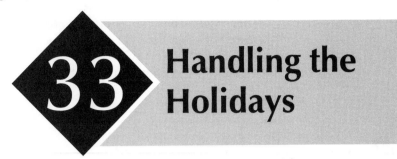

33 Handling the Holidays

For many fibromyalgia patients, the worst time of the year is the holiday season, starting in late November and hitting full peak in December. Return visits for increased fibromyalgia pain and flare-ups are common. I actually see most of these patients in January because they are hurting after the holidays.

There are numerous reasons why fibromyalgia is so susceptible to flaring up during the holiday season. The most prevalent reason is the increased stress at this time of the year.

The extra stresses are a problem for women especially since they are traditionally the ones responsible for preparing for the holidays. Extra duties of buying gifts, wrapping, cooking, baking, decorating, entertaining, and transporting various family members to and from school and related activities are superimposed on the everyday responsibilities — a good recipe for a fibromyalgia flare-up.

Various **physical stresses** during the holidays include:

1) The shopping required with prolonged standing, walking, and carrying.

2) The cookie baking and other cooking involved. Somehow the holiday pans are always in the highest shelves, and there seems to be some sort of relationship between the heavier the pan, the higher and the more out of reach it will be.

3) The holiday decorations, putting up lights, Christmas trees, and the hundreds of other items that get arranged throughout the house and yard to prepare for the holidays.

4) Increased job demands during the holidays, particularly with factory workers and retailers who may work many overtime hours.

5) Increased school and social activities demand more physical effort. This includes our children's school holiday plays and activities, all the holiday parties and get-togethers.

In addition to physical reasons, there is increased stress caused by **weather changes**. By now the weather is changing to cold and damp, particularly for those of us who live in the northern part of the country. There is less sunlight as the days get progressively shorter, and this combination disrupts our fibromyalgia baselines. Seasonal affective disorder (SAD) is a form of depression caused by lack of sunlight.

There are also plenty of **mental stresses** during the holiday season:

1) Family relations are often strained as everyone is experiencing a higher level of stress. Numerous family get-togethers, out-of-town visitors staying over, and

other events that brings families together for lengthy periods of time may create both anticipated and unexpected stresses.

2) Depression is common during the holidays. Multiple factors are involved, but it seems that everywhere you go happy Christmas music and decorations abound, and everyone appears to be joyous and excited... but you hurt more.

One patient had so much stress and worry about getting all of the gifts that she simply forgot where she put them. I suggested to her that she create a special temporary space for the holidays. In this space, whether it be a closet or a corner of the room, she will have her gifts, gift wrap, and accessories needed to wrap the gifts. She can get bankers' boxes and label them and stack them neatly, and she knows that this is her temporary holiday special space.

3) Procrastination is a mental stress and can lead to an overwhelming sense that everything will not get done in time. I tell my family members to make sure they've bought my presents first...and then they can procrastinate!

4) Worries about finances abound at this time of year with extra holiday expenses, savings depletions, tax concerns, and more.

Another cause of feeling bad around the holidays is the **change in our usual eating patterns**. From Thanksgiving to New Years, many of us eat large quantities of refined sugar. We may eat out more and eat more fatty foods, gourmet foods, or unusual foods that are not a part of our routine diet. The altered eating and over-eating disrupts our usual gastrointestinal balance, and may aggravate fibromyalgia by draining energy, aggravating irritable bowel symptoms, or simply causing us to not feel like ourselves.

Holidays happen at predictable times, so don't act surprised when they come, and don't assume you have no control over this situation. You can recognize potential stresses and take specific steps to decrease your risk of a flare-up.

Here are some tips on handling the holidays:

Stress: Don't forget to practice your stress management techniques. Recognize that the holidays are a difficult time of the year, but the higher stress level is temporary. One patient told me she got particularly upset because she literally lost all of her purchased Christmas gifts. She had so much stress and worry about getting all of the gifts that she simply forgot where she put them. I saw her in early January and I reassured her that the gifts would probably be found in some closet she never knew she had! I suggested to her that she create a special temporary space for the holidays. In this space, whether it be a closet or a corner of the room, she will have her gifts, gift wrap, and accessories needed to wrap the gifts. She can get bankers' boxes and label them and stack them neatly, and she knows that this is her temporary holiday special space.

Weather changes may force you to revise your schedules suddenly, so don't worry if you don't get everything done. Be glad you got ANYTHING done. Make an extra effort to follow through with your exercise program.

Shopping: Start your shopping in July. Order your gifts from catalogs or from the numerous computer on-line shopping sites instead of going out and physically shopping. First do mental shopping and know what you want to buy for everyone, then go out and buy the presents. Don't spend hours on your feet looking for them. If you are in the malls or stores, take frequent rest breaks and actually sit down for at least five to ten minutes for every hour of shopping. Carefully organize your time so that you do not find yourself spending several hours on your feet before your realize so much time has passed.

Be careful about carrying packages through the store as these assorted boxes of different weights quickly multiply and become a burden to your  One of my patients "recycles" cookies. She puts cookies others have given her on a nice plate and takes them somewhere else! You can freeze your extra cookies to use over the next few months when you have company.

muscles, making it difficult to follow proper fibronomics. Take advantage of shopping carts to haul your merchandise around. Ask the stores if you can store your newly purchased items behind the counter while you finish your shopping, then gather up all the packages in one final sweep. Get two oversized shopping bags and distribute packages evenly between the bags, carrying one in each arm to balance the weight on your body.

Watch out for the mall parking where the only available parking spot is practically in a different city. It is a good idea to have a non-fibromyalgia person drop you off at the mall's main entrance so you can avoid the long walking. Shop during low volume times at the stores (early morning) so you can park closer and spend less time waiting in line. Remember where you park.

Instead of wrapping all your gifts, take advantage of the free gift-wrapping at the stores or use decorative gift bags or boxes that require no wrapping. I bribe my daughter to do my gift wrapping. If I wrap my own gifts, I definitely leave my perfectionist tendencies in the other room!

Baking: When baking or cooking, make sure that you practice your fibronomics. Instead of baking cookies, try buying them or paying someone else to bake. By the time you figure the time and cost, particularly the intangible costs of increased pain/flare-up, you would be amazed that buying your cookies will be cost-effective.

Make sure your kitchen work area is ergonomically efficient; that is, you are not putting yourself into prolonged unnatural positions to accomplish a task. Store the pans where they can be reached easily. Have someone else get the heavy pots and pans down from the high shelves or bring them up from the basement.

One of my patients "recycles" cookies. She puts cookies others have given her on a nice plate and takes them somewhere else! You can freeze your extra cookies to use over the next few months when you have company.

Decorating: Spread out your decorations over a two-week period instead of trying to cram it into one day. Use ladders to put your body and arms closer to your decorations. Be creative to maintain fibronomics: place decorations at lower levels instead of up high, use decorations that wrap instead of those that need to be hung, clipped or nailed. Hire your neighbor's kid to put up your outside lights while you supervise. Have someone carry up your holiday boxes from the basement. Get a smaller tree; it's a lot less work but still gives the Christmas

Don't forget to enjoy the holidays! Just because you have fibromyalgia does not automatically mean you will be miserable. You can take some active steps in preparing for the holidays and assuring that you have as much control of your fibromyalgia as possible during this difficult time.

spirit. It's exciting to put up decorations; but remember they will have to come back down in January, so plan ahead.

Job: Be particularly attentive to your job's fibronomics. If possible, schedule vacation time, or at least schedule a long weekend. Try to protect your weekends as much as possible so that you do not find yourself working six or seven days a week. If you can, bring some of your work duties home to a less stressful environment.

Parties: Prioritize the parties that you must attend. Do not commit yourself to any party you don't feel you need to attend. If you go to parties, avoid prolonged standing and take frequent sitting breaks. If you are unable to sit in a chair, make sure that you take frequent bathroom breaks and sit on the commode for a few minutes, even if you don't have to go! It's okay to leave the party early (or go to the party fashionably late). For your own parties, try to do pot-luck instead of assuming all the responsibility. If you are able, hire a caterer to handle your party.

Dressing: Dress warmly, making sure that the neck and hands are covered. If it is icy, make sure you have one free hand at all times to hold on to something. Wear good traction shoes or boots. Try to soak up any sunlight, as it can be invigorating. Plan a vacation to a hot, dry area!

Family: Pay special attention to family stresses and family needs. Keep communication open. Schedule a private night out with your spouse for just the two of you. Take family time-outs where everyone takes a break from their hectic schedules, catches up, and relaxes.

Depression: Watch for depression. See your doctor or counselor if it develops. Antidepressant medications may be necessary. Attend support group meetings, and discuss with others problems and strategies for handling the holidays.

Procrastination: To avoid procrastination, buy a monthly planner calendar and write your necessary events, highlighting those areas, and committing only to those dates. Get together with a group of your fibromyalgia friends and plan a shopping outing as a group in July. Make a list of things that you absolutely must do and eliminate those things that are not really necessary.

Finances: Set financial limits on what you will spend during the holidays. Participate in your bank's Christmas Saver's Club to save throughout the year. Don't be tempted by such offers as "90 days, same as cash," since, if you can't afford it now, you can't afford it in 90 days. Plan how much you will spend for each gift. Be careful with your credit cards. Force yourself to add to your savings account in the month of December, rather than depleting it.

Eating: Instead of eating large amounts of everything, eat less and have more frequent, smaller meals. Promise yourself that you will not gain any weight over the holiday season. Don't neglect your exercise program since you need to burn off calories. If you are increasing your carbohydrate consumption, make sure you eat adequate protein as well to minimize the chance of hypoglycemia and carbo craving. So if you are eating sugar cookies, eat some cottage cheese also. Heck, try dipping your sugar cookies in cottage cheese!

Don't forget to enjoy the holidays! Just because you have fibromyalgia does not automatically mean you will be miserable. You can take some active steps in preparing for the holidays and assuring that you have as much control of your fibromyalgia as possible during this difficult time.

Chapter 33 — Survival Strategies

1) Reduce physical stress during the holidays as much as possible.

2) Plan (on paper) for gifts and schedules so you are better prepared.

3) Avoid procrastinating to avoid being overwhelmed by too many projects.

4) Stay on budget.

5) Shop early.

6) Don't worry if you don't get everything done. Your new motto is, "Be glad you get ANYTHING done."

7) Continue your home program without interruption from the holidays.

8) Follow good eating habits.

34 Your Car and Fibromyalgia

Many of us spend considerable time in our cars every day. Commuting to and from work, running errands, traveling, and repeated trips to our doctors (!) give us the opportunity to know our car very well. We should not buy a vehicle based on how it looks, but how functional it is for our fibromyalgia. If you have the opportunity to shop around, some important features of a car may help decrease your fibromyalgia pain, or help prevent it from being aggravated while you are traveling.

I think an important preventive feature is an **adequate headrest**. As you may know, whiplash injury commonly occurs after a rear-end collision and is one of the most common causes of post-traumatic fibromyalgia. A good headrest can help reduce the severity of a whiplash injury during a rear-end collision, although this has never been proven with studies. Headrests do not prevent whiplash injuries, nor do they help in head-on or side collisions.

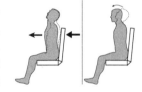

How does whiplash happen? The person sitting in a stopped car that is suddenly rear-ended will experience forward movement of the body. The head acts as an independent 10 pound object which initially stays in the same position because of inertia. The body moving forward causes the head to vigorously hyperextend or jerk back. The sudden hyperextension activates stretch reflexes in the front muscles of the neck which cause the head to jerk forward (or hyperflex) to catch up with the rest of the body. These jerking movements are the whiplash effects.

The body reacts by tightening up the strong neck muscles in a brief protective spasm, thereby supporting the spine and head and absorbing the transmitted forces from the collision. Although these heroic protective efforts by the cervical, spinal, and shoulder muscles are usually successful in preventing serious neurologic injuries, stretches and tears in the neck muscles and injuries to the ligaments often occur.

Unequal injuries in different parts of the neck depend on the position of the head at the time of the collision and the angle of the impact. Not all strains that occur from whiplash ultimately result in post-traumatic fibromyalgia. Also, there is usually no correlation between the severity of the rear-end collision and whether or not a person develops a severe whiplash injury. The key cause of the injury is the actual whiplash reaction, which can be triggered by any impact, whether minor or major.

Is there any way to prevent a few split seconds of trauma from causing a lifetime of pain? Obviously, we cannot avoid rear-end collisions, but we can try to minimize the amount of jerking that the head experiences by having a proper sturdy headrest. Many times the car headrest is not in the right position, is all the way down, or it is not designed well. Many of my patients who have been involved in rear-end collisions and then developed post-traumatic fibromyalgia reported that the headrest broke off during the accident. Because of my experience with so many people suffering from whiplash injuries, I make certain that my vehicles have an adequate headrest for the driver

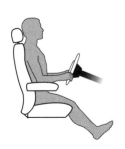

and all the passengers. Very few vehicles, especially the larger ones (mini-vans, trucks, SUVs) meet this criteria.

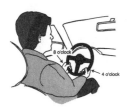

When you are seated in the car, the headrest should rest just behind the middle of your head. When you move your head backwards, it should come against the headrest very quickly. Make certain that the headrest has strong supports even if it is raised into the upper position so it won't snap off in the event of a rear-end collision. Ask questions and do your research so you can make knowledgeable choices. Make sure you keep the headrest up whenever you are driving or riding.

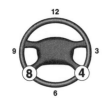

Another important feature is **armrests**. There should be armrests on both sides of us, whether we are drivers or passengers. Prolonged driving with unsupported arms is a major cause of fatigue in the arms and upper back area. Armrests on both sides enable us to unload the upper back muscle by supporting our arms while we maintain safe control of the steering wheel. Make sure the armrests have adequate padding so as not to put pressure over the bony elbows or nerves inside the elbow. I find my arms are most comfortably positioned when the steering wheel is held in the 4 o'clock and 8 o'clock spots.

We need to adequately support our spine. Cars should have **adjustable seats and backs.** Power controls are better than manual devices, allowing you to make adjustments while you are driving. This feature not only enables us to find an individual comfortable position, but to adjust position while driving if needed. I have a favorite adjustment of my car seat, but I will change this position several times a week depending on whether my upper back or lower back is bothering me more. A more reclined position helps decrease my lower back pain. Each person needs to experiment in order to find the right balance of back/pelvic/leg angles. Keeping the seat as close to the steering wheel as possible helps prevent painful reaching to hold the wheel, and it also better positions feet and knees to unload the back.

If you move your seat too close to the steering wheel, you may have to disable your air bag to avoid air bag injury in case of a collision. Check with the law enforcement officials in your state before doing this. The highway patrol officials I've talked with tell me air bags save lives and disabling them could increase your risk of serious injury.

Some cars are equipped with lumbar supports, which can be helpful if low back pain is a problem. Avoid very deep seats that you sink into, which make it difficult to get in and out. You may have a favorite lumbar roll or cushion that you can bring into your car for more comfortable seating while you are driving or traveling.

A **good climate control system** is mandatory in a car. Without an air conditioner, we must rely on open windows for air circulation during hot days, and this invites the humidity, dust, pollen and drafts which all can irritate our sensitive skin and muscles. If you can control the air, you can keep some control of your condition. Make sure that the heating and air conditioning units are functioning properly.

Car vents should be adjusted so as to redirect the cold air away from the body. Direct cold air hitting the skin can trigger reflexes that cause muscle spasms and flare-ups. Warm air from defrosters can cause nausea or stuffiness if it directly hits your face, especially for those of us who are sensitive to odors and fumes and have overactive nasal responses. Adjust the vents so air does not hit you directly. If some vents cannot be adjusted to redirect the air, they can be closed.

Mirrors are also important; make sure there are lots of them so you can scan the outside world without turning your head too far. When you are comfortable in the driver's seat, you should be able to glance into the rear view mirror and the side mirrors by moving your eyes mostly to see easily everything that is happening beside and behind us. When you turn your head to the left to see in your blind spot, be sure

that your properly positioned headrest is not obstructing the view or causing you to strain your neck. Power mirrors let you make more adjustment choices and are worth the money.

Be sure your car has an **automatic drive**. No stick shifts or clutches allowed unless you want your right

When you are seated in the car, the headrest should rest just behind the middle of your head. When you move your head backwards, it should come against the headrest very quickly. Make certain that the headrest has strong supports even if it is raised into the upper position so it won't snap off in the event of a rear-end collision. Ask questions and do your research so you can make knowledgeable choices. Make sure you keep the headrest up whenever you are driving or riding.

shoulder and left leg to fall off! One patient thought a stick shift would be good exercise for her arm; she quickly learned that it caused bad flare-ups instead. Let your car do as much work for you as possible.

Be careful about twisting and reaching for items that always manage to be just beyond a comfortable reach. I am talking about items that end up on the floor such as tapes, sunglasses, pens, or snow scrapers. One of my patients uses an assisting device called a reacher/grabber which she keeps in the front seat and uses to retrieve those impossible-to-reach items. This enables proper body mechanics. The reacher/grabber can also be used in the trunk to retrieve items and prevent risky bending.

In general, the bigger and roomier the vehicle, the easier it will be on fibromyalgia posture. We need to be able to easily step into the vehicle. It's better to climb up a little to get into the car; getting out will then be simple. If you have to drop down into your car seat, it will be hard for you to lift yourself up and out of the car. Let gravity work for you when you get out of your car, not when you get into your car.

Chapter 34 — Survival Strategies

1) Shop for a car that is fibro-friendly.

2) Purchase a car based on how functional it is, not on how it looks.

3) Check for adequate headrests to minimize whiplash injuries.

4) Choose a car with adequate arm rests, preferably for both arms.

5) Consider a car with a good climate control system.

6) Test the car's mirrors to see if your view is good without straining your neck.

7) Buy a car with an automatic transmission. Let the car do as much work for you as possible.

35 Handling Flare-ups

Every individual with fibromyalgia will experience flare-ups from time to time. We can't stop them from happening; they are a fact of fibro! We strive for a stable baseline as long as possible, but inevitably, the ugly flare-up head will rear itself. Some have frequent flare-ups, others stay in remission practically all the time (and they'd better not brag about it if they want to stay in remission!). All flare-ups have a cause even if we don't know the cause for a particular one. Usually, we can identify a specific cause of our increased pain, but if we can't find a specific reason, the flare-up may be called "spontaneous" or "idiopathic." One of the most frustrating complaints I hear is that flare-ups occur in spite of doing "everything" right. We must simply deal with them as they occur and try to accept these periodic, uncontrolled intrusions as part of this condition.

What exactly is a flare-up? How does one know if it is a flare-up due to fibromyalgia or if it is a new problem? What should we do during a flare-up; should we exercise, do our regular work duties, attend social events? These are frequent questions asked by individuals suffering from fibromyalgia. This chapter is a detailed guide to assist you in successfully overcoming a fibromyalgia flare-up.

My definition of a fibromyalgia flare-up is as follows: Increased regional or generalized pain or fatigue, when compared to a stable baseline level, that persists for at least 3 consecutive days and interferes with usual daily activities. General causes of flare-ups include:

1) Physical factors: physical activities, trauma, too little activity, severe fatigue

2) Infections: colds, flu syndromes, bladder infections, yeast infections

3) Hormonal factors: menstrual cycle, menopause, thyroid or growth hormone changes

4) Environmental factors: cold damp weather, hot humid weather, air conditioner drafts

5) Psychosocial stresses: job changes, marital stresses, depression

Flare-up causes can also be causes of the initial fibromyalgia. Many of my patients have the misfortune of having two injuries impacting their fibromyalgia. The first injury caused the fibromyalgia, then a later injury made it permanently worse.

A stable baseline is not a perfect state. We all experience increased pain on a daily basis. Fluctuations above and below our baseline state are typical — some days we feel better, other days we feel worse, and our pain moves around to different locations. Certain activities may cause a person to hurt more for a few days, but if the pain resolves or decreases to baseline, we would not consider this a flare-up. Each of us has a unique realistic baseline.

Our tender points always have some degree of spontaneous soreness responsible for that constant ache. Palpation of these tender points will cause increased pain, or certain activities will increase the pain, but the pain should quickly return to baseline. Flare-ups occur when the tender points

My definition of a fibromyalgia flare-up is as follows: Increased regional or generalized pain or fatigue, when compared to a stable baseline level, that persists for at least 3 consecutive days and interferes with usual daily activities.

become more persistently and painfully sore. We need to specifically address our flare-up and ask various questions:

1) **Describe the pain.** Where is the pain? Is it localized to a region or is the whole body affected?

   When does it hurt? Is the pain constant or intermittent? If the pain is intermittent, does it occur regularly in the morning, during the day, after exercise or at night? Intermittent pain can still meet the definition of a flare-up if it is "persistently intermittent" and interferes with daily functions.

2) **What caused this increased pain?** Many factors can cause flare-up including physical, emotional, environmental and idiopathic reasons. Not all pain is related to fibromyalgia, as other unrelated conditions can be present. If the pain is mostly in the morning, the factors may be related to poor sleep or poor sleep positioning. Increased pain during the day may reflect work activities, household activities, improper body mechanics. Pain after exercise may indicate that the person is overdoing or doing new and unusual activities or not adequately stretching and warming up before the exercise. Increased pain at night might reflect accumulated strains during the day from job activity, or may reflect strenuous leisure activity. Increased fatigue at night often causes increased pain. A person in constant pain may have a combination of multiple factors involved.

3) **What type of treatments can the individual do on his or her own?** If the cause or causes can be identified, they should be removed, altered or modified. Various stretches and exercises, resting certain body parts and restricting certain activities are all a part of the personal strategies in dealing with a flare-up. Increasing the use of home remedies or over-the-counter medications may help.

4) **When should your doctor be consulted?** The patient can consult with the doctor at any time he or she has increased pain. People who have had fibromyalgia for a while may decide to try a home program first. However, even experienced fibromyalgia sufferers will get new pains or problems that require further medical evaluations, so one is never discouraged from consulting with his or her doctor. If you first try to manage the flare-up on your own and it does not improve, you will need to follow-up with your doctor.

When I evaluate increased symptoms in my patients, I always try to determine the answer to a basic question: Is this a fibromyalgia flare-up, or is a new condition involved? I perform a clinical evaluation and determine if any specific diagnostic tests are needed. My doctor-directed treatment might include prescription medicines, trigger point injections, therapy orders, manipulations, adjustments and specific instructions. Hopefully, the program instituted will resolve the flare-up, reestablish a stable baseline, and enable the home program to be resumed successfully.

When should your doctor be consulted? The patient can consult with the doctor at any time he or she has increased pain. People who have had fibromyalgia for a while may decide to try a home program first. However, even experienced fibromyalgia sufferers will get new pains or problems that require further medical evaluations, so one is never discouraged from consulting with his or her doctor. If you first try to manage the flare-up on your own and it does not improve, you will need to follow-up with your doctor.

I have just described a basic approach to handling a fibromyalgia flare- up. The following sections of this chapter are descriptions and strategies using this general format:

1) Where is the pain/flare-up?

2) Conditions that can cause the flare-up whether they may be related or possibly related to fibromyalgia, or may be unrelated to fibromyalgia

3) Treatments to do on your own to resolve flare-up

4) Doctor strategies to resolve flare-up

Each section represents a different part of the body.

Headache

Conditions related or possibly related to fibromyalgia

1) Tension/migraine headaches (the majority of fibromyalgia patients have these). Causes include:

a) Increased stress (personal relationship difficulties, job pressure, financial concerns, etc.)

b) Exposure to bright lights, loud noises

c) Dietary factors; certain foods such as cheese, chocolate, lunch meat, beans, alcohol, caffeine, and milk can trigger migraines. Cold foods ("ice cream" headache)

d) Strenuous exercise-induced headaches

e) Exposure to strong odors, chemicals, perfumes, fumes, exhaust from buses/cars

2) Temporomandibular joint (TMJ) dysfunction (causes jaw pain, dizziness, and head pains; a common condition associated with fibromyalgia). Causes include:

a) Grinding teeth at night (called bruxism)

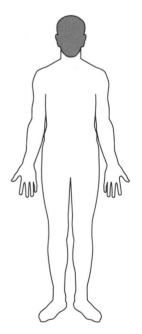

b) Chewing gum, hard candy, hard foods

c) Jaw strain from excessive talking

d) Yawning injury or "big bite" injury

3) Post-concussive syndrome (residual headaches, neck pain, difficulty concentrating after a concussion, often part of post-traumatic fibromyalgia and severe whiplash injury). Causes include:

a) Head injury from fall or car accident

b) More sensitivity to migraine headaches (see above)

c) Usually coexisting neck muscle injury and pain

4) Allergy flare-up with congestion or cold symptoms (allergies are more common in people with fibromyalgia). Causes include:

a) Exposure to pollens, molds, dust, etc.

b) Sinus congestion or infection

c) Sensitivity to fumes, smells, viruses

5) Referred pain from tender/trigger points in neck and shoulder area. Causes include:

a) Strenuous physical activity (new job duties, move to new house, too much computer time)

b) Weather-related problems (cold, damp weather, shoveling snow, falling on ice)

c) Spontaneous flare-up of tender/trigger points

d) Bad pillow

6) Side effects from medications used to treat fibromyalgia (examples: tricyclic antidepressants, beta-blockers, migraine medicines, muscle relaxants. Consider:

a) Many medicines can cause headaches as side effects; new medicine or change in dosage

b) Some medicines cause rebound headaches if they are stopped suddenly

c) Fibromyalgia persons are usually more sensitive to any medicine

7) Hormonal changes in women (women with fibromyalgia commonly experience more intense headaches as part of premenstrual syndrome (PMS) or menopause). Causes include:

a) Water retention phase of menstrual cycle causes exaggerated PMS (premenstrual syndrome) headaches in women with fibromyalgia.

b) Menopause

c) Estrogen medicines

8) Dry eyes syndrome (common in fibromyalgia; may cause eye irritation and headaches). Causes include:

   a) Dry, dirty environment

   b) Contact lenses

   c) Sunlight sensitivity

   d) Chemical fumes sensitivity

   e) Cigarette smoke overexposure

9) Eye strain. Causes include:

   a) Prolonged reading

   b) Incorrect eyeglass strength

   c) Poor, artificial lighting

10) Conditions unrelated to fibromyalgia (but may cause headaches)

   a) Hypertension

   b) Renal disorder

   c) Infection

   d) Eye disease

   e) Cervical osteoarthritis (may cause secondary fibromyalgia)

   f) Vasculitis (inflammation of blood vessels)

   g) Cerebral hemorrhage

   h) Brain tumor

   i) Birth control pills

Treatments to Do on Your Own

1) Practice deep breathing and relaxation techniques; seek positive outcomes and strategies in dealing with stress or stressful relationships.

2) Dampen and remove noises, use natural lighting especially in settings where a lot of reading and studying is required.

3) Proper dietary habits, avoid skipping meals or prolonged fasting. Eliminate foods that you are sensitive to; be careful with food additives, caffeine and alcohol.

4) Use over-the-counter medications such as aspirin, acetaminophen, ibuprofen, naproxen; use medicines not only to treat pain but as a preventive measure (for example, take over-the-counter medicine one hour before exercise or a

bothersome activity; women can take ibuprofen or a diuretic during the painful phase of menstrual cycle).

5) Perform stretching and light conditioning exercises; avoid strenuous, heavy strengthening exercises. Place particular emphasis on stretching the neck and trapezius muscles.

6) If dry eyes are the problem, avoid wearing contact lenses; use artificial tears frequently, especially in smoky areas or dry environments. Review medications which may be causing dry eyes as a side effect. Stop smoking!

7) Eye checkup. Determine if a change is needed in eye glasses. Change reading habits to avoid prolonged reading time, especially if eye strain is a factor in causing headaches.

8) Moist heat or ice to the back of the head and neck area

9) Self-massage to work out soreness in the scalp, jaw, and neck muscles.

10) If the flare-up does not return to baseline with these measures, see your doctor.

Doctor Strategies

The doctor will discuss causes of headaches and conduct a physical examination focused on the nerves and soft tissues in the head and neck. The neurologic exam makes sure the reflexes, sensations, strength, eye muscles, visual acuity, face sensation, pupil reaction, hearing, swallowing, memory and orientation are all within normal limits. The palpation of the head and neck muscles to determine tender areas and testing neck and jaw range of motion to look for stiffness are also important components of the exam.

Your doctor may order additional diagnostic testing, which could include a head CT scan, EEG, head MRI, memory/cognitive testing, X-rays of the sinus, TMJ, neck areas, and an eye examination. If the doctor feels that the headaches are due to flare-up of fibromyalgia or fibromyalgia-related factors, specific treatments directed at the headache can be instituted.

If TMJ dysfunction is suspected, a referral to an appropriate dental specialist may be considered. TMJ treatment may include customized bite splints, crown and bridges as part of a restorative procedure, especially if there is a malocclusion (bad bite).

If eye-related headaches are a problem, a referral to an eye doctor may be needed. The eye doctor will evaluate vision and determine if glasses or adjustments are necessary. Vision therapy for strengthening the eye muscles can be helpful if headaches are induced by reading or eye strain.

If allergies are involved, your doctor may prescribe a decongestant and an antibiotic. You may need to see an allergy specialist for specific testing or allergy shots.

A variety of medicines may be used to treat headaches: analgesics, anti-inflammatories, muscle relaxants, antianxiety medicines, or antidepressants. Prescription anti-migraine medicines such as Midrin, ergotamine tartrate, and an injectable medicine called sumatriptan can be very effective.

Trigger point injections might be tried, especially if trigger regions are identified as the cause of the headache. The posterior occipital and cervical regions, which flare up frequently and cause headaches, may respond very well to a trigger point injection.

Therapy modalities may be prescribed and might include hot packs, ultrasound, massage, craniosacral techniques, or electric stimulation. Chiropractic treatment is helpful and includes manual therapy and adjustments.

Biofeedback can help patients learn relaxation and control body responses that lead to headaches. Individuals can usually learn this technique after a few sessions.

Neck Pain

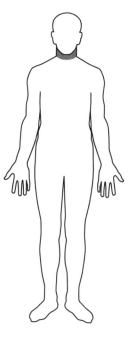

Neck pain often accompanies headaches. Many people describe their headaches as in the back of their neck, radiating up to the base of their skull. However, a flare-up in the neck area may not necessarily associated with headaches.

Conditions related or possibly related to fibromyalgia

1) Cervical strain and sprain. Consider:

    a) Trauma such as an automobile accident where whiplash injury occurs; work injury; sports injury

    b) Physical activities such as prolonged reading, driving, studying, looking up, or looking sideways. Examples: riding a bike with Ram's horn handle bars looking up, talking on the phone hand-free by holding the phone with your head against your shoulder

    c) Weather changes, particularly cold, damp weather; or increased stress, both physical and emotional

2) Referred pain from shoulder strain. Causes:

    a) Repetitive reaching, overhead use of arms

    b) Lifting, shoveling, throwing, etc.

Conditions unrelated to fibromyalgia

1) Cervical disc disease such as degeneration or herniation

2) Torticollis (wry neck or twisting of the neck due to abnormal muscles)

3) Cervical osteoarthritis (may cause secondary fibromyalgia, though)

Treatments to Do on Your Own

Identify any physical causes and try to remove or modify these activities. Certain head positions at work may require modification, such as turning your head to the right to look at a computer monitor or tilting your head to the side to hold a phone while you type. Make the necessary changes, such as rearranging workstations so that the monitor is directly in front of you; get head phones if your job involves answering phones.

Practice proper posture and fibronomics. Alternate various positions so as not to strain the neck muscles. Try to be consciously aware of the proper neutral position of the neck at all times.

Continue a regular exercise program but emphasize neck stretching and range of motion. Do these exercises as warm-ups before starting a daily job or household chore.

Take over-the-counter medicines including acetaminophen, ibuprofen, or Naproxen. Use muscle creams that give either heat or cold sensation. Use topical anesthetics such as capsaicin ointment.

Use heat packs or ice packs and self-massage. Self-massage can make the muscles "hurt good." A soft cervical collar worn for short periods of time such as when driving or reading may help relieve the neck muscle pain.

If the flare-up does not return to baseline with these measures, see your doctor.

Doctor Strategies

Your doctor will examine you with emphasis on the neck muscles, neck range of motion, and neurologic exam. If there is concern for underlying disc or arthritic disease, additional diagnostic tests may be ordered (cervical spine X-rays, cervical CAT scan, MRI, or electrodiagnostic testing).

Specific treatments directed toward increased fibromyalgia-related neck pain may include prescription medicine such as analgesics, anti-inflammatories, and muscle relaxants. Trigger point injections using local anesthetic and cortisone combination may also be necessary, particularly if painful tender and trigger points are the major sources of the pain.

Work restrictions may be needed to avoid repetitive neck movements from side to side or looking up or down. Your doctor will instruct you on proper neck posture.

Specific therapies may include hot pack, ultrasound, massage, adjustments, cervical collar, and neck exercises. Traction can sometimes help, but many people with fibromyalgia find that cervical traction increases their neck pain. A therapy course may average three times a week for a month as needed. Chiropractic treatments may help.

Shoulder Pain

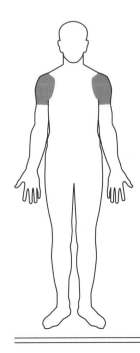

Conditions related to or possibly related to fibromyalgia

1) Shoulder strain, rotator cuff tendinitis (tendinitis is common in fibromyalgia patients)

2) Biceps tendinitis (inflammation of tendon in upper arm flexion muscle)

3) Shoulder bursitis (inflammation of bursa or fluid-filled sac in shoulder)

4) Shoulder adhesive capsulitis (inflammation and tightening of the shoulder joint lining also called frozen shoulder)

5) Reflex sympathetic dystrophy (painful condition where the small sympathetic nerves to the arm become overstimulated). Various causes include:

a) Physical activities that involve a lot of reaching or use of the arms in out stretched or overhead position. Example: cleaning windows, painting

b) Activities requiring throwing or lifting such as bowling, softball, weight lifting, shoveling snow

c) Seat belt trauma following an accident

d) Shoulder pressure from a heavy backpack or narrow bra strap

e) Driving a car with a stick shift; prolonged driving

f) Throwing, weight-lifting, shooting activities

g) Repetitive reaching or pushing on the job

h) Yard work requiring clipping and trimming

i) Putting up holiday decorations

j) Fall on outstretched arms (rotator cuff injury)

Conditions unrelated to fibromyalgia

1) Rotator cuff tear

2) Referred neurological pain from radiculopathy (inflamed nerve root), brachial plexus injury (shoulder nerve group), or shoulder nerve entrapment (pinched nerve)

3) Shoulder dislocation

4) Shoulder arthritis

Treatments to Do on Your Own

Remove or modify physical activities that are causing shoulder pain. Reevaluate your work station or house duties to minimize reaching, lifting, or overhead use.

Follow proper fibronomics; remember to keep the arms close to your body when performing tasks involving reaching or overhead use of the arms.

Perform regular shoulder stretching and flexibility exercises. Examples:

1) Reach your arms overhead as far as possible and hold for three seconds.

2) Perform shoulder rolls for 15 seconds each side several times a day to loosen the shoulder soft tissues.

3) Do corner stretches. Stand in a corner and put each hand on the wall at shoulder level and do a reverse push-up into the corner, feeling the muscles between the shoulders stretch and "hurt good".

Wear a strapless bra or a bra with wider straps to minimize focused strain and pressure on the trapezius muscles.

Use moist heat, try an ice pack, use muscle creams and self-massages frequently to shoulder muscles.

Continue a regular exercise program but emphasize neck stretching and range of motion. Do these exercises as warm-ups before starting a daily job or household chore.

Take over-the-counter medicines both to treat the pain and as a preventive measure. Take the medicine one hour before performing activities that may aggravate your shoulder; that way, the medicine will be absorbed and start to work when you need it.

Avoid using a sling as this increases the tendency for stiffness and weakness in the shoulder and makes the rehabilitation process more difficult.

If the flare-up does not return to baseline with these measures, see your doctor.

Doctor Strategies

Your doctor will focus on the shoulder exam, which will include shoulder palpation, checking range of motion, and evaluating shoulder stability. He will check whether or not there is any impingement or tear of the rotator cuff. The shoulder muscles will be examined for muscle spasms, painful tender points or swelling. In addition, the neurological exam (reflexes, sensation, and strength) will be evaluated for any underlying nerve damage.

Depending on the exam results, the doctor may order additional diagnostic testing including shoulder X-ray, shoulder arthrogram, shoulder MRI, and electrodiagnostic testing.

If the increased shoulder pain is thought to be related to fibromyalgia, specific treatment including medications (analgesics, anti-inflammatories, and muscle relaxants) can be tried.

Trigger point and shoulder injections can be helpful. Injections into muscle, joint space, tendon or bursa can help, depending on the location of the pain. "Spray and Stretch" is a good technique for shoulder pain. A vapor-coolant is sprayed onto the skin followed by stretching and manipulative therapy. Chiropractic treatments such as manual therapy and adjustments are also helpful.

Therapies emphasizing the shoulder area can include hot pack, ultrasound, electric stimulation, iontophoresis (using electric current to deliver medicines beneath the skin), massage, shoulder stretching, strengthening, and mobility exercises.

Work restrictions may be necessary, which would include avoiding and minimizing repetitive reaching and overhead work, decreased lifting with the arms, and decreased operation of hand controls.

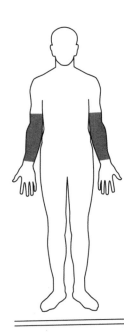

Elbow and Arm Pain

The dominant side will flare up more often than the non-dominant side.

Conditions related to or possibly related to fibromyalgia

1) Lateral epicondylitis (tennis elbow or pain outside elbow)

2) Medial epicondylitis (golfer's elbow or pain inside elbow)

3) Elbow strain

4) Forearm strain

Various causes of the above include:

   a) Playing tennis

   b) Repeatedly gripping hand tools

   c) New job activities requiring more forearm stress such as squeezing objects, bending the wrist back, or using computers.

   d) Playing golf

   e) Gripping objects with the wrist bent in (wrist flexion)

   f) Any new or unusual physical activity involving the arm (job, hobby). Examples: writing numerous letters or bills, ironing for a few hours, chairs without arm rests.

Conditions unrelated to fibromyalgia

1) Cervical radiculopathy (inflamed nerve root in neck) which refers pain to elbow

2) Brachial plexopathy (irritated shoulder nerve group)

3) Carpal tunnel syndrome (pinched nerve in wrist)

4) Ulnar nerve entrapment (pinched nerve in elbow)

5) Fractures

Treatments to Do on Your Own

1) Remove or modify activities that cause or aggravate the symptoms.

2) Use the unaffected arm to make up for some of the usual function of the painful arm.

3) Continue a regular exercise program but emphasize stretching the elbow and forearm, especially before any activity, and range of motion.

4) Do these exercises as warm-ups before starting a daily job or household chore.

5) Use over-the-counter medications for increased pain as a preventive measure.

6) Soak the arm in very warm water and stretch; use ice.

7) Do self-massage with pressure and rubbing of the tender regions of the elbow and forearm; use muscle creams and get either a hot or cool effect along with the massage.

8) Follow fibronomics and proper body mechanics.

If the flare-up does not return to baseline with these measures, see your doctor.

Doctor Strategies

Your doctor will examine you and pay particular attention to the elbow and forearm area. The palpation exam will cover the epicondyle area (tennis elbow and golfer's elbow regions), as well as palpation of the forearm muscles. Range of motion will be checked in the elbow and wrist joints to determine if there is any inflammation. The neurologic exam (reflexes, sensation, strength, and coordination) will also be tested to make sure there is no underlying neurologic disorder or nerve entrapment.

Certain tests may be considered including X-rays and electrodiagnostic testing. If inflammation is present and thought to represent an underlying inflammatory disease, laboratory studies may be ordered.

If the flare-up is thought to be from fibromyalgia, specific doctor treatments may include instruction on ways to rest and exercise the affected area. There may be job restrictions that limit the use of the affected arm or arms or specifically limit the amount a person may lift, grasp, or operate hand controls. Your doctor will reinforce the need to use the unaffected side to compensate for the affected side until the pain quiets down, but also to be careful not to overuse the good side and cause pain there also.

Medications to be considered include anti-inflammatories, pain medicines, and muscle relaxants. Injections may also be appropriate, particularly into painful or trigger areas.

Specific therapies may include ultrasound, electrical stimulation, friction massage, elbow braces (such as a tennis elbow brace) and specific stretching and strengthening exercises. Chiropractic adjustments of the neck and elbow may also be effective.

Wrist and Hand Pain

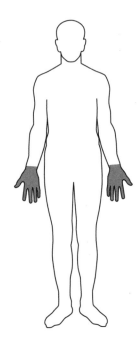

Conditions related or possibly related to fibromyalgia

1) Writer's cramp

2) Wrist strain

3) Wrist and hand tendinitis

4) Autonomic nerve hypersensitivity (small sensory nerves are easily irritated especially in hand and cause pain, burning, swelling, itching, etc.)

Causes include:

1) Repetitive job activity, particularly those that require a lot of gripping or grasping, operating tools, and repetitive wrist movement, such as increased writing, typing, or computer-keyboard operation

2) Exposure to cold temperature or changes in temperature; not wearing gloves in winter

Conditions unrelated to fibromyalgia

1) Carpal tunnel syndrome (pinched nerve in wrist)

2) Peripheral neuropathy (disease of the small nerves causing numbness, weakness and loss of reflexes)

3) Cervical radiculopathy (inflamed nerve root in neck)

4) Fracture

5) Rupture of tendon

6) Arthritic conditions

7) Dupuytren's contracture (tightening and scarring of the connective tissue in the palm)

8) Upper motor neuron disease (disease of the brain or spinal cord)

Treatments to Do on Your Own

1) Remove or modify the activities that cause the pain.

2) If unable to remove or modify the activities, alternate between various tasks or use the less affected arm as often as possible without causing increased pain on that side.

3) Do specific exercises for the wrist and hand. Maintain proper body mechanics and fibronomics.

4) If cold temperature aggravates the symptoms, wear gloves when working outdoors in cool, wet environments.

5) Use over-the-counter medicines to treat pain or as a preventive measure 1 hour before the offending activity.

6) Continue a regular exercise program but emphasize neck stretching and range of motion. Do these exercises as warm-ups before starting a daily job or household chore.

7) Use muscle creams if they do not cause increased sensitivity.

8) Use hot or ice water or alternate between the two to create your own contrast bath. Prepare a bowl of each. Dip painful hand into bowls, alternating one minute of heat with 30 seconds of cold for a total of 10 minutes. Do this twice a day.

9) If the flare-up does not return to baseline with these measures, see your doctor.

Doctor Strategies

Your doctor will perform an examination that emphasizes your wrist and hand areas. The exam will consist of examining the joints to see if there is any evidence of swelling or limitation of motion. There will be an examination to see if there are trigger points where the fingers lock in a bent position. The neurologic exam will be important to make sure there is no evidence of carpal tunnel syndrome, radiculopathy, or other nerve problems that can cause hand pain.

Further testing may include laboratory studies, X-rays, electrodiagnostic testing, or a bone scan. Specific treatments related to fibromyalgia may include medications such as analgesics, anti-inflammatories, or muscle relaxants.

Injection of the wrist or carpal tunnel area with cortisone may help. Bracing of the wrist in the neutral position can be helpful particularly if wrist strain or tendinitis is a major problem.

Various therapies that may be useful include heat, electric stimulation, massage, stretching, exercise programs, more bracing. Chiropractic adjustments of the wrist have been effective.

Epidural blocks or sympathetic blockade are two anesthesiology techniques that may be appropriate, particularly if there is extreme autonomic (small nerve pain) hypersensitivity. Shoulder-hand syndrome or reflex sympathetic dystrophy can occur. This condition is characterized by overactive autonomic and small sensory nerves that cause extreme pain, burning and swelling in the hand especially.

Chest Pains

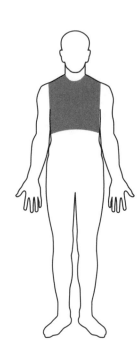

Conditions related to or possibly related to fibromyalgia

1) Costochondritis (rib pain)

2) Pectoralis (chest muscle) strain

3) Mitral valve prolapse (bulging of one of the heart valves)

4) Anxiety/panic attacks

5) Referred symptoms from irritable bowel syndrome

6) Fibrocystic breast disease

7) Sensitivity to environmental allergens/asthma

Various causes include:

1) Coughing-induced flare-up of chest wall muscle

2) Smoking

3) Increased physical activities involving a lot of reaching, twisting, or pulling; example: washing the car

4) Breast pain from pregnancy, large breasts, or breast implants

5) Lactating breasts, causing increased strain/irritation of breast tissue/muscles

6) Anything that provokes anxiety attacks such as stress, sensitivities to certain foods or beverages, exercise, chemicals

7) Anything that aggravates allergies, such as ragweed, pollen, chemicals, fumes, and dust

8) Eating certain foods (greasy, spicy), drinking carbonated beverages, overeating.

Conditions unrelated to fibromyalgia

1) Coronary artery disease

2) Hiatal hernia

3) Esophagitis (inflammation of the esophagus)

4) Pneumonia

5) Bronchitis

6) Asthma

7) Peptic ulcer disease

Treatments to Do on Your Own

1) Identify, remove and modify any causes; for example, if a new job activity requires a lot of reaching forward with the arms outstretched, modify the work area so that excessive reaching and subsequent chest irritation does not occur.

2) Add stretching exercises that focus on the chest wall and pectoral muscles.

3) Practice deep breathing exercises and relaxation techniques.

Chest pain is usually very disturbing to patients, especially if it is a new symptom. Although there are many ways it can be attributed to fibromyalgia, many people feel that there is a problem with the heart and will see their doctor immediately. If you are having new onset of chest pain, always see your doctor at once. If you have previously had chest pain attributed to your fibromyalgia and you have a flare-up, you may try these techniques first. If your pain is not returning to baseline with the measures you try on your own, see your doctor.

Doctor Strategies

Your doctor will focus on your chest exam, which includes listening to the lungs and the heart, checking blood pressure, pulse, respiration, and palpating the chest muscle areas. Additional specialist referral may need to be considered (cardiologist, pulmonologist, gastroenterologist or gynecologist).

Testing that could be considered includes laboratory studies, chest X-ray, EKG, cardiac echogram, cardiac stress test, cardiac angiogram, pulmonary function test, bone scan, thoracic spine x-rays, mammogram, allergy testing.

If the chest pain is thought to be related to the fibromyalgia, specific treatments may include allergy shots (if allergies are a problem) and such medications as analgesics, anti-inflammatories, muscle relaxants, antianxiety and anti-depressants. These treatments may help decrease the conditions (allergies, anxiety, muscle spasm, etc.) that cause chest/breathing difficulties.

The patient will often have soreness in the chest wall area, particularly the designated tender point of the second rib, and an explanation that this is not the heart may help decrease some of the anxiety associated with these chest symptoms.

Injections into the costochondral regions using a combination of local anesthetic and cortisone can be helpful. Prolotherapy can help as well. Chiropractic adjustments have been effective. Therapy that include chest wall exercises can help. Stretching and strengthening exercises using therabands have been particularly effective for decreasing chest wall pain by increasing chest muscle flexibility and strength. If anxiety attacks are a particular problem, referrals for biofeedback and stress management may be considered in addition to the other treatments.

Back Pain

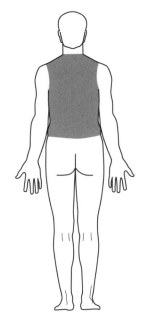

Conditions related to or possibly related to fibromyalgia

1) Strain of back or hip muscles

Causes include:

a) A new or unusual physical activity that requires bending, twisting or lifting, whether at work or at home

b) Prolonged walking or standing, especially on hard surfaces

c) A recent long car ride without any rest stops, especially if driving

d) Playing an unusual sporting activity, such as a basketball game or volleyball

e) Sleeping in a different bed on a surface that was either too hard or too soft; sleeping on stomach

f) A specific trauma from heavy lifting or improper body mechanics

g) Coughing or sneezing spells

h) Poorly fitting shoes or high heels

2) Scoliosis (frequently seen in fibromyalgia patients)

3) Irritable bowel syndrome (which can cause referred pain to the low back and sides)

4) Flareup of tender point and trigger point in the back

Causes include:

a) Weather changes, especially cold, damp weather

b) Recent flu or a viral infection

c) Increased emotional stress

Conditions unrelated to fibromyalgia

1) Osteoarthritis/osteoporosis (may cause secondary fibromyalgia, though)

2) Degenerative disc disease

3) Herniated disc (ruptured disc)

4) Intervertebral disc dysfunction (internal disc damage)

5) Spinal stenosis (narrowing of the spinal canal)

6) Spondylolisthesis (forward displacement of one vertebrae upon another)

7) Compression fracture

8) Subluxation syndrome (imbalance of vertebral, soft tissue, and nerve positions)

9) Thoracolumbar junction syndrome (pain from the facet joints in the middle and low back)

10) Bone tumor

11) Scarring from previous back surgery

12) Connective tissue disease (such as lupus)

13) Foot/leg problems causing bad alignment

Treatments to Do on Your Own

1) Remove or modify the offending physical activities, if possible.

2) Evaluate the workstation and make changes to reduce back strain.

3) Pay attention to proper body mechanics and fibronomics.

4) Alternate between various positions such as walking, standing or sitting and avoid being in one position for too long. Sit whenever possible at work.

5) Review your exercise program and continue exercises that emphasize back stretching.

6) Use modalities, particularly a hot tub or moist heat to the painful back muscles; sometimes ice works well. Use these modalities as frequently as needed.

7) Have a spouse or significant other rub muscle cream into the back or do a massage.

8) Do your own back massage by rubbing your back against a door knob or a golf ball on the floor, or devices to provide deep trigger point pressure.

9) Take over-the-counter medicine as a preventive and therapeutic measure; that is, take it one hour before an "offending" activity to try to prevent pain, or take it when you have more pain.

10) Continue a regular exercise program but emphasize neck stretching and range of motion. Do these exercises as warm-ups before starting a daily job or household chore.

11) Temporarily wear a back brace, and if work particularly aggravates back pain, consider using a back support for work only.

12) Consider a cushioned insert in the shoes to absorb some of the ground reactive forces and prevent them from aggravating the back. Orthotics or special foot braces may help.

13) Stand on a rubberized mat at work to reduce some of the force from the hard surface.

14) Try to eliminate excessive body weight, particularly in the abdominal area, as abdominal obesity is a major cause of increased strain on the lumbar muscles.

15) Make sure you are sleeping on a comfortable bed that supports your back, paying attention to a proper sleeping position to enable the back to rest at night.

16) Get extra rest during the day for acute back flare-up.

17) If the flare-up does not return to baseline with these measures, see your doctor.

Doctor Strategies

Back pain is one of the most common symptoms a doctor evaluates. Your doctor will examine you particularly to rule out some serious causes of back pain, such as a herniated disc or radiculopathy. The exam will include palpation of the spine and spinal muscles and measuring the back's flexibility and range of motion. The neurological exam performed will assess reflexes, sensations, muscle strength and coordination to look for nerve damage. Straight leg raising is a technique that can sometimes help to determine if there is acute nerve root irritation.

Depending on the exam findings, additional testing may be necessary. Some testing may include laboratory studies, back X-rays, back CAT scan, lumbosacral MRI, electrodiagnostic testing, bone scan, myelogram.

If the condition is thought to be related to fibromyalgia, specific treatment will likely include instruction on proper rest, exercise, and activity. Work restrictions may be necessary, such as restricting the amount of weight able to be lifted, restricting bending and twisting, or requiring alternating between various positions. Lighter duty work may be necessary on a temporary basis. Depending on the severity of the flare-up, time off work for recovery and therapy may be recommended.

Various medications including analgesics, non-steroids and muscle relaxants may be considered. Trigger point injections, spray and stretch techniques, and lumbar epidurals are additional ways of providing pain relief.

A therapy program may be prescribed to include:

a) Modalities such as hot packs, ultrasound, electric stimulation and ice

b) Massage and massotherapy

c) Back stretching and conditioning exercises

d) Instruction on a home program

Chiropractic manual adjustments may also be helpful. Often a combination of all of the above works best.

Hopefully, these doctor measures will reduce the pain to return to a more stable and functional baseline so you will be able to continue with your home program.

Hip/Pelvis Pain

Conditions related to or possibly related to fibromyalgia

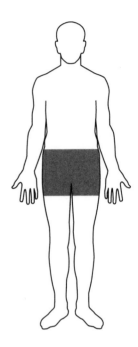

1) Sacroiliac strain

2) Gluteal strain (buttock muscle)

3) Lumbosacral pelvic dysfunction (back-pelvic muscle imbalance)

4) Tension myalgia of the pelvic floor (tight pelvic muscles)

5) Greater trochanteric bursitis (hip bursa irritation)

6) Ischial tuberosity bursitis (buttock bursa irritation)

7) Coccygodynia (tailbone pain)

Various causes of the above include:

　　a) Excessive bending or twisting due to various physical activities that may be occurring on the job or at home. Example: carrying boxes up and down steps

　　b) Prolonged walking and standing, especially on concrete surfaces or uneven surfaces

　　c) Hamstring tightness, which alters the lumbosacral pelvic balance and rhythm

　　d) Prolonged sitting, especially on a low seat

　　e) Excessive climbing, especially stairs

　　f) Standing on ladders for long periods of time

　　g) Sleeping on stomach or poor sleep positions

8) Irritable bowel syndrome (refers pain to pelvic area)

9) Dysmennorhea (abnormal menstrual periods)

10) Endometriosis (refers pain to pelvic area)

11) Irritable bladder (can cause pelvic pain)

12) Vulvodynia (vaginal pain)

Conditions unrelated to fibromyalgia

1) Hip osteoarthritis

2) Avascular necrosis (deterioration of the hip joint due to lack of blood supply)

3) Radiculopathy, plexopathy or other nerve irritation in lumbosacral area

4) Abdominal and pelvic diseases

5) Hernia (inguinal, femoral, umbilical)

Treatments to Do on Your Own

1) Identify offending activities and try to remove or modify them.

2) Emphasize back and pelvic stretching exercises. Work on the hamstrings to get them as stretched out as possible, as the more flexible they are, the better the lumbosacral pelvic joints can be balanced.

3) Use heat, such as hot packs, hot baths, hot tubs; or try ice.

4) Participate in an aquatics exercise program in a heated pool, emphasizing stretching and walking for preventive and therapeutic treatment.

5) Continue a regular exercise program, but emphasize neck stretching and range of motion. Do these exercises as warm-ups before starting a daily job or household chore.

6) Take over-the-counter medicines.

7) Use cushioned shoe inserts.

8) While working, use a tight, wide belt to stabilize the sacroiliac joints (leather weight-lifting belt can work well).

9) If coccygodynia or tailbone pain is a problem, try sitting on a ring or donut cushion and take it wherever you go for your chairs and car seat.

10) If endometriosis pain is a problem particularly during the water retention phase of menstrual cycle, try taking an over-the-counter diuretic along with ibuprofen.

11) If these measure are not helping your flare-up return to baseline level, see your doctor.

Doctor Strategies

Your doctor will examine you with emphasis on the low back, hip and pelvic areas. Particular attention will be paid to the sacroiliac area to see if it is in proper alignment, or if it is out of balance and demonstrates increased pain when various sacroiliac stressing maneuvers are performed. Palpation of the back and hip bones and muscles to see if there is particular increased tenderness, as well as palpation of the gluteus maximus (buttock muscle) tender points and other muscles is emphasized. Referral to an obstetrician or gastroenterologist may be necessary for pelvic or abdominal problems. Sometimes a hernia can be present, which can require referral to a surgeon. If a urologic disorder is suspected, a referral to a urologist may be recommended.

Additional testing can include pelvic and hip X-rays, bone scans, pelvic CAT scan, electrodiagnostic testing, pelvic ultrasound, and abdominal studies.

If the pain is directly related to fibromyalgia, specific treatment program may include:

1) Medication (anti-inflammatories, non-steroidals, muscle relaxants)

2) Trigger point injections and specific sacroiliac injection

3) A therapy program including ultrasound, hot packs, electric stimulation, iontophoresis

4) A sacroiliac corset and manual adjustments may help stabilize the low back and pelvis and help realign the sacroiliac joint.

5) Lumbosacral pelvic stretching and strengthening exercises are often useful to help tight muscles to relax and strengthen weaker muscles to stabilize the lumbosacral rhythm.

6) Aquatic exercises are particularly effective.

Hopefully, these doctor measures will help reduce the flare-up to a more stable baseline that you can manage on your own.

Knee/Leg Pain

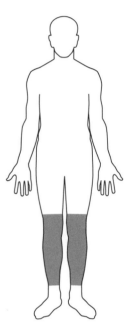

Conditions related to or possibly related to fibromyalgia

1) Knee strains, bursitis or tendinitis

2) Tender or trigger point flareup in knees or legs

3) Restless leg syndrome (leg pain and restlessness, especially at night)

4) Referred pain from myofascial regions and back, hip and sacroiliac regions

Causes include:

1) Increased hill climbing, walking, standing, kneeling or crawling.

2) Increased running activities as can occur when one begins a jogging, walking, or bicycling program, or uses a stair machine.

3) Increased squatting; example: playing volleyball at a picnic causes thigh pain.

Conditions unrelated to fibromyalgia

1) Deep venous thrombosis (blood clot in legs)

2) Peripheral vascular disease (blood vessel hardening or blockage)

3) Neurologic irritation in leg

4) Chondromalacia patella (knee cap pain from arthritis or degeneration)

5) Osteoarthritis

6) Knee ligament, cartilage, or meniscus injury

7) Bone fracture

Treatments to Do on Your Own

1) Avoid or modify activities that are aggravating the condition; reduce the amount of time spent on your feet.

2) Avoid running activities; decrease your running and walking program in half until baseline level is achieved. Then gradually increase the program again, but not to the point where you had been before so as not to cause another flare-up.

3) Wear a neoprene knee brace when more active on feet.

4) Review the exercise program and focus exercises on stretching the knees and calf muscles.

5) Try foot orthotics and wear good supportive shoes for work and exercise.

6) Use over-the-counter medicines for preventive and therapeutic pain control.

7) Continue a regular exercise program but emphasize leg stretching and range of motion. Do these exercises as warm-ups, before starting a daily job or household chore.

8) Rub legs at night and move legs around, especially if restless leg syndrome is a problem.

9) Use modalities such as hot packs or whirlpool, or ice the knees especially after activity.

If these measures are not helping your pain return to baseline level, see your doctor.

Doctor Strategies

The knee exam involves palpating for any tender areas, swelling, or heat. The knee joint itself is examined for any evidence of instability that might indicate an internal derangement or ligament strain. Testing the knee motion and searching for any unusual clicking or grinding is performed. Your doctor will make sure there is no swelling in the calf or veins, and check for adequate pulses and nerve function.

Depending on your doctor's concerns, additional testing may include venus duplex scan to look for a blood clot, vascular studies to measure for arterial disease, knee and leg X-rays, or knee arthroscopy.

If the condition is related to fibromyalgia, specific doctor treatments may include direction on proper exercises. Certain restrictions such as avoiding bending at the knees, kneeling, and repetitive stair climbing may be necessary. A therapy program that includes knee strengthening exercises may be instituted. Knee braces can be ordered, and knee injections and various medicines, especially anti-inflammatories and analgesics, may be tried. For Restless Leg syndrome, drugs such as Klonopin or Sinemet may be tried.

Hopefully, these doctor measures will help decrease the pain to a stable baseline that you can manage again on your own.

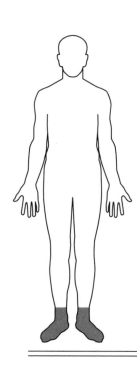

Ankle/Foot Pain

Conditions related to or possibly related to fibromyalgia

1) Ankle sprains and tendinitis

2) Foot tendinitis

3) Plantar fasciitis (bottom of foot)

4) Autonomic nerve hypersensitivity in feet (causes pain, burning, numbness)

5) Spontaneous flareup of tender or trigger points

6) Referred pain from painful back, hip, leg areas

Causes of above include:

a) Walking for long periods of time, and walking on hard surfaces, such as concrete or uneven surfaces; example: mall shopping for hours

b) Running activities (jogging, sprinting)

c) Prolonged standing (shopping, waiting in line, job)

d) Jumping activities (volleyball, basketball)

e) Trauma to the feet (dropping something on the foot or twisting foot on stone)

f) New shoes or poorly fitting shoes

Conditions unrelated to fibromyalgia

1) Referred pain from radiculopathy or other nerve lesions

2) Tarsal tunnel syndrome (pinched nerve at the ankle)

3) Peripheral neuropathy (disease of the smaller nerves causing numbness, weakness, loss of reflexes)

4) Morton's neuroma (a painful nerve "scar" between the toes)

5) Plantar warts

6) Athlete's foot

7) Stress fracture

8) Arthritis, bunions, spurs

9) Connective tissue disease

10) Vascular disease

Treatments to Do on Your Own

1) Modify or remove aggravating activities. Get off feet as much as possible.

2) Wear cushioned inserts, heel pads or metatarsal pads.

3) Try home modalities, such as heat, alternately dipping the feet between warm and cold water, foot whirlpool.

4) Continue a regular exercise program but emphasize stretching and range of motion. Do these exercises as a warm-ups before starting a daily job or household chore.

5) Rest, specifically get off your feet and elevate them.

6) Wear comfortable shoes that have been broken in.

7) If these measures do not reduce the pain to baseline, see your doctor.

Doctor Strategies

Examination of the ankle and feet will include checking pulses and skin to look for any vascular disease. Palpation of the ankle and foot tendons to look for specific areas of soreness, making sure that the joints move to their full range, and making sure that the sensations, strength and reflexes are all normal, are key components of the examination. Specific testing might include X-rays and bone scan. A podiatry referral may help.

Various treatments include:

1) Instruction on exercises and rest

2) Medications

3) Orthotics, whether they be soft cushioned ones or more firm supportive ones

4) Therapies including ultrasound, electric stimulation, and massage may be helpful.

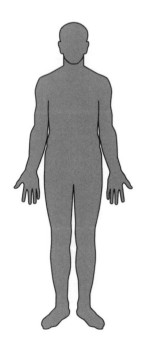

Whole Body Flare-Up

Patients will more often complain of the whole body flaring up rather than one specific region. The overall pain can be overwhelming. The combination of increased pain and fatigue can be particularly difficult for people to cope with and try to maintain their daily functional activities.

Causes of whole body flare-up include:

1) Increased emotional stress [new job, job promotion (with additional responsibilities), job transfer, job termination, new house, divorce, newborn, death in family, illness in family].

2) Increase or decrease in physical activities; new job duty, "weekend athlete," "weekend yard warrior," decreased usual exercise program, illness.

3) Weather changes: In my practice I see flare-ups occurring most commonly in the fall, then winter, then spring, and least often in summer. There may be no other cause except for cold, damp weather. The fall is a particular problem because warm days end with cold, damp evenings. These extremes of temperature fluctuations cause problems in fibromyalgia because the weather change actually "stresses" the muscles and small nerves (autonomic nerves) and causes a flare-up. Another major fall fibromyalgia enemy is the holidays with its associated physical and emotional stresses that make us particularly prone to flare-ups.

4) Trauma. This can be a localized strain which ultimately causes a generalized flare-up, or it can be an unrelated trauma such as a fracture, which heals, but that region becomes more painful and contributes to a generalized flare-up.

5) Surgery. Surgery for any reason can cause flare-up. This is probably due to various factors including stress, strains related to all the required positioning that is unusual for the body, and possibly from general anesthesia. A temporary bedridden state and a relative deconditioning can occur due to inactivity caused by surgery.

Carpal tunnel surgery, knee surgery, and hip surgery are common procedures that often flare up fibromyalgia. Any surgery and surgery-related restrictions on activities or weight-bearing will disrupt the "baseline" body mechanics and put patients at risk for a generalized fibromyalgia flare-up. I have seen patients with generalized flare-ups occurring after silicone breast implant surgery and rupture of the implants, presumably due to an inflammatory reaction against the silicone.

6) Infection. (Flu, cold, bronchitis, etc.) Getting a flu shot has caused flare-ups in many patients of mine.

7) A flare-up of allergies, especially in people who have multiple environmental allergies; allergy flare-ups can occur with exposure to dusts, pollens, weeds, chemicals, fumes, sprays, etc. Flare up risks increase during allergy seasons such as Spring and Fall.

8) In women, flare-ups can be associated with hormonal changes related to the menstrual cycle or menopause.

9) Depression: Depression is common in fibromyalgia and can contribute to a generalized persistent flare-up.

10) Seizures: I have several patients with seizure disorders and fibromyalgia who experience flare-ups after having a generalized seizure. The resulting muscle spasms during the actual seizure causes increased muscle strain and pain.

11) Pregnancy (see Chapter 30)

Treatments to Do on Your Own

I think it is important to try to isolate your worst area or areas and focus on them according to the guidelines described for different areas.

- If you are anticipating a situation that could cause a flare-up such as an upcoming surgery or pregnancy, try to prepare yourself for this "event" by paying extra attention to stretching and light conditioning exercises to get your muscles in as good shape as possible. Ask your doctor what to expect physically: position required during surgery; how long; post-surgery limitations, etc. so you can best prepare yourself and avoid "surprises."

- However, if you are reading this now, chances are you are already experiencing a flare-up and don't have much use for preventive measures at this point. You can try to remember the preventive measures the next time! Identify emotional stresses and practice relaxation techniques and stress reduction strategies. Make a list of all your daily physical activities and look at each one individually to try to determine whether there has been any recent change in this type of activity that may be a factor in causing or contributing to your pain. If you can identify specific activities, try to remove or modify them temporarily. More importantly, make permanent adaptive changes in these activities.

In menstruating women who have problems during the water retention phase, take a diuretic and anti-inflammatory medicine, such as ibuprofen, during your worst week of the menstrual cycle.

- Take over-the-counter medicines regularly until your flare-up is under control, then try to minimize your need for medications.

- Soak in a hot tub or take hot baths or frequent long, hot showers; self-massage your most sore muscles.

- Massotherapy for extra work on the muscle spasms and pain.

- Try soft tissue and muscle nutritional supplements, particularly those that contain supplementary doses of magnesium, malic acid, manganese, vitamin B1 and vitamin B6.

- Continue your routine exercise program at a reduced level if necessary. It is very important to continue with your stretching and conditioning exercises no matter how bad you feel. It is okay to reduce the intensity of your usual programs; say, for example you decrease by one-half the time and number of repetitions. Not doing anything will cause the muscles to suddenly experience a deconditioned state which contributes to even more muscle pain in addition to your current flare-up.

- If these measures and strategies indicated in the other sections for specific areas are not helping you return to your baseline, see your doctor.

Doctor Strategies

- Your doctor will want to make certain that you are not experiencing pain due to another problem. Various disease can aggravate preexisting fibromyalgia, and fibromyalgia can be secondary to an underlying connective tissue disease, thyroid problem, inflammatory arthritis, or other problem. Attention will be paid on the exam to various tender points and whether or not there is any evidence of inflammation, spasm, or neuralgic problem. If there is concern about an underlying medical problem other than fibromyalgia, various testing, including laboratory and X-rays may be ordered. Further consultants may be involved, and if depression is a problem, there may be a referral to a psychiatrist or psychologist.

- Various doctor strategies for managing a flare-up include worker activity restrictions, instruction on exercises, medications, manual therapy, and other therapy programs that include modalities, myofascial release techniques, massage, exercise, and development of a successful home program. If specific areas are identified as more troublesome and more painful, these particular areas will probably receive extra attention. The goal is to try to get the pain reduced as quickly as possible, and then to reactivate the muscles to get them to their functional baseline and keep them there.

Summary

Flare-ups are a part of fibromyalgia, probably the most aggravating part (no pun intended!). These flare-ups unpredictably (sometimes predictably) come to visit us from time to time. Our job is to make their visit as short as possible!

Chapter 35 — Survival Strategies

1) Don't panic with the onset of new pain. Remaining calm and thinking clearly will help the most.

2) Try to recall recent activities that might be responsible for your pain.

3) Consult your doctor if you feel your symptoms warrant investigation.

4) Manage your pain with a home program first. If it continues for more than 3 days above the baseline, consider getting a doctor's opinion.

5) Keep a few good books on fibromyalgia in your home. You can have access to info at any time of the day or night.

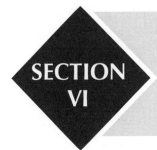

SECTION VI

FIBROMYALGIA INTO THE NEW MILLENNIUM

What can we expect as we move into the new millennium? Will our body's internal computer pretend we don't have fibromyalgia anymore? Not this millennium! I think it will probably happen by the year 3000, so hopefully we can hang around a little bit longer! This section summarizes some of my thoughts about the future and fibromyalgia. As long as we are able to be fibromyalgia survivors in the present, we should be able to handle anything the future holds for us.

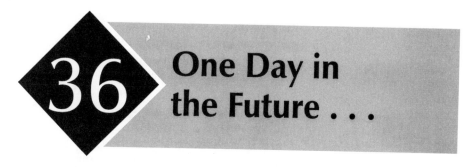

36 One Day in the Future . . .

One Day in the Future . . . (with apologies to all the real science fiction writers)

Dr. Nestor was concerned. Something didn't seem right, didn't feel right. He studied the information on the computer screen and re-calibrated the thermal setting. "System normal," the screen read. He entered several more queries and each time the system read, "Normal."

He turned and scanned the vast computer room at NASA where dozens of engineers and scientists manned their stations, talking and checking their instruments. The scurrying movements of the personnel, the blinking lights of the equipment, and the reverberating noise in no way indicated chaos; this was the most organized operation in the history of NASA.

"Like ants in a colony," thought Dr. Nestor.

In 15 minutes, Project Pain-Free would be launched into outer space to complete a most remarkable two-year journey. Everything appeared on schedule to Dr. Nestor, yet he was still concerned.

Dr. Nestor was appointed Director of Scientific Operations two years ago after Project Pain-Free was approved by Congress. This project was given the highest priority by President Arlene Jenkins and billions of funding dollars materialized, seemingly from a bottomless pit. A project of this magnitude cost a lot and required tens of thousands of health professionals recruited worldwide who were able to miraculously accomplish this project in two years. Two years, and now in a few minutes, human pain would be permanently removed from the face of the Earth, and launched into deep outer space.

Dr. Nestor paused to reflect on the whirlwind of events that roared through the world in the five years since he discovered PS-22. While he was studying advanced pain physiology at The University where he had already published numerous studies on the physiology of pain, he identified a derivative of substance P that neutralized human pain. He named this protein-like substance Pain Specific 22, after the year of the discovery. PS-22 chemically binds to the pain-causing proteins and neutralizes them, abolishing pain. This chemical binding produced a larger protein complex that was found to be highly unstable. This complex protein compound was water soluble, however, so it was dissolved in the urine and eliminated from the body with urination. However, the dissolved compound in the urine was so unstable that if it came into contact with water vapor in the air, it would quickly break up into the pain proteins and PS 22 again, and the pain proteins would reenter the body through the skin pores.

Within hours of this exposure, pain was reestablished, usually more severe than the pain prior to PS-22 treatment.

Dr. Nestor was able to perfect a technique where he injected a dose of PS-22 into the person's arm and collected the first urine (which contained 99.9% of the crystallite) using a sealed container free of any water vapor. He could centrifuge the urine under high pressure, remove the liquid, and seal the remaining crystallite in a saline gel solution. This process prevented the unstable compound from being reabsorbed into the air moisture and reentering any human in contact with this moisture.

The benefits were miraculous. Dr. Nestor's mother had fibromyalgia and was one of the first persons to benefit from PS-22. Her pain, any pain, was completely eliminated from her body. Millions of fibromyalgia suffers in the world hailed this as a miracle. PS-22 became affectionately known as "the P Shot." People who took the PS-22 treatment could still experience warning signals recognized as pain, but severe pain was completely eliminated, permanently.

Dr. Nestor was awarded the Nobel.com Award and the Internet Scientific International Award, the only living person ever to receive these awards. To receive both awards truly elevated Dr. Nestor to a hero's status.

The ease of this technology quickly led to widespread applications. Self-injection techniques were popularized by the EMS-Hologram health care delivery system. Collection facilities sprung up practically on every street corner. These collection facilities, known as P Centers, soon became the most popular franchise in the history of the world, surpassing even the "Lipo and Tuck" Shops. The collected concentrate was stored in holding facilities utilizing nuclear waste protocols originally described in the late-1900's.

Then the government stepped in with an ambitious project, dubbed Project Pain-Free, to eradicate pain from the world. Not since the smallpox vaccination a century ago had such an enormous project been attempted. It took fifty years to eradicate smallpox from the world; Project Pain-Free was completed in two years. Mass inoculations of PS-22 by government health care workers, special command centers, processing and purification equipment, super semi trucks which transported the saline concentrate to holding facilities; the rapidity of the deployment, and the results were simply mind-boggling.

There were some problems along the way, however. Right-to-Hurt activists held numerous demonstrations and attempted to sabotage medical operations. They viewed pain as a privilege and did not want to remove it. Also, some accidents occurred. In one instance a health worker accidentally fell into a tank of concentrated PS-22 crystallite and experienced immediate horrible pain. This particular accident revealed that reinoculation with PS-22 did not work. It appeared that the pain mutated once the person was re-exposed and, thus, did not respond to another attempt to remove pain with PS-22. As a result of this accident and realization, strict security was enforced and the United States military oversaw Project Pain-Free worldwide.

Dr. Nestor himself questioned whether this was the right thing to do, but everything moved so fast. He never had a chance to catch his breath, much less stop and think about any moral ramifications.

Now the final step of the project, the rocket ship launching, was only a few minutes away. The rocket itself was of monstrous proportions. It was the single largest rocket ever built, the length of 3 Lacrosse fields. In its central holding tank were 1.7 billion gallons of concentrated PS-22 crystallite, representing 99.9% of the world's pain. As expected, a small number of people could not be inoculated due to political or military reasons causing inaccessibility. These numbers could have been higher had not the Antarctican Civil Wars come to a timely cease-fire a few months before the project's completion date.

The smaller prototype rocket performed beautifully during its launch and flight trial, so the confidence level was high. Everyone expected this rocket giant to gracefully sail up into space, never to return. The words from a recent hit song, "I sent part of me all that way into space, not expecting it ever to return..." sung by the Back Street Grandpas, seemed to describe this upcoming moment.

Dr. Nestor felt his role today was symbolic; his work ended when the last batch was collected in Australia and secured in headquarters in Cape Kennedy, Florida. Dr. Nestor's job was to oversee the collection and storage of the PS-22 concentrate, and to advise on the scientific issues. So many incredible minds were involved to promote science and technology for this project.

Dr. Nestor's computer monitored temperature, pH, and stability of the concentrate; all remained flawlessly normal throughout the prelaunch operation. So why did he think something wasn't right? Dr. Nestor felt a slight twinge in his left chest wall. He noticed his PFE button (Pain-Free Earth) had become unhooked. Dr. Nestor realized that the pin had worked its way into the tissue of his left pectoralis major muscle. He removed the pin and fixed the button, once again appreciating the benefits of his PS-22 treatment.

"Dr. Nestor? Dr. Nestor?" Commander Zach Jones, the overall project commander, was calling him. "We're ready. Please join me in the launch control center."

Dr. Nestor surveyed the room, performed one last check of his instruments, and walked with Commander Jones to the central module in the heart of the launch center. "This is it," thought Dr. Nestor. "I'm standing at the podium next to the conductor as he prepares to lead this scientific orchestra." Commander Jones' voice boomed out, "Okay, let's go now people. Give me a go for launch. Boosters?"

"Go."

"Retro?"

"Go."

"Guidance?"

"Go."

Dr. Nestor felt his pulse quickening, the adrenaline was surging.

"FAO?"

"Go."

"Network?"

"Go."

"Cap Com?"

"Go."

"Launch control, we are ready to go! Start the launch sequence!"

"T minus 60 seconds and counting."

"We are go for launch." Commander Jones gave Dr. Nestor a thumbs-up sign. The chattering on the radio and intercom provided a steady flow of information. Finally the intercom announced, "10-9-8-7-6-5-4-3-2-1-lift off!"

"We have a lift off" roared Commander Jones.

A cheer arose from the control room.

"How are we looking?" asked Commander Jones.

The launch coordinator answered, "Everything looks good, the tower has been cleared and altitude and velocity are online."

"Beautiful," roared Commander Jones.

Dr. Nestor was in awe of this display of technical proficiency. His legs actually began trembling and he held onto the rail for support. Suddenly, another voice called out, "Commander, we got a glitch."

"Talk to me, Freddy," barked the Commander.

"We're getting a pressure buildup inside the P storage tank. The P is expanding."

"Let's activate the autovents to try to relieve the pressure," ordered the Commander.

"Roger that," said Freddy.

A hush had fallen over the control room as everyone waited.

"Venting is occurring," announced Freddy, "but expansion is occurring more rapidly than we can vent. The pressure is rising out of control. If this continues, the main storage tank will explode."

"We need to get that damn rocket out of the atmosphere," said Commander Jones. "How much time until she clears?"

"Twenty-five seconds."

"Mark that time."

"25-24-23..."

Dr. Nestor couldn't believe it. The PS-22 compound must be expanding due to the thin air and high velocity. But how come the prototype flight went so well? How could anyone have predicted this? He looked around the room and did not find any answers on the concerned faces.

"11-10-9..."

"The pressure's still rising; she's going to blow!"

"4-3-2..." The deafening noise of a huge explosion filled the room. Dr. Nestor gripped the rail tighter, for it felt as if the whole room was shaking.

Then there was complete silence. After what seemed to be an eternity, Commander Jones' voice broke through the silence.

"Did it make it out?"

"I'm not sure," another voice answered.

Dr. Nestor walked away from the center podium in stunned disbelief. He knew what everyone else feared. If the solution reentered the atmosphere, it would disperse worldwide and re-infect everyone. He prayed that the ship made it out of the atmosphere before the explosion.

But he still had that bad feeling.

Dr. Nestor walked down the stairway and stepped outside. The crisp October air surged into his nostrils, bringing a hint of a burned fuel smell. He looked up into the blue sky. There was not a cloud in sight. "What a beautiful sky," Dr. Nestor found himself thinking.

A drop splashed on Dr. Nestor's forehead. Then he felt a few more drops. He took a few steps back into the doorway and watched.

The drops began to fall steadily from the sky, like rain.

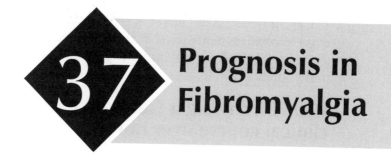

37 Prognosis in Fibromyalgia

We do everything we can to try to keep fibromyalgia from bothering us. We educate ourselves on this condition, we follow through with medical treatments, we think up mental strategies and physical strategies and try to consistently apply them to our home program. We do all of this in an attempt to grab that most precious gem of them all, a stable baseline! We do all of these things, but we still need to ask, "What can we expect with our fibromyalgia?"

I am frequently asked what to expect; what is the prognosis regarding fibromyalgia? Determining a prognosis is one of the most important, yet most difficult, aspects in the practice of medicine. Prognosis is defined as a forecast of the probable outcome of a medical condition. Doctors try to determine whether there will be a recovery, a worsening, or complications by studying the nature and particular features of the medical condition. In determining any given prognosis, doctors must rely on knowledge of an individual's condition, symptoms, physical findings, natural progression of the pain, combined with his or her experience in treating individuals with fibromyalgia.

If a condition is expected to become worse over time, or if no cure is available, the prognosis may be "poor" or "guarded." If full recovery is expected, the prognosis would be "excellent." If improvement occurs, but the condition may persist, the prognosis may be "fair" or "good." Chronic conditions often have "poor" prognoses because there is no cure, even though they may not be life threatening.

Prognosis can be applied to different aspects of fibromyalgia. For example, we can talk about the prognosis of curing fibromyalgia, the prognosis of fibromyalgia's clinical course over time, the prognosis of successful response to treatment, the prognosis of whether fibromyalgia will cause disability, and more. For each component of fibromyalgia, we try to make a medical forecast or prediction based on the probability that a particular outcome will occur.

I have tried to determine the prognosis in fibromyalgia based upon my knowledge and experience combined with my understanding of the scientific literature (at least what I can remember of it!). Based on this, I will review prognosis for different components of fibromyalgia, from my point of view.

Will Fibromyalgia Ever Go Away? (Is there a cure?)

Fibromyalgia is a chronic and permanent condition. Once this condition has developed and is clinically measurable upon examination, it will be present for the remainder of the person's life. I am aware of no cure for fibromyalgia at the present time. Therefore, the prognosis is "poor" that a given individual's fibromyalgia will ever be completely cured. Even though the prognosis is "poor" for a cure, the prognosis is "good" that one can improve (or heal!).

Certainly we can feel better in spite of our fibromyalgia and some are lucky enough to get a complete remission, but the fibromyalgia doesn't go away. We are working on a cure, and I think we will find one someday, but in the meantime, let's live our lives to the fullest possible.

Will Fibromyalgia Get Worse over Time? (What is the clinical course over time?)

Fibromyalgia symptoms can improve. There may be less pain over time and some-times fibromyalgia can go into remission. The prognosis for stabilization or improvement in most people over time is good, however, even though fibromyalgia is still present.

To explain what happens to a group of patients with fibromyalgia over time, I use the "*1/3 Rule*" to explain prognosis. In a group of people with fibromyalgia, the 1/3 rule means that:

1/3 of the people will do better over time
1/3 of the people will stay the same over time
1/3 of the people will do worse over time.

This means that at least 2/3 of the people will do better or not get worse over time; hence, the prognosis for most people with fibromyalgia to be stable or improve is good.

The 1/3 rule applies to a group of people with fibromyalgia. It is difficult to look at any one individual and accurately predict how that person will do over time. However, there are some characteristics that may help determine who would do more or less favorably over time.

Those who do better or at least not worse are most likely to have the following characteristics:

1) Early diagnosis of fibromyalgia after symptoms began

2) Younger age when diagnosed

3) Successful response to treatments

4) Few associated conditions

5) Have flexible job situations

6) Follow through with a home program

The 1/3 that get worse are more likely to have the following characteristics:

1) A delayed diagnosis after symptoms develop

2) No response to treatments or non-compliant with treatments

3) Numerous associated conditions that cause additional impairment

4) Stressful and physically demanding job

5) Men whose fibromyalgia came on rapidly and caused early disability

There are various reasons why the 1/3 group gets worse over time. Injuries or secondary conditions may have developed that caused an overall worsening of the fibromyalgia. For example, an individual with fibromyalgia may be involved in a motor vehicle accident and sustain a severe whiplash injury that permanently worsens the fibromyalgia and causes it to be more painful. Or a person may develop progressive osteoarthritis or an inflammatory arthritis, which causes fibromyalgia to worsen in addition to causing "separate" pain. I suspect some people are just "destined" to get worse with fibromyalgia regardless of whether or not intervening circumstances occur and whether or not the person had appropriate treatments.

Nearly everyone with fibromyalgia will experience flare-ups from time to time as part of the natural long-term course of fibromyalgia. In most, however, these flare-ups are a temporary aggravation of the baseline level that can last anywhere from days to weeks before the pain returns to the previous stable baseline. In some, however, flare-ups seem to lead to progressive worsening of the fibromyalgia and the previous stable baseline is never reached.

Although we know flare-ups will occur, we cannot predict when or how frequently. My patients have an average of two major flare-ups per year, and the average duration of each flare-up is about a month. These figures were determined by a retrospective review of patients, but there was a wide disparity among individual patients. Some people may have flare-ups every month, while others may not flare up for over a year. As we have reviewed in the flare-up chapter, there are a variety of reasons why flare-ups happen, and those who are "exposed" to more of these flare-up risks will certainly experience more flare-ups over time.

Although a third of the people report that they get worse over time, I think everyone diagnosed with fibromyalgia who has had some opportunities for positive intervention with fibromyalgia treatments will have the potential to do better over time. Even those who report feeling worse pain over time may be more flexible and more functional than they were prior to their diagnosis. The patients may be more aware of the fibromyalgia and notice if the pain worsens. Yet they may still be successfully maintaining their functional abilities even with noticeably worse pain.

A way to understand how positive interventions can help one do better over time, compared to no treatment at all, is demonstrated in the following diagram. The diagram shows a patient's pain level over time with no treatment. You can see that the pain level became worse from the time of diagnosis and continues to get worse at a steady rate over time.

Now, suppose the same patient were treated for pain over time. She still became worse overall; however, she did not get as bad as she would have without treatment. So, if we compare the difference between the two, as noted in the diagram, we can see that the patient actually did a little better over time with treatment than without.

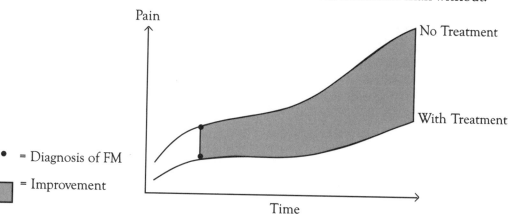

Pain

No Treatment

With Treatment

• = Diagnosis of FM

▨ = Improvement

Time

Thus, positive intervention did help this patient even though the pain got worse over time. So, hopefully we can say that the diagnosis and treatment of fibromyalgia will help a person over time, even if one feels worse. And if one feels worse, hopefully the functional abilities remain good despite the worsening pain.

Will Fibromyalgia Cause Disability?

Fibromyalgia causes impairment in everyone. An impairment is any abnormality of anatomic structure or physiological function. Tender points are impairments because they are soft tissue abnormalities in our bodies. Thus, everyone with fibromyalgia has an impairment.

Any restriction or lack of ability to perform a normal activity is considered a disability. The vast majority of people with fibromyalgia will have some type of disability or restriction as defined above. These restrictions include difficulty performing repetitive reaching, bending, twisting or standing, or difficulty with concentration and memory. By definition, fibromyalgia causes impairment in everyone and disabilities in almost everyone. Some people with fibromyalgia do not have any disabilities (and their last names aren't Ripley!).

Individuals whose fibromyalgia worsens over time have a higher probability (unfavorable prognosis) that they will have more functional impairment, disability or inability to perform various daily activities or job duties.

Will Treatments Help Fibromyalgia?

Treatments DO help!

Treatments help reduce the pain, resolve a flare-up and return the condition to a stable baseline. The prognosis is good for getting some type of successful response to treatment. I am always reviewing treatment responses in patients to determine if they are improving and to make any changes needed in the program to achieve the best treatment response possible.

Treatments do not eliminate fibromyalgia, and they may only last a short while. I believe that a supervised medical treatment program which includes instruction on a home program can help control long-term symptoms. I do not encourage ongoing indefinite supervised medical treatment. Rather, I promote individual responsibility for following through with an independent, unsupervised home program to control chronic problems associated with fibromyalgia.

So, we're stuck with fibromyalgia, but we certainly have some control over how well we can do. We learn to accept the things we can control, but most importantly we also have to accept the things that we cannot control. As I look into my crystal ball to see what the future holds, I notice that there is a lot of ... fog. Lots and lots of fog. Now isn't that typical?

Chapter 37 — Survival Strategies

1) Accept that once you have been diagnosed with fibromyalgia, it will be present the remainder of your life. How you deal with it is up to you.

2) It is normal to have flare-ups from time to time.

3) Participate and control your symptoms as much as possible.

4) Remind yourself that your treatment goals are to reduce pain, resolve the flare-up, and return to a stable baseline, not eliminate fibromyalgia.

5) Learn to accept the things we can control.

6) Learn to accept the things we cannot control.

7) Learn the difference between the two.

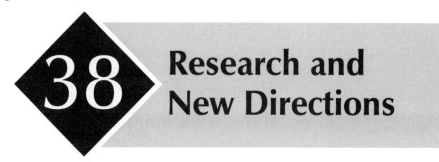

Research and New Directions

We have come a long way with fibromyalgia in the last one hundred years. I don't mean that we feel like we are a hundred years old with fibromyalgia, although that's usually the case, too! Fibromyalgia was "discovered" about a hundred years ago. In the past thirty years, we have a better understanding of pain mechanisms, and fibromyalgia. We also have a controversy regarding any twelve-letter words that begin with "fibro" and ends with "myalgia!"

Controversies are not unique to fibromyalgia. Any condition that affects a lot of people and is undergoing a lot of scientific research will be faced with controversy. Controversies are helpful and "therapeutic" as they encourage medical professionals to look at all sides of the picture and reach a better understanding and clarification. In fibromyalgia's case, doctors may choose to better understand fibromyalgia, accept it, and incorporate it into their medical thinking. Some individual doctors may choose not to accept fibromyalgia based upon their individual opinions.

Ongoing Controversies

Most of the controversies have been mentioned in this book, but I will summarize some of the current controversial points in a Point-Counterpoint fashion.

Point	Counterpoint
No obvious pathology in fibromyalgia.	We know a lot about the pathophysiology and have objective tender point abnormalities.
Therapy does not cure fibromyalgia.	Treatments can heal fibromyalgia even if there is no cure.
Treatments are costly.	What is the price of improving the quality of life?
No proof that trauma causes fibromyalgia.	Much evidence that trauma causes fibromyalgia. No proof that trauma DOESN'T cause fibromyalgia.
Legal system too involved in fibromyalgia.	This country has laws regarding trauma and liability.
Labeling people with fibromyalgia has gotten out of control.	Fibromyalgia is a legitimate, valid medical diagnosis.
It is a syndrome, not a disease.	It is a disease of pain perception.

We should limit treatments of fibromyalgia.	We should teach home programs and personal responsibility.
A few people use most of the care.	Some require more treatments to achieve a better outcome.
Fibromyalgia is overdiagnosed.	Fibromyalgia is undertreated.
There should be no disability awards for fibromyalgia.	Each person's situation is unique and decisions regarding disability should be individualized.
Illness magnified by medical model of care.	Illness helped by chronic pain approaches.

I expect controversies to persist well into the new millennium. I also expect that we will continue to learn more about fibromyalgia. Ongoing funding and research of this complicated condition will result in further understanding. Here are some of my predictions.

Research Projections:

1) More specific identification of fibromyalgia subgroups and better delineation of the overall fibromyalgia spectrum.

2) Further research into the causes and mechanisms of fibromyalgia to better understand the actual pathologic mechanism and learn what specifically triggers fibromyalgia from a microscopic or cellular level.

3) The ability to predict who will get fibromyalgia and what happens over time, and to understand the risks. We'll study individuals with fibromyalgia to determine what happens in response to long-term treatment, and whether other conditions develop. We'll further understand the prognosis. We may even find that aliens from outer space also have fibromyalgia!

4) New medications to treat pain and fibromyalgia-specific medications will probably be developed. Medications that are more selective and specific for controlling neurotransmitters and protein factors involved in pain will become available. The ideal medication would be one that is tolerated, not addictive, and does not cause serious side effects such as impaired cognition or sedation. The medicine must continue to work over time. A major problem for people with fibromyalgia is that medicines are often not tolerated and/or have numerous side effects. Many who are lucky enough to find a medicine that will work are often frustrated that the medicine stops working over time. There are currently no magical pills.

A multicenter study is currently being done on a drug, Pregabalin, which works by blocking substance P, the neurotransmitter found in very high concentrations in fibromyalgia patients. Any drug that successfully quiets the pain-mediating activity of substance P will be a welcome one for fibromyalgia people.

Powerful painkillers can be developed from natural toxins. The venom from snakes, poisons from frogs, and chemicals from sea creatures can be turned into powerful painkillers. Drug researchers can modify the molecular structures to remove the toxicity while enhancing the analgesic effect (develop molecular "smart bombs"). We may not be pain-free, but we may find medicines that significantly relieve the "irritating" component of pain. If we were pain-free, we would still have to complain about something!

5) The delivery of medications will be refined over time. Those of us with fibromyalgia are very sensitive to medicines, and especially oral medicines, which cause our stomachs to speak in languages different from our native tongue! Anything that can bypass our overly sensitive stomachs should help. Various new delivery systems that may be applied to fibromyalgia treatment would include the use of microneedles which can painlessly break through the skin and enter the subcutaneous space for delivery of medicine, or lasers that can create painless holes for medicines to enter the bloodstream. We already uses patches to deliver medicine transdermally, and we can refine that method for pain treatment. Sublingual medicine can be absorbed under the tongue and enter the bloodstream. Inhalants can also bypass the stomach by being absorbed directly into the bloodstream through the nasal blood vessels. Perhaps someday we will be able to take a shower and have medicine absorbed into our skin from the soap! If this happens, people with fibromyalgia would certainly be the cleanest group of people in the world!

> Powerful painkillers can be developed from natural toxins. The venom from snakes, poisons from frogs, and chemicals from sea creatures can be turned into powerful painkillers. Drug researchers can modify the molecular structures to remove the toxicity while enhancing the analgesic effect (develop molecular "smart bombs"). We may not be pain-free, but we may find medicines that significantly relieve the "irritating" component of pain.

6) New forms of treatment may be discovered. Genetic research may identify more specific gene markers and result in specific gene therapy. Perhaps fibromyalgia expression genes can be identified and blocked. Immunotherapy may evolve and give us new allergy treatments, using manufactured proteins or vaccines. Immunotherapy could reduce inflammation and boost the immune system or enhance the neurotransmitter function.

Growth factor therapy may be developed. We have discovered nerve growth factors and the role they may play in fibromyalgia. Perhaps nerve growth factor therapy may help reduce fibromyalgia pain. Perhaps we may find ligament growth factors or muscle growth factors. Ligament or muscle growth factors, if discovered and refined, may have applications in treatment of acute trauma, especially for acute whiplash injuries. If these treatments could reduce the damage to soft tissue structures and encourage healing, they would play a major role in acute soft tissue injury treatment strategies. Perhaps future emergency room/stat care strategies would include the injection of standard doses of soft tissue growth factors for all patients with acute musculoskeletal injuries.

I expect that nutritional medicines will be further refined and will play a major role. Prolotherapy or treatments that try to repair and restore tissues could play a bigger role in fibromyalgia treatment over time.

Insurance Trends

Having health insurance will not guarantee that one's pain problems will be covered in the future. As many patients have discovered, more and more insurance plans make it very difficult and in some cases impossible to obtain necessary medical treatment for fibromyalgia. I have been in private practice for over ten years now, and I have observed a number of trends concerning the insurance industry.

1) Insurance industries are a "big business."

Health insurance is the lifeblood of reimbursement for fibromyalgia. In our country, health insurance is usually provided by employers. Over the years I have met many people who work in the health insurance industry. These individuals are great people who try to do the best job they can, and who try to have fulfilling and enjoyable careers. Many in the insurance industry who are also my patients can appreciate seeing "both sides of the fence." I have no problem with individuals who work in the health insurance field, or the health insurance field in general.

My concerns (and frustrations!) have to do with the health insurance BUSINESS. Specifically, the insurance industry is a for-profit business, and thus is interested in making profits, lots of them. I don't have a problem with businesses making profits, but it seems that the health insurance business has a unique philosophical problem in their business. It is what I would call the health insurance paradox. The health insurance industry wants to make large profits, and to increase profits, they need to decrease spending. Yet the very nature of this industry is to spend money on its clients who require medical care. Whatever care is necessary, the clients who purchase insurance expect that this care will be provided. The paradox is that insurance companies want to spend less money on their clients and do less for them so they can make more money. When chronically painful conditions such as fibromyalgia are diagnosed, this paradox can lead to an antagonistic relationship; that is, the insurance companies may try to avoid treating chronically painful problems because of the perception that it is too costly and will reduce profits. We pay the insurance company to act in our best interests, yet they may selectively choose not to do that.

It would be like agreeing to purchase a new Cadillac and make payments, but when you go to get the Cadillac, the car dealership won't give it to you. They give you a Yugo instead! And the owner of the car dealership is driving your Cadillac!

2) Difficulty getting treatments approved.

Necessary treatments, when requested, are often denied by the insurance company. The insurance company may request more information, or send the request off for medical review before it can "decide" on our request for treatments. This creates delays in starting the needed treatments.

Treatments may be approved at first, but later are denied. The insurance policy may state the treatments are covered and approval given, but it's not a guarantee that they will be actually paid! The patient's treatments are done, but may be denied at a later time. Some of the usual reasons given by the insurance company for denial of a covered service include:

- Treatments are not medically necessary.
- The patient's condition is no longer an acute problem.
- The treatments are considered experimental.

I appeal, send letters and talk to the insurance company's medical director to try to get denials overturned.

I feel as if all of my doctoring services are being arbitrarily denied from time to time for no consistent or valid reasons. And I am not even talking about fibromyalgia yet!

I educate insurance personnel about chronic conditions such as fibromyalgia which are characterized by acute exacerbations that need definite medical treatments. I, the treating physician, can determine when the patient has reached maximum benefit and when the condition is no longer acute. I am much more competent and capable of doing of this than a non-physician insurance clerk who is being instructed to deny certain services and requests.

Many times patients will complete a treatment program and accomplish their goals only to receive notification from their insurance company that essentially says, "Oh, by the way, we're not covering any of these services." Talk about a stress-related flare-up! We are always told by health insurance companies that we can appeal any denials. We do, and guess what usually happens?

3) Restriction of services.

Physical therapy services have been getting hit particularly hard over the past several years. Many insurance companies have begun cutting services altogether, limiting services, or making it difficult to qualify for any of these services. Some insurances companies will acknowledge the diagnosis of fibromyalgia but won't allow any treatments for it. Essentially, they are saying, "Yes, you can see a doctor for the legitimate condition of fibromyalgia, but we won't pay for any treatments of this legitimate condition."

Another restriction is to allow therapy to be performed only by a licensed physical therapist or a physician. This means that any ancillary medical professionals who are working under the guidance of a physician or physical therapist cannot treat the patient, including physical therapy assistants, therapy aides, massotherapists, nurses, or athletic trainers. The only ones who can "lay on the hands" are the physical therapist or the doctor. Insurance companies know that there are only a limited number of people who can be treated by these limited number of physical therapists or doctors, and thus, are restricting access of their clients to therapy services.

Workers' Compensation Trends

Workers' Compensation insurance for work related injuries also has several trends that often interfere with fibromyalgia treatment.

Only "allowed conditions" can be treated. This following common example will demonstrate how frustrating it can be for a physician treating a Workers' Compensation problem.

Mary injures her back at work. She goes to the emergency room and is diagnosed with a lumbosacral sprain and strain. This diagnosis becomes the Workers' Compensation "allowed condition." Mary does not get better. She has severe low back pain radiating to the right hip and down the leg with numbness and weakness in her right leg. She sees a specialist who diagnoses her with lumbar disc disease and lumbar radiculopathy due to the work injury. The physician also acknowledges that a lumbosacral sprain and strain is also present, but the main Workers' Compensation problems causing Mary's problems are the disc disease and associated nerve root irritation.

What do you think happens at this point? Does Workers' Compensation allow the physician to treat Mary's actual problems? What usually happens at this point is that Workers' Compensation will deny any treatment request for lumbar disc disease or radiculopathy. Furthermore, Workers' Compensation will not even pay for the visit to the specialist since the main conditions are something other than the "allowed condition" of lumbosacral sprain and strain. Mary hasn't done anything different since she first hurt herself. She didn't re-injure herself. She still is the same person with the same problems and the same injury, yet Workers' Compensation only recognized her lumbosacral sprain and strain. Sure, Mary can try to get these other conditions (the actual conditions that are bothering her) allowed as additional conditions, but she probably will have to get an attorney and go through a lengthy process to do so. This is an example of how actual conditions (including post-traumatic fibromyalgia) can be "invisible" in the eyes of Workers' Compensation.

The frustrating part of these independent medical examinations is that they are held as the "gospel truth" by Workers' Compensation. The treating physician (*i.e.*, me) has examined the patient on multiple occasions and has tried to come up with a plan to help the patient. Yet Workers' Compensation will usually place more emphasis on the report of the independent medical examiner who sometimes has spent as little as ten minutes with these patients. If the independent examiner doesn't recommend treatments, then Workers' Compensation will deny any further treatments for the injured worker. The injured worker must resort to hiring an attorney and go through the appeals process to try to get the medically necessary treatments approved. Many of them don't have the resources or stamina to go through this process.

Most treatments must be pre-authorized. Like other medical health insurances, most treatment in the Workers' Compensation system must have prior authorization before it can be carried out. If we carry out treatments without prior authorization, the chances are very high that Workers' Compensation will not pay. However, it is not unusual to have to wait a few months to receive the authorization. Meanwhile, the patient remains in severe pain without any therapies authorized. Some Ohio Workers' Compensation managed care organizations do an excellent job of responding very quickly to requests for treatments, but many are very slow.

Independent medical examinations (the "hired gun"). Workers' Compensation (and insurance companies and defense attorneys) will contract with physicians to independently examine an injured worker and render an "independent" opinion. The independent examiner is asked if the requested treatments are appropriate and medically necessary. After performing this exam and submitting a report, the independent medical examiner is promptly paid by Workers' Compensation. Many independent medical examiners derive a large portion of their income from performing independent medical examinations.

Do you see the problem here? How can an exam be completely "independent" when the physician is being paid by the same company requesting the exam? If the physician writes a report that Workers' Compensation doesn't like (*i.e.*, the examiner agrees with the requested treatments), then Workers' Compensation will not likely use that physician again. And if the physician is expecting a certain number of referrals (and income) from Workers' Compensation, there is at least a suggestion of a bias that the physician would want to keep the referring source happy.

Another potential bias occurs when the independent medical examiner is a direct competitor of the physician requesting the treatments. The independent medical examiner may be less likely to respond in a favorable manner to the requesting physician's program if the independent examining physician is trying to increase his business by decreasing someone else's business. Over ninety-nine percent of my patients who have seen one of these Workers' Compensation hired guns have received reports that state my requested program is not medically necessary and would not be helpful. I don't believe that I can be so completely wrong that many times!

The frustrating part of these independent medical examinations is that they are held as the "gospel truth" by Workers' Compensation. The treating physician (*i.e.*, me) has examined the patient on multiple occasions and has tried to come up with a plan to help the patient. Yet Workers' Compensation will usually place more emphasis on the report of the independent medical examiner who sometimes has spent as little as ten minutes with these patients. If the independent examiner doesn't recommend treatments, then Workers' Compensation will deny any further treatments for the injured worker. The injured worker must resort to hiring an attorney and go through the appeals process to try to get the medically necessary treatments approved. Many of them don't have the resources or stamina to go through this process.

Private insurance companies and defense attorneys also use independent medical exams to "clarify" a diagnosis or request for treatment. In my experience, this usually means the insurance company doesn't like my diagnosis or doesn't want to approve my proposed treatments, so they send the patient to a doctor who will "predictably" disagree with my findings.

I have observed a trend in which Workers' Compensation has shifted the pendulum more in favor of the employers and less in favor of the injured workers when it comes to a chronic pain problem such as fibromyalgia. Workers' Compensation appears to disapprove of any chronic conditions, and whenever any condition is not completely healed within four to six weeks, the injured worker faces a lot of difficulties in getting conditions and treatments approved. I certainly hope that the pendulum swings back the other way. For this to happen, there will need to be political interventions in favor of the injured worker. Perhaps we need to elect people who have post traumatic fibromyalgia as a result of work injuries, especially the ones who were denied treatments!

As more difficulties arise with insurance coverage and reimbursement for fibromyalgia, more and more people are privately paying for medical services, particularly alternative or complementary treatments. Invariably, many patients who would benefit from treatments or frequent treatments cannot afford to pay for them, and thus, may get far fewer treatments than they actually need. Hopefully, more and more people with fibromyalgia will be winning lotteries, inheriting large sums of money, inventing popular devices, and winning at slot machines!

The health insurance trend regarding fibromyalgia is a discouraging one. It is getting harder and harder to get medically necessary treatments. The insurance companies tell me that they cannot afford to treat fibromyalgia on an indefinite basis. Fibromyalgia is their worst nightmare; it is chronic and there is no cure. I explain my treatment philosophy to teach individual self-responsibility to manage fibromyalgia more effectively and try to decrease the need for health services over time. I hope that the pendulum does shift into the patients' corner where necessary services will be provided.

Doctor Trends

The medical profession continues to change. The most significant change I have noticed over the past ten years is the steady loss of control by the doctors. Medical care is now controlled by the health insurance industry whose medical reviewers are often non-physicians without intensive training. In the new millennium, we may soon have new high school graduates making decisions regarding medical care!

Patients often have to see doctors not by choice but because they are the only ones covered by insurance. Many physicians who have not been able to thrive as private practitioners must join larger groups or become salaried employees of large medical companies. The ongoing changes in the medical industry have threatened the physician's independence and income, and most importantly, their treatment ideals. Many doctors are leaving the profession because they are so frustrated by the changes that have directly impaired their ability to care for patients effectively.

It is unfortunate when doctors who have gained valuable knowledge and experience, and can be so effective and helpful to patients, decide to leave their careers because of seemingly senseless changes in the medical industry. Physicians have groups such as the American Medical Association (AMA) that lobby for our interests, but sometimes individual physicians still feel helpless in the big picture. Politics are a necessary part of medicine, yet I feel that the more time I spend on politics, the less time I have available for my patients, so I try to minimize politics in my medical practice. In spite of the trends, the medical profession is still a professionally and personally rewarding one. I still love what I am doing, but I am still a youngster! (A middle aged one!)

The AMA wants to organize their doctor members into a union primarily to address the issues of control. Doctors want control of the way their patients are treated and what they are allowed to prescribe. Doctors want patients to be able to see them or the doctors of the patients' choice, not the insurance companies' choice. I believe a physician's union for better patent care will help fibromyalgia patients obtain the best quality treatments.

I am pleased to see that medical schools are now teaching about fibromyalgia. Nearly every medical student gets an opportunity to see patients with fibromyalgia and learn about this disorder in his or her training. If medical students and doctors don't read about fibromyalgia in the scientific journals, they can read about it in the consumer magazines. They'll probably be seeing it in the grocery store tabloids soon!

Many physicians are promoting themselves as pain specialists and I expect as they gain more experience in treating fibromyalgia, more and more physicians will be able to offer comprehensive treatments. Chronic pain does not disappear with expensive medical care, but it can decrease and the quality of life can improve. We are seeing more blending of traditional and alternative/complementary medical care in hospitals and clinics. Many pain centers offer a wide range of treatments and specialists, as does my clinic. Currently we have three physicians who specialize in different aspects of pain management. We offer a wide variety of diagnostic and treatment services as they relate to fibromyalgia and other pain disorders. Patients appreciate the quality, convenience, efficiency and cost-effectiveness of a comprehensive pain program under one roof. We work closely with other medical professionals and use the team concept. We also try to be creative in designing treatment programs that fit the individual's particular personal and financial situation. Our challenge is to be able to offer comprehensive services to all patients who medically qualify regardless of the individual's financial situation. As I have met with numerous physicians across the country, I see a lot of positive trends in developing specialized pain centers that are helping patients with fibromyalgia.

Legislative Trends

We are seeing more legislation as it regards pain management. Like anything else in politics, some of the legislation isn't so favorable! Medicare cutbacks have made it more difficult for older patients with fibromyalgia to get treatment. The Balanced Budget Act of 1997 cut Medicare benefits by placing a cap on physical therapies. The new law has forced some Medicare patients to curtail their therapies, thus reducing their quality of life, especially those who have multiple therapy needs for multiple problems, including fibromyalgia.

Medicare changes are guided by legislation, but the trend has been for insurance companies to follow Medicare's lead, especially if it means cost reduction and potentially increased profits, and they may be reducing their therapy benefits. As I have previously mentioned, an ongoing problem is the steady erosion of therapy benefits for patients with fibromyalgia. Currently several different bills aimed at changing or removing the caps in Medicare treatment are working their way through Congress and, hopefully, the health care industry and patients will get some relief soon, literally and legislatively!

In recent years, favorable legislation has been passed that protects physicians who prescribe narcotic medications for patients with chronic pain. This trend should help remove some of the fears of physicians, specifically fears that they may be

As long as there is pain, there will be legislation that directly or indirectly affects those who have pain. Pain is certainly not a political problem, but there is no way to keep politics and future legislation out of pain. Perhaps we need a prominent politician who has fibromyalgia to get the legislative momentum rolling in our direction!

"red-flagged" whenever they prescribe narcotic medication. Physicians who specialize in pain management are expected to see a higher percentage of patients who may benefit from narcotic medications. Physicians still need to prescribe all medicines responsibly and appropriately, but allowing the physicians to make unbiased decisions on what is best for patients is certainly preferred and encouraged.

As long as there is pain, there will be legislation that directly or indirectly affects those who have pain. Pain is certainly not a political problem, but there is no way to keep politics and future legislation out of pain. Perhaps we need a prominent politician who has fibromyalgia to get the legislative momentum rolling in our direction!

There doesn't appear to be any magic pill for fibromyalgia in the immediate future. No PS-22 is foreseeable at this time. Don't underestimate the scientific potential, however. If you look at how far we've come with our understanding of fibromyalgia in just a few short years, we can certainly comprehend a major breakthrough or a series of mini-breakthroughs over the years to come that will make fibromyalgia far more manageable and far less a nuisance for our children. Instead of feeling that we're passing on a burden to our children, let's hope that our children will be able to appreciate the burden being completely lifted. And let's hope we're still around to see this happen!

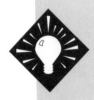

Chapter 38 — Survivor Strategies

1) Remember that controversies about medical conditions are not limited to just fibromyalgia.

2) Remember that health insurance is a business and the bottom line is profit.

3) Denial of payment is not a personal decision against you — it's strictly a profit decision.

4) Avoid an antagonistic relationship with your insurance company, but be persistent and firm.

5) Network with other patients on the same plan. Learn the intricate details of how to get treatment approved.

6) Pay for complementary treatments that you can afford. Research as a consumer and do not commit to treatments you cannot afford.

7) Encourage your medical professional to look at all sides of the picture.

8) Seek medical professionals who are open minded and educated about fibromyalgia.

9) Advocate treatment for chronic pain patients through your legislature.

10) Keep the hope that new discoveries will make fibromyalgia more manageable.

39 Hope for a Better Tomorrow

Fibromyalgia can be a scary condition. It is not life-threatening, but the pain it causes can lead to severe problems with everyday functioning. One can be overwhelmed with the difficulties of dealing with fibromyalgia, from understanding and living with the diagnosis each day, to wondering what will happen tomorrow and the next year. Physicians try to help fibromyalgia patients by prescribing medicines, therapies, and anything that we think may work. We have an unlimited array of treatments we can try, but I believe the most important thing we can prescribe for fibromyalgia patients is hope.

Hope: to cherish a desire with the expectation of fulfillment.

Hope means something different to each of us. Each person's interpretation of hope is shaped by that individual's experiences, backgrounds, and influences. Like our fibromyalgia, hope is unique for each individual.

Everyone has "basic" experiences and influences such as growing up, puberty, school, family, and heritage. Many share common experiences and backgrounds that impart a general flavor to this "hope recipe," but each adds secret ingredients that ultimately give hope its unique individual flavor.

My three secret ingredients to my hope recipe which provide me with unique influences and experiences, are: (1) hearing impairment; (2) fibromyalgia; (3) rehabilitation specialty. Each give me a different perspective on the meaning of hope and have defined for me my expectation to be fulfilled.

I have a hearing impairment. Specifically, I have a form of nerve deafness caused by damage from an antibiotic, Streptomycin. I lost most of my hearing at a young age, but fortunately I was born with normal hearing and was able to develop language skills before I lost most of my hearing. Also, I have enough residual hearing that allowed me to benefit from hearing aids. I have worn hearing aids since I was 14 years old (about 10 years ago...I think!). My hearing impairment has taught me that understanding is helpful.

My hearing impairment has taught me that *understanding* is hope. I literally strive to understand what is being said because I can't hear well. When someone speaks to me, I hope I can understand what was said so I can effectively communicate. My association of hope with understanding began at a young age when I first lost most of my hearing.

When I listen to songs on the radio, I can hear music and voices, but I cannot quite understand the words. If I could only turn the "clarity notch" up just a bit more so that I could understand the words and symbolically understand the music of life. Each day I hope to understand the words to the songs.

My fibromyalgia has taught me that *knowledge* is hope. Unknown pains can trigger the worst fears. Knowing about fibromyalgia, knowing that it is not life-threatening, deforming, or paralyzing, starts the education process. With education and knowledge come opportunity to improve the pain, to gain successful experiences, and to accept the fibromyalgia.

My emphasis has been on educating people about their fibromyalgia. The diagnosis of fibromyalgia is the start of the education; finding successful treatments is continuing the education process. Knowing as much as possible about fibromyalgia and educating others on fibromyalgia allows me to have hope. If we understand more, we fear less, do better and have hope. Someday I hope all of our combined knowledge will lead to a cure for fibromyalgia.

My rehabilitation specialty has taught me that *ability* is hope. Disabilities, or focusing on what we can't do, are the opposite of hope. Focusing on our abilities is hopeful, for it motivates us to do what we can. It also lets us anticipate that we can do even more, that we have the ability to improve.

Ability as hope can help erase the negative stereotypical comments, "There's nothing to do for your fibromyalgia," "You just have to learn to live with your pain," "You can't do this anymore," or "You'll probably get worse." Use your abilities to achieve positive rewarding goals.

I have taken my hope "ingredients" and realized my individual hope definition or hope philosophy: learn and understand everything you can about your fibromyalgia. Apply this knowledge to improve your quality of life, and expect even better knowledge, abilities and understanding tomorrow.

Our fibromyalgia is painful and it interferes with everyday routine activities and function. It creates a burden and can make a person feel all alone.

I am not alone and you are not alone. We do not have to bear the burden alone. Whatever our backgrounds, whatever our differences, we all share the same painful problem. Because we live each day facing the same challenges and the same obstacles, we have developed a unique understanding of each other, despite never having met one another!

When people with fibromyalgia first meet each other, there is almost a magical ability to immediately open the doors that lead to our most innermost sensitivities, fears, and hopes. On the outside we may be perfect strangers, but given the opportunity to look inside and help each other, we may find that we are indeed perfect friends.

Fibromyalgia has caused a lot of changes in our lives. Living with fibromyalgia has given us very personal experiences. Indeed, fibromyalgia is very personal for us and we need to remind each other that we are not alone, that we understand the pain, that we can do better even if we hurt, that the sun can shine brighter tomorrow, and that there is hope for a better tomorrow.

Chapter 39—Survivor Strategies

1) Work with your doctor to take an active role in managing your fibromyalgia.

2) Strive to keep a sense of hope and well-being through understanding, knowledge, and ability.

3) Use your abilities to achieve positive rewarding goals.

4) Learn and understand everything you can about your fibromyalgia.

5) Apply this knowledge to improve your quality of life.

6) Expect even better knowledge, abilities and understanding tomorrow.

7) You are not alone.

8) Interact with other fibromyalgia patients. They have developed a unique understanding of your condition. You can help them — they can help you.

9) Never give up hope!

Index